# SARS-CoV-2 Origin and COVID-19 Pandemic Across the Globe

*Edited by Vijay Kumar*

Published in London, United Kingdom

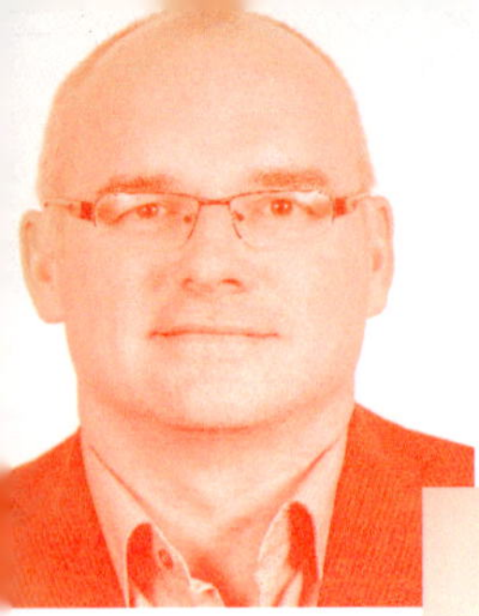
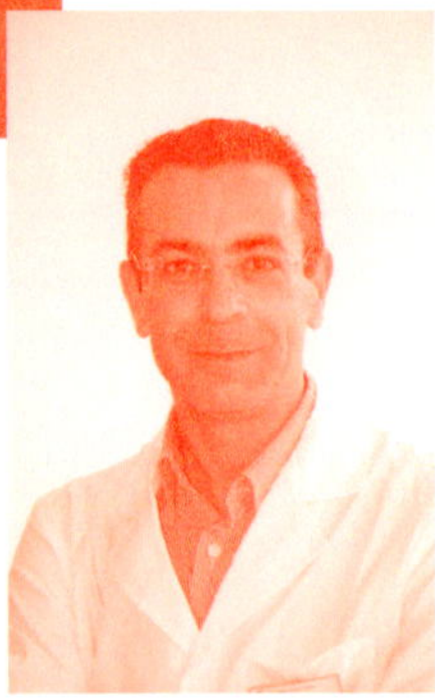
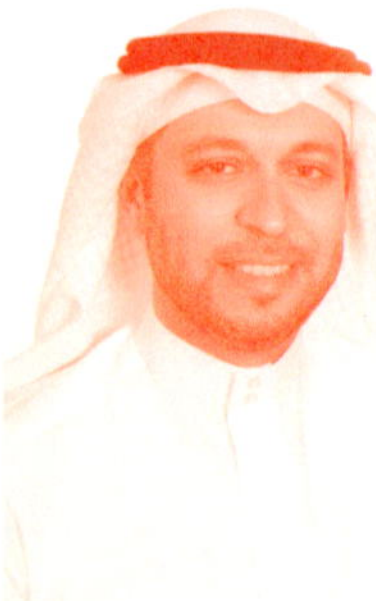
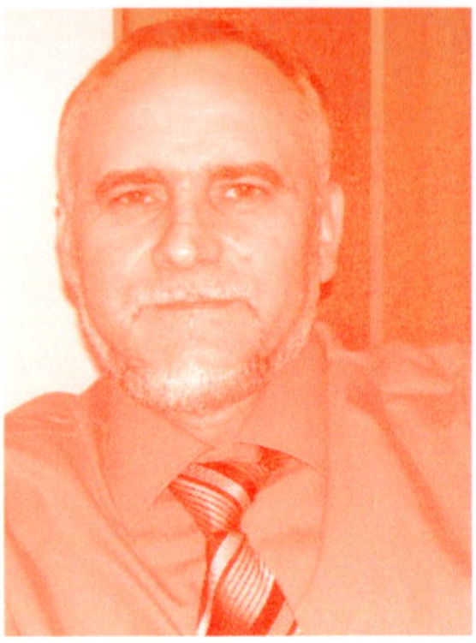
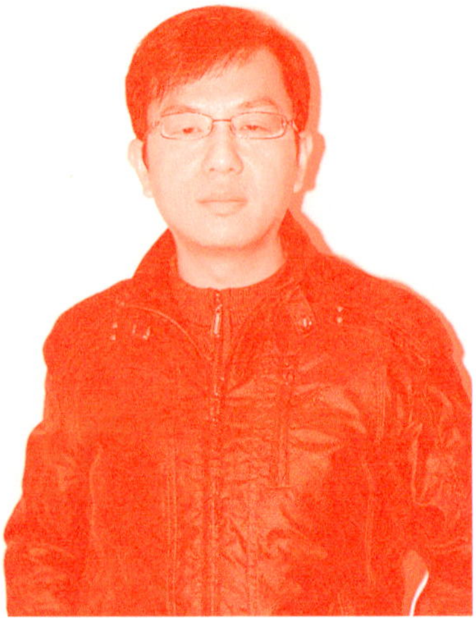
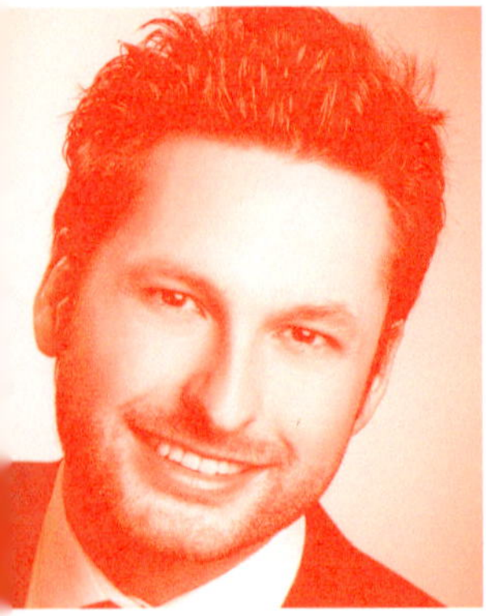
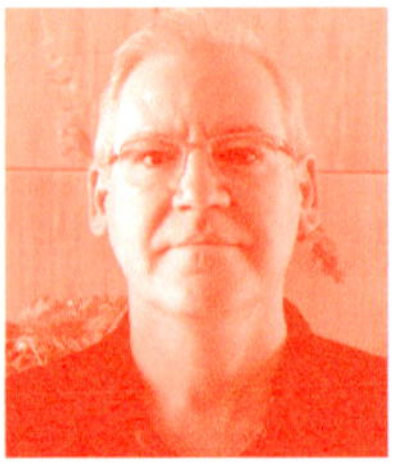

IntechOpen

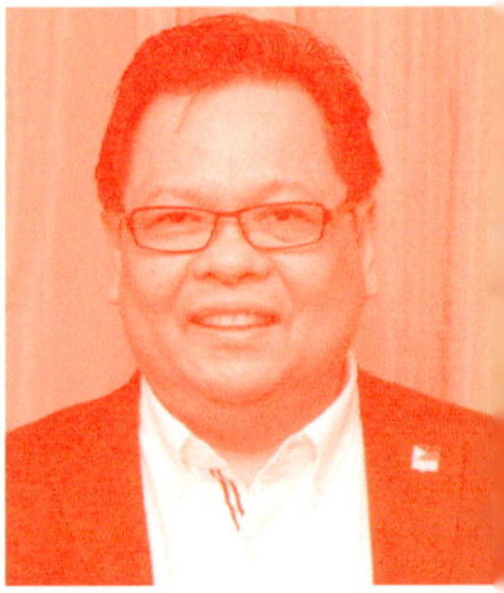
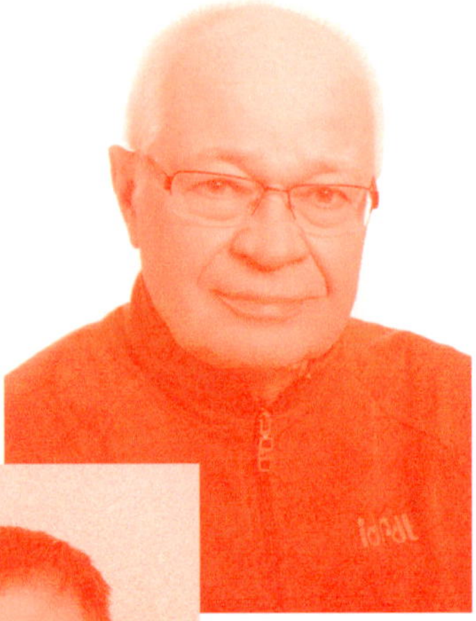
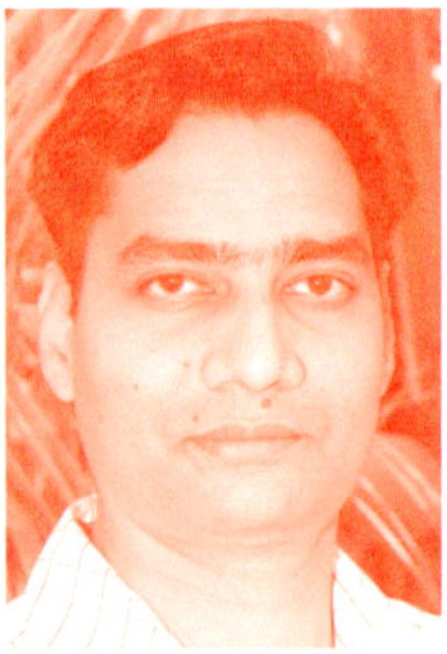
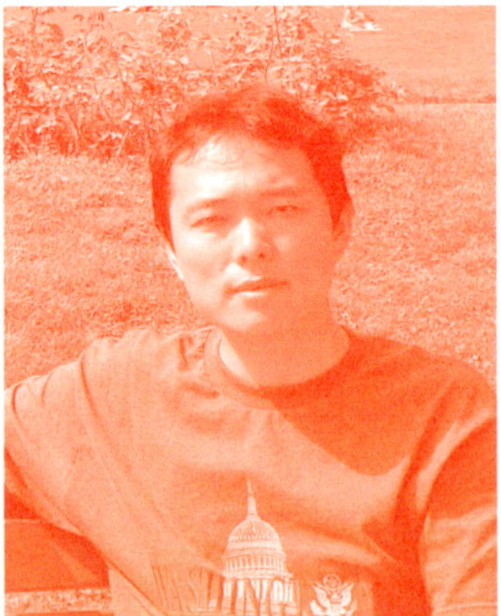
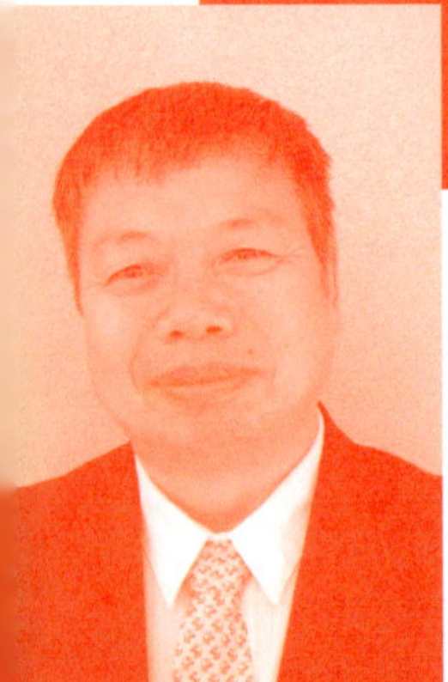
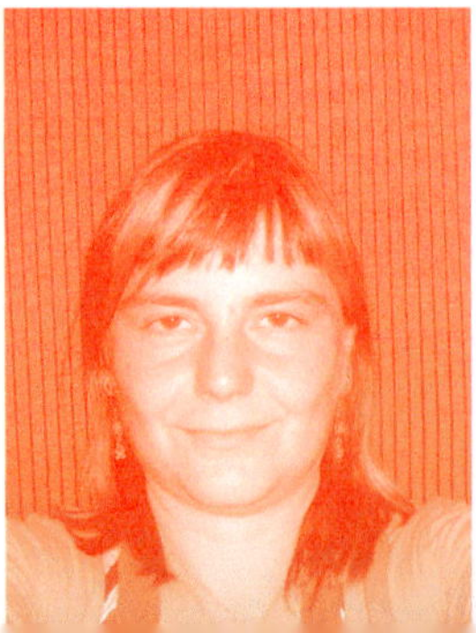

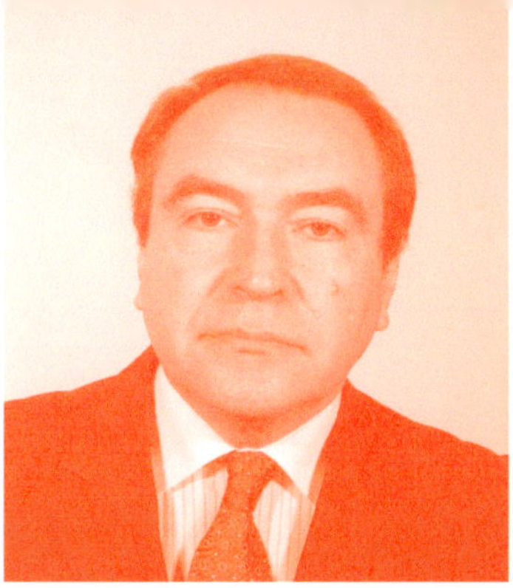
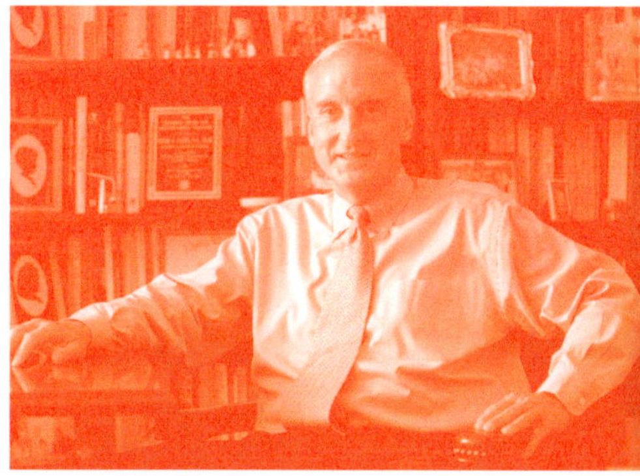
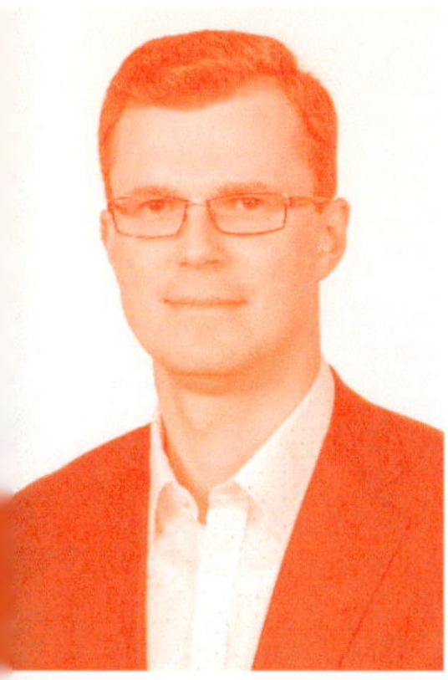
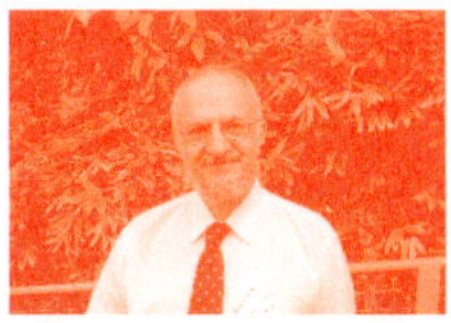
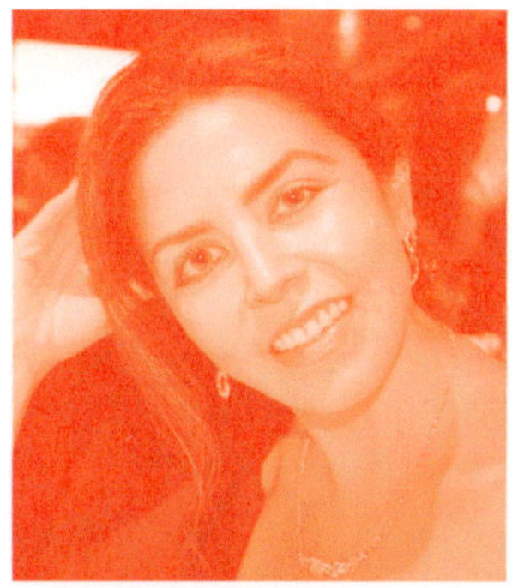

*Supporting open minds since 2005*

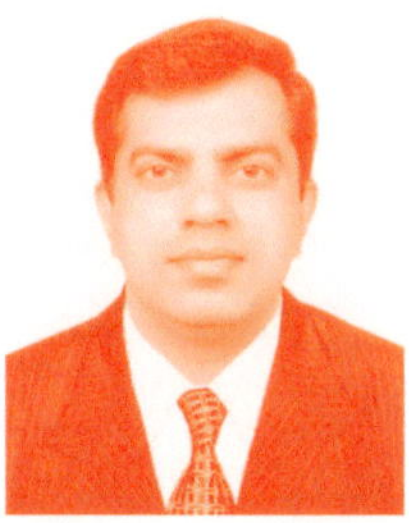
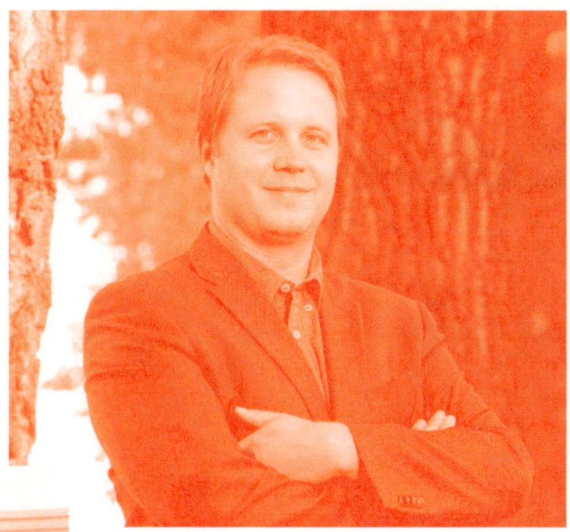
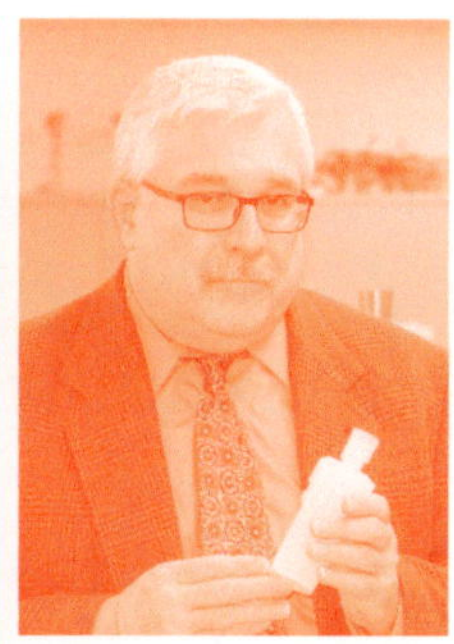
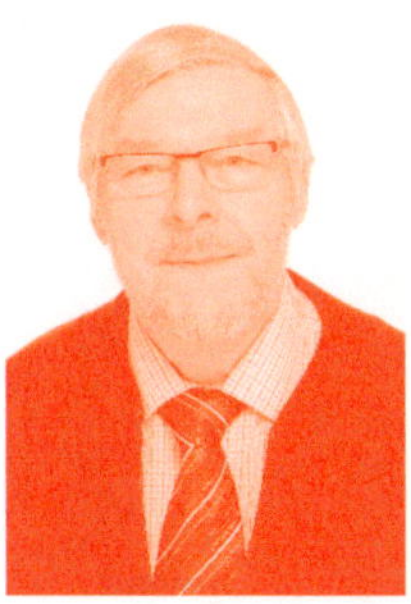
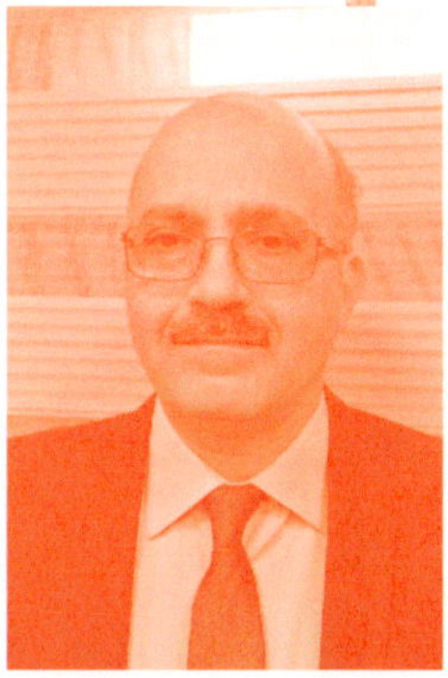
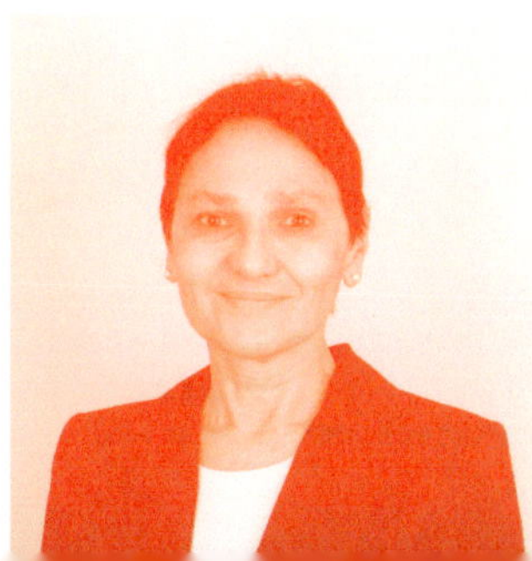
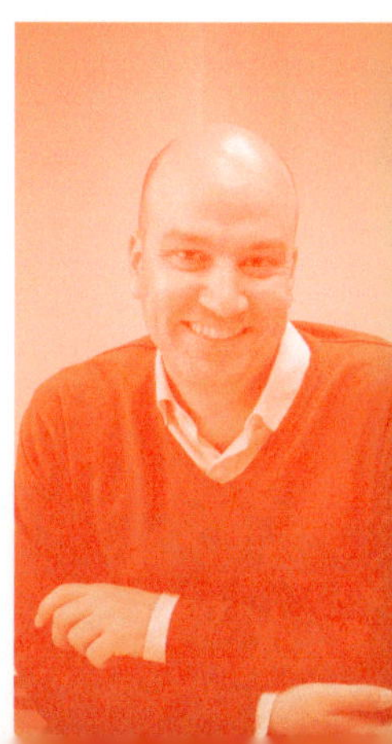

SARS-CoV-2 Origin and COVID-19 Pandemic Across the Globe
http://dx.doi.org/10.5772/intechopen.92909
Edited by Vijay Kumar

Contributors
Mario Pérez-Sayáns García, Alba Pérez González, Cintia Micaela Chamorro Petronacci, Karem Lopez Ortega, Eva M. Otero Rey, Charles M. Lepkowsky, Tean Zaheer, Muhammad Imran, Aqsa Ahmed, Amjad Islam Aqib, Sadia Muneer, Muhammad Imran Arshad, Iqra Zaheer, Gaffar Sarwar Sarwar Zaman, Mesfer Al Shahrani, Shankar Das, Julie Richards, Ömür Baysal, Ragıp Soner Silme, Vijay Kumar, Tullia Penna, Sergey Mosolov, Dmitry Sosin, Ekaterina Mosolova, Arshed Hussain Hussain Parry, Abdul Haseeb Wani, Sharon Attipoe-Dorcoo, Rigoberto Delgado, Vishwas Tripathi, Nisha Nair, amaresh mishra, Pratima Solanki, Jaseela Majeed, Amit K Yadav, Tej Prakash Sinha, Brunda RL, Sakshi Yadav, Sanjeev Bhoi, irena mitevska, Bogdan Andrei Fezi, Hatice Mine Cakmak, Manash K. Paul, Ria Sanyal



First published in London, United Kingdom, 2021 by IntechOpen
IntechOpen is the global imprint of INTECHOPEN LIMITED, registered in England and Wales, registration number: 11086078, 5 Princes Gate Court, London, SW7 2QJ, United Kingdom
Printed in Croatia

British Library Cataloguing-in-Publication Data
A catalogue record for this book is available from the British Library

Additional hard and PDF copies can be obtained from orders@intechopen.com

SARS-CoV-2 Origin and COVID-19 Pandemic Across the Globe
Edited by Vijay Kumar
p. cm.
Print ISBN 978-1-83968-755-6
Online ISBN 978-1-83968-756-3
eBook (PDF) ISBN 978-1-83968-757-0

For EU product safety concerns:
IN TECH d.o.o., Prolaz Marije Krucifikse Kozulić 3, 51000 Rijeka, Croatia, info@intechopen.com or visit our website at intechopen.com.

# Meet the editor

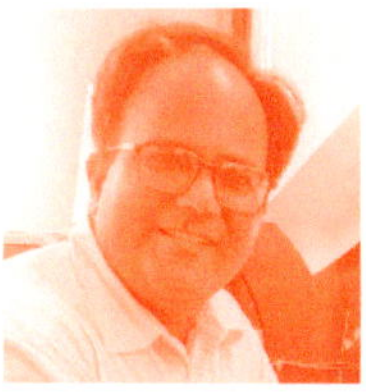

Dr. Vijay Kumar, Ph.D., has more than sixteen years of research experience in the field of bacterial infections, including sepsis and pneumonia, innate immunity, immunopharmacology, immunomodulation, and inflammation. He obtained his Ph.D. in June 2009 from the Department of Microbiology, Panjab University, Chandigarh, India. Dr. Kumar is the recipient of the prestigious "Piero Periti review article award" for 2008, awarded by the *Journal of Chemotherapy* in the field of immunomodulation and antimicrobials for the article entitled "Innate immunity in sepsis pathogenesis and its modulation: new immunomodulatory targets revealed." He was the recipient of a junior research and a senior research fellowship (2004–2009) offered by the Indian Council for Medical Research (ICMR), New Delhi, India. He has been awarded seventeen international travel awards to attend various international conferences in the field of infection and immunity. He has seventy publications in peer-reviewed international journals to his credit. To date, he has achieved more than 2100 citations and an h-index of 21. He has contributed five peer-reviewed articles in the field of SARS-CoV-2 infection/COVID-19, including an invited editorial on COVID-19 in *Expert Review of Proteomics.* Dr. Kumar is an associate editor for *Frontiers in Immunology* (Inflammation section), executive guest editor for *Coronaviruses*, and editorial board member of *Frontiers in Biosciences* and other journals. He is also an invited reviewer for several immunology journals, including *Scientific Reports, British Journal of Pharmacology, Pharmacological Reports, Frontiers in Immunology, Frontiers in Medicine, Journal of Inflammation Research, Cellular and Molecular Immunology, Immunology, Innate Immunity*, and others.

# Contents

# Preface

Coronaviruses (CoVs) were first identified in humans in the early 1960s. Depending on their serological and genetic characteristics, they can be classified into four major genera: (1) Alphacoronaviruses (α-CoVs), (2) Betacoronavirsues (β-CoVs), (3) Gammacoronaviruses (γ-CoVs), and (4) Deltacoronaviruses (δ-CoVs). These four groups of CoVs diverged from each other around 240–3000 BC, infecting and circulating in animals depending on their hosts. Severe acute respiratory syndrome (SARS) originated from SARS–coronavirus (SARS-CoV) in November 2002 in Foshan municipality, Guangdong Province, China. It spread to at least twenty-nine countries, including China, Hong Kong, Taiwan, Singapore, Vietnam, Canada, the United Kingdom, United States, and several European countries. Worldwide, SARS-CoV infected more than 8000 people and killed more than 770 people, with a case fatality rate (CFR) of 11% by the end of the epidemic (June 2003). It was also a zoonotic infection and SARS-CoV had been isolated from Himalayan palm civets (Paguma larvata), and evidence of infection has been found in a raccoon dog (Nyctereutes procyonoides) and a Chinese ferret-badger (Melogale moschata). However, it took fourteen years (December 2017) to establish that the major animal reservoir of SARS-CoV is a horseshoe bat (family, Rhinolophidae, genus Rhinolophus). The coronavirus isolated from these bats has the same genetic material as the SARS-CoV that triggered the SARS epidemic in 2002–2003. Of note, phylogenetic analysis and sequence comparisons have shown that SARS-CoV causing SARS did not closely relate to the previously known human and animal CoVs. However, after almost ten years of the SARS epidemic, another epidemic due to CoVs, Middle East respiratory syndrome (MERS) caused by MERS-CoV, originated in Jordan in April 2012. It was first reported in September 2012 in Saudi Arabia and rapidly spread to twenty-seven countries, including the United States, United Kingdom, Netherlands, Philippines, South Korea, and Kenya, and killed at least 845 people. MERS is also considered a zoonotic disease. However, we still do not know its exact animal reservoir.

The major emphasis of this book is COVID-19 caused by SARS-CoV-2 infection that originated in Wuhan, China in December 2019. The CoVs causing all the three major outbreaks belong to the subgroup (Sarbecovirus) of β-CoVs. COVID-19 has become one of the biggest infectious disease pandemics of the 21st century, infecting more than 219 million people and killing 4.55 million people worldwide as of October 8, 2021. Over seven sections and seventeen chapters, this book comprehensively reviews COVID-19, including information on the virus that causes it, pathogenesis, impact on human health and socioeconomics, and much more.

Chapter 1, "Learning from Bats to Escape from Potent or Severe Viral Infections," discusses the different bat species and their immunological adaptations preventing them from becoming severely infected by potential viral pathogens, including CoVs, but making them a potential source of infection transmission. This chapter adds to the understanding of bat immunological adaptations to maintain the virus at harmless levels. We can develop novel immunomodulatory therapeutics for humans through a deeper understanding of bat immunity and translating those findings into humans.

Chapter 2, "Epidemiology, Zoonotic and Reverse Zoonotic Potential of COVID-19", examines potential roadmaps to prevent future outbreaks of COVID-19 through the tools of epidemiological studies, the transmission of the disease, and public health safety measures.

Chapter 3, "Coronavirus Disease 2019 (COVID-19): Origin, Impact, and Drug Development", discusses the origin of COVID-19 and its relations with SARS and MERS along with the availability of current treatment approaches and drug repurposing.

Chapter 4, "Utilization from Computational Methods and Omics Data for Antiviral Drug Discovery to Control of SARS-CoV-2", discusses the design of potent antiviral drugs against SARS-CoV-2 to protect against COVID-19 utilizing computational methods and omics studies.

Chapter 5, "Organoid Technology and the COVID Pandemic", discusses the recently developed organoid technology to study COVID-19 pathogenesis and drug targeting.

Chapter 6, "Chest Imaging in Coronavirus Disease-19 (COVID-19)", discusses the role of chest imaging techniques for diagnosis and effective management of thoracic complications, which are one of the primary complications of COVID-19 patients.

Chapter 7, "COVID-19 and Cardiovascular Disease: Mechanisms and Implications", discusses the impact of COVID-19 on the cardiovascular system, its mechanisms, and implications to prevent further damage.

Chapter 8, "Management of Covid-19 Disease in Pediatric Oncology Patients", discusses the management of COVID-19 in pediatric cancer patients. Although children typically experience a mild course of COVID-19, children with cancer experience more severe disease.

Chapter 9, "Economic, Health-Care and Teaching-Learning Impact of COVID-19 (SARS-CoV-2) on Dentistry", talks about the impact of COVID-19 on all aspects of dental medicine practice, including economics, healthcare, and teaching-learning.

Chapter 10, "COVID-19, Telehealth and Access to Care", discusses the emergence of telemedicine during the COVID-19 pandemic and its limitations for older patients who may be naïve or less fluent in using information technology and apps.

Chapter 11, "Mobile Clinics in the United States and the COVID-19 Pandemic: A Response Strategy Model", discusses the emergence of mobile clinics in the United States and their role in dealing with COVID-19.

Chapter 12, "Practice Changing Innovations for Emergency Care during the COVID-19 Pandemic in Resource Limited Settings", discusses the COVID-19 pandemic in resource-limited countries and how these countries prepare different medical equipment and PPE kits to combat the virus.

Chapter 13, "Origin and Impact of COVID-19 on Socioeconomic Status," considers the impact of COVID-19 on the socioeconomic status of people around the world.

Chapter 14, "Psychosocial Effects and Public Health Challenges of COVID-19 Pandemic in India", investigates the psychosocial effect of COVID-19 on the population of India and the challenges faced by its public health sector.

Chapter 15, "Stress, Anxiety, Depression and Burnout in Frontline Healthcare Workers during COVID-19 Pandemic in Russia", assesses the impact of COVID-19 on the life of frontline healthcare workers in Russia.

Chapter 16, "The Role of Architecture and Urbanism in Preventing Pandemics", discusses the importance of architecture and urbanism in preventing future pandemics.

Finally, Chapter 17, "Why a Bioethical Approach is Needed in Addressing Health Risks Stemming from Pandemics Due to Zoonoses Linked to Human Impact on Biodiversity?", presents bioethical approaches to deal with pandemics/epidemics arising through zoonosis as human invasion/impact on the natural habitats of different wild animals invites the emergence of infectious diseases, including HIV-1 infection (AIDS), Ebola virus infection and the current COVID-19 pandemic.

**Vijay Kumar**
Department of Pharmaceutical Sciences,
College of Pharmacy,
University of Tennessee Health Science Center (UTHSC),
Memphis, TN, USA

Section 1

# Bats and Zoonotic Viral Infection

Chapter 1

# Learning from Bats to Escape from Potent or Severe Viral Infections

*Vijay Kumar*


## Abstract

The COVID-19 pandemic that started in December 2019 in Wuhan city, China has created chaos all over the world with over 185 million infection cases and 4 million deaths world-wide. The pathogen behind COVID-19 has been identified as severe acute respiratory syndrome Coronavirus 2 (SARS-CoV-2) that is more close to the previous SARS-CoV responsible for SARS epidemic 2002–2003. Although, SARS-CoV-2 also differs from SARS-CoV in many aspects as indicated by genetic studies. For example, SARS-CoV does not have a furin binding domain or site, whereas its presence in SARS-CoV-2 spike (S) protein increases its potential for infectivity. The horseshoe bats (Rhinolphus species) from China are considered as primary animal reservoirs for SARS-CoV and SARS-CoV-2. However, along with CoVs, bats also harbor many other viral pathogens (Ebola, Nipah, and Hendra viruses) without having serious infections. The bat physiology plays a crucial role in harboring these viruses along with adaptations to longevity and slow aging process. The immune system plays a crucial role in the clearance or establishment of the infection. Present chapter discusses different immunological aspects (innate immune response comprising the virus recognizing pattern recognition receptors (PRRs), type 1 interferon production, pro- and anti-inflammatory immune response, and adaptive immune response) that help bats to control viral infection without getting a severe infection as compared to other mammals, including humans.


**Keywords:** Bats, innate immunity, autophagy, infection, IFNs, adaptive immunity

## 1. Introduction

Bats and flying foxes, including large flying foxes (*Pteropus vampyrus*) and variable flying foxes (*P. hypomelanus*) are the mammals belonging to the order *Chiroptera* (hand wing). This order contains 1232 species of bats and flying foxes constituting a more diverse and important order of mammals after rodents. They evolved approximately 52 million years ago [1, 2]. Taxonomically, bats represent approximately 20% of mammalian diversity [3]. They are the real flying mammals and come out for prey in the night time (nocturnal aerial predators). Many species of bats are frugivorous (fruit eating), insectivorous (insect eating), and some feed on blood of other animals (hematophagous). Some species of bats fly long distances during seasonal migration with a speed of 100 miles per hour, making them the fastest mammal (free-flying Brazilian free-tailed bats or *Tadarida brasiliensis*) on earth [4]. Some species of bats fly during night and some are diurnal or crepuscular. Bats are found in all continents, except Antarctica. They live in caves or in other dark spaces in large groups or colonies and some are solitary in nature. Besides playing a crucial role in maintaining biodiversity or ecological balance through their different roles (insects eating, pollination, and seed dispersal etc.), they remain crucial to researchers due to their strange characteristics and reservoir for different pathogens [2]. For example, the advancing knowledge in bat biology has implicated them (the tropical frugivorous Honduran white bat *Ectophylla alba*) to be studied as a mammalian model for skin carotenoid metabolism [5].

Bats are crucial primary reservoirs for emerging viral infections that can be transferred to humans or cross the species barrier to infect other wild or domesticated animals through spill over [6]. Studies have indicated that they harbor higher numbers of zoonotic viruses per species than rodents [7]. Even they have higher (3.9 times stronger) sympatry than bats and sympatry within a taxonomic order serves as a most crucial host trait for zoonotic virus enrichment [7]. Of note, despite harboring more zoonotic viruses per species than rodents, the total number of zoonotic viruses found in bats (61) are lower than rodents (68) due to double the number of rodent species than bat species. However, bats are the primary host for more virulent viruses than other mammals, including rodents [8]. Before, the emergence of recent virus infections, including severe acute respiratory syndrome (SARS), middle-eastern respiratory syndrome (MERS), Ebola virus infection, and most recent Coronavirus disease 19 (COVID-19) pandemic caused by SARS-CoV-2, MERS-CoV, Ebola virus or *Zaire Ebolavirus* (three different species of Ebola viruses have been found in greater long-fingered bat (*Miniopterus inflatus* or *M. inflatus*) in Liberia's Sanniquellie-Mahn District that borders to Guinea and insect-eating bat, *M. schreibersii*), and SARS-CoV-2, the studies of natural histories of bats, their importance as primary reservoirs for different zoonotic viral diseases have been largely underappreciated, underrated, and underfunded [9–12]. Although, they (vampire bats or *Desmodus rotundus murinua* found only in the Latin America) were considered for their role in the rabies transmission called vampire bat rabies as suggested first in 1959 [13–16].

Fruit bats, including *Hypsignathus monstrosus*, *Epomops franqueti*, and *Myonycteris torquate* have also been suggested as potential reservoirs for *Zaire Ebolavirus* [12, 17]. In addition to these zoonotic viral infections, bats also serve as potential reservoirs for other viruses responsible for infections in humans that include Nipah, Hendra, Marburg, Hepadna (able to infect human hepatocytes), and Lyssa viruses etc. Thus, different viruses of 23 virus families have been detected in different bat species (196) in 69 countries all over the world [3, 18]. The mortality among bats due to bacterial or viral infection has been the least observed cause of death [19]. In comparison to humans, where 7% of the genome encodes for the immune or related genes (1562 immune genes recorded in humans as of 1st October 2004 by the immunogenetic related information source or IRIS), only less than 4% of the bat (Australian flying fox or *Pteropus alecto*) genome encodes from immune related genes (about 500) [20, 21]. For example, Jamaican fruit bat or *Artibeus jamaicensis* has 466 immune-related genes (IRGs) and the Egyptian Rousette bat (*Rousettus aegyptiacus*), a common fruit bat species has 407 or 2.75% IRGs of their total genome [22, 23]. Thus, either bats have lower numbers of IRGs as compared to humans or we need further studies in other potential bat species harboring potent virus pathogens that can infect humans directly or indirectly through secondary reservoir hosts.

Also, Panamanian Seba's short-tailed bats (*Carollia perspicillata*), a widely distributed neotropical species shows individual and population-specific diversity in their major-histocompatibility complex 1 or MHC-1 genes with an unique genotype in each individual comparable to passerine or perching or singing birds [24]. The MHC-II diversity is also correlated with the geographic origin and population admixture in *Carollia perspicillata* and *Molossus molossus*, and in *Desmodus rotundus* MHC-II DRB gene diversity depends on the environment only [25]. The MHC diversity in bats may impact their defense against different reservoir viruses inducing resistance against them and providing an opportunity or a perfect animal niche for the virus evolution that may infect other hosts, including humans severely [24]. The Egyptian Rousette or fruit bat does not support the productive growth or replication of the Nipah virus [26]. No seroconversion against Nipah virus glycoprotein has been reported in these bats. Hence, only specific bat species serve as potential reservoirs for Nipah viruses. This may be true for other viruses too. The *in vitro* study based on bat cells (RoNi/7.1 (*Rousettus aegyptiacus*) and PaKiT01 (*P. alecto*) cells) lines has indicated the enhanced interferon (IFN)-mediated antiviral immune response generation of either constitutive or induced form that allows a rapid cell to cell virus transmission rate (β) within the host [27]. The IFN-induced antiviral state protects live cells from apoptotic or other forms of cell death *in vitro* that (the *in vitro* epidemic or extended life of the cells) enhances the probability of developing and establishing a long-term persistent infection [27]. This phenotype of infection and associated host-pathogen interaction response is absent in Vero cells (a cell line derived from the kidneys of African green monkeys) due to the genetic defect in the IFN production [27, 28]. Hence, viruses evolved in bats as reservoirs have an increased IFN capabilities that helps to achieve a rapid within-host transmission rates without inducing clinical symptoms of the disease. Thus these rapidly reproducing viruses in bats may become more virulence upon spillover to hosts, including humans lacking similar immune capabilities like bats. Hence, understanding the bat immune function or response becomes crucial to understand. The present chapter describes the immunological aspects or features of bats preparing them to harbor a wide range of viruses without severe disease causing mortality.

## 2. Innate immune adaptation of bats as preventing to develop severe infections

The innate immune system is primary or first line of the defense against invading pathogens. The pattern recognition receptors (PRRs), including toll-like receptors (TLRs), Nod-like receptors (NLRs), absent in melanoma-2 (AIM2)-like receptors (ALRs), retinoic acid-inducible gene-1 (RIG-1)-like receptors (RLRs, RIG-1 and melanoma differentiation-associated protein 5 or MDA5), C-type lectin receptors (CLRs), and cyclic GMP (guanosine monophosphate)–AMP (adenosine monophosphate) synthase (cGAS) and stimulator of interferon genes (STING) signaling pathways play a crucial role in the host defense and the generation of pro-inflammatory immune response (cytokine, chemokines, reactive oxygen and nitrogen species (ROS and RNS), and type 1 interferon (IFN) production) [29–34]. TLR4 is a crucial PRR to recognize Gram-negative bacterial lipopolysaccharide (LPS) as a potent microbial or pathogen-associated molecular pattern (MAMP or PAMP) to induce a potent pro-inflammatory immune response to clear the infection. However, its overactivation may cause severe inflammation. Pallas's mastiff bats (*Molossus molossus*) upon exposure to the *Escherichia coli* (*E. coli*)-derived LPS do not develop leucocytosis and hyperthermia or fever independent of their sex (**Figure 1**) [35]. However, they show weight loss upon exposure to the LPS. This study indicates the presence of defective TLR4 signaling responsible for the NF-κB-dependent pyrogenic cytokines (IL-1 and IL-6) (**Figure 1**). This defect may also prevent the further activation of cytosolic NLRP3-dependent inflammasomes responsible for generating IL-1β and IL-18. Bat (little brown bat or *Myotis lucifugus*) mitochondria produce lesser ROS (a potent inducer of NLRP3 activation) [36].

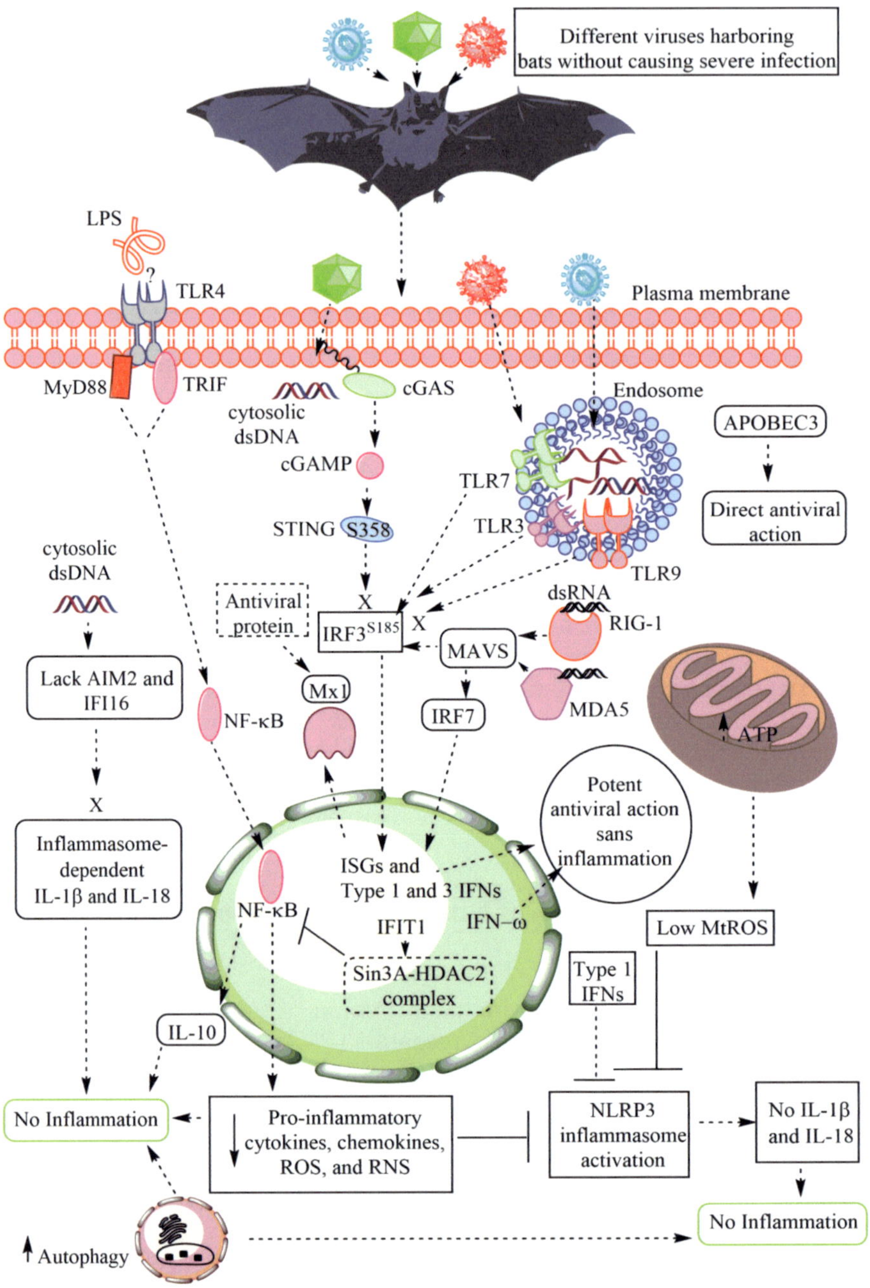


**Figure 1.**
*Schematic representation of immune response in bats preventing development of severe infection and inflammation. The gram-negative bacteria or its PAMP (LPS) recognition in bats do not stimulate pro-inflammatory cytokine production through NF-κB activation and increase in body temperature. The increase in autophagy further increases cellular longevity, acts as an antiviral mechanism to clear or control the infection, decreases or suppresses inflammation. The PYHIN domain containing AIM2 and IFI16 inflammasomes are absent and hence, do not take part in cytosolic DNA recognition as DAMP to inflammasome activation-based maturation of IL-1β and IL-18. This further decreases the incidence of inflammation and associated tissue damage. The cGAS-STING-based signaling mechanism recognizing cytosolic dsDNA as DAMP also does not work in bats due to the presence of serine at 358 AA position in STING that is unable to activate IRF3 and type 1 IFN production. Hence, this further prevents inflammatory events in response to the self-DNA. Only the cytosolic RNAs activate different PRRs (RIG-1, MDA5, and TLR3) that via IRF3 and IRF7 activation synthesize type 1 and 3 IFNs, which exert antiviral action, but damp pro-inflammatory action of NRLP3 and NLRP1 inflammasomes. Mx1 is an IFN-inducible antiviral protein with a GTPase activity. APOBEC3 also directly acts as an antiviral host factor without inducing inflammation. Hence, only protective antiviral immune response works in bats to control their number without inducing severe inflammation.*

The reduced mitochondrial ROS (mtROS) production in Seba's short-tailed bats involves a mild depolarization of the inner mitochondrial membrane that decreases the membrane potential to a level sufficient to produce ATP molecules but insufficient to synthesize mtROS (**Figure 1**) [37]. This mechanism decreases with age in mice but remains intact in these bats. For example, in 2.5 years old mice this mechanism of mild mitochondrial depolarization disappears in different organs (lungs, liver, spleen, skeletal muscles, heart, brain, and kidneys). Hence, mtROS-mediated DNA and protein damage is seen in mice or other mammals but not in bats.

The immune challenge among bats does not alter their oxidative stress irrespective of their pre-migration and migration seasons [38]. However, bats have higher baseline leukocytes but lower neutrophil numbers during their migratory seasons as compared to their pre-migratory season. Their plasma haptoglobin (a humoral innate immune component) levels also remain same during both seasons [38]. However, plasma haptoglobin level of migratory bats increases upon an immune (LPS) challenge that remains unchanged in non-migratory or pre-migratory bats under the same immunogenic stimulation. Of note, bats do not upregulate genes associated with chronic inflammation with the advancement of age that is seen in other mammals, including humans [39]. Hence, this protects them from age related inflammatory diseases and predisposes them towards healthy aging and longevity along with tolerance to infections, including Ebola, Nipah, and many more. Also, the bat microbiota (Firmicutes and Proteobacteria are dominant bacteria) differs from other terrestrial mammals (strict anaerobic phylum Bacteroidetes in mice and humans), and remains intact throughout their life that further protects them from age-associated inflammation and inflammatory diseases [40, 41]. On the other hand in mice and humans gut microbiota changes with time and aging that predispose them to age-associated inflammatory diseases associated with gut bacteria dysbiosis [42–44].

A study has shown the TLR3, TLR7, and TLR9 expression at mRNA levels in different organs of Leschenault's Rousette bats (*Rousettus leschenaulti*) [45]. Another study has shown the expression of full length mRNA transcripts of TLR1-TLR10 in the Australian flying fox or *P. alecto* [46]. This bat species also expresses the pseudogene for TLR13. However, their functional protein level expression in different bat species needs further investigation. The evolutionary studies have shown that the bats evolved under the influence of positive selection for TLR7, TLR8, and TLR9 that is highest for TLR9 and lowest for TLR7 [47]. The TLR3 in bats has evolved under a negative selection process. This study indicates the adaptation of host-pathogen interaction in bats, particularly in bat TLR9. The bat TLR8 has an extensive sequence variation within them that separates them from other mammals, including humans [48]. Bat TLRs are evolving slowly under purifying selection in response to the functional constraints with a divergence process that is overall congruent with the species tree [49]. The bat TLRs show unique mutations in their ligand-binding domains even involving their non-conservative amino acid (AA) change and/or targets of positive selection. These changes can modify the binding of the corresponding TLR ligands. Hence, bat TLRs may vary in recognizing the same ligand recognized by other mammalian or human TLRs.

Flying fox bats (*P. alecto*) have other cytosolic dsRNA recognizing receptors called RLRs, including RIG-1, MDA5, and laboratory of genetics and physiology 2 (LGP2), like humans that upon recognizing cytosolic dsRNA induce the type 1 IFN production [50]. LGP2 synergy with MDA5 to generate antiviral immune response during RLR-dependent dsRNA recognition [51]. LGP2 interacts with the IFN-inducible, dsRNA binding protein PACT (a cofactor of DICER in the processing of microRNAs) through its regulatory C-terminal domain that inhibits RIG-1-dependent signaling but promotes MDA5-dependent antiviral immune response [52]. TLR3, RLRs (RIG-1), and MDA5 serve as potent antiviral immune response inducers in bats to protect them from severe infection caused by Encephalomyocarditis virus (EMCV) and Japanese encephalitis virus (JEV) (**Figure 1**) [53]. The functionally conserved RLR adaptor called mitochondrial antiviral signaling (MAVS) protein has been demonstrated in the Chinese rufous horseshoe bat (*Rhinolophus sinicus*) and straw-colored fruit bat (*Eidolon helvum*) that upon RLR (RIG-1 and MDA5)-based activation transmits signals to produce type 1 IFNs (IFN-β) and interferon stimulated gene (ISG) called IFN-induced protein with tetratricopeptide repeats 1 (IFIT1) that further enhances IFN gene program (IFN-β, IRF7, and OAS1 or 2′-5'oligadenylate synthase 1), which activates ISGs, immune homeostasis, and cell's internal antiviral immune response (**Figure 1**) [54–56].

The activation of MAVS involves the RIG-1 and MDA5 dimer formation [57]. Also, the IFIT1 generated exerts an anti-inflammatory action via suppressing TLR-dependent NF-κB-mediated pro-inflammatory cytokines (TNF-α, IL-1β) and chemokines (CCL3) through activating Sin3A-histone deacetylase 2 (HDAC2) transcriptional regulatory complex containing SAP25 that has an inhibitory action (**Figure 1**) [56]. Hence, these PRRs protect bats from developing severe viral infections through increased type 1 IFN production but low tissue damaging pro-inflammatory immune response. It should be interesting to observe that viruses harboring bats as their primary reservoirs may have evolved strategies to escape this innate immune mechanism to recognize cytosolic dsRNA viruses or bats have developed other mechanisms to escape from exaggerated pro-inflammatory innate immune response upon recognizing cytosolic dsRNA viruses. The MERS-CoV replicates efficiently in Jamaican fruit bats (*Artibeus jamaicensis*) without causing a productive infection with clinical signs of the disease [58]. The interferon regulatory factor (IRF3) transcription factor activation plays a crucial role in generating the potent antiviral immune response in the bat (*Eptesicus fuscus*) against MERS-CoV (**Figure 1**) [59]. In comparison to humans or other mammals, MERS-CoV fails to subvert the IRF3 activation and dependent type 1 IFN response generation in *E. fuscus*. The IRF3 in bats differs from humans due to the presence of serine185 (S185) that provides an enhanced antiviral protection (**Figure 1**) [60]. The S185 insertion in the human IRF3 increases its antiviral action. Hence, the positive selection of S185 in the bat IRF3 increases its antiviral action. Also, the bats persistently infected with MERS-CoV have increased type 1 IFN levels than non-infected ones and its disruption increases the virus replication [61].

The bat cells repeatedly select for the mutant MERS-CoV called delta open reading frame (ΔORF5) MERS-CoV and are resistant to superinfection by wild type (WT) MERS-CoV due to deficiency of MERS-CoV binding receptor dipeptidyl peptidase 4 (DPP4) and increased type 1 IFN levels [61]. Additionally, the Australian black flying foxes in response the cytosolic TLRs and RLRs recognizing viral PAMPs (dsRNA) also activate IRF7, which also induces type 1 IFNs mediated antiviral immune response (**Figure 1**) [62]. The deficiency or the defective activation of IRF7 in bats enhances viral replication and the development of the productive infection. Of note, virus (bat paramyxovirus, Tioman virus) infection to bats also induces protective type III IFN production that further provides protection from the development of productive infection (**Figure 1**) [63]. Egyptian rousette bats (*Rousettus aegyptiacus*) are the naturally harbor Marburg virus (MARV) and do not develop clinical symptoms of the disease as compared to humans due to generation of IFN-based immune response by DCs and suppressing pro-inflammatory immune response [64, 65]. This is because these bats secrete IFN-ω, which have antiviral action against RNA viruses (**Figure 1**). Also, the 13% of genes induced by IFN-ω in bats are not found in the interferome and other ISG databases, indicating their uniqueness to bats [64].

Bat immune cells exert protective type 1 (IFN-α, β, and ω) type II (IFN-γ) IFNs against Filoviruses (Marburg and Ebola viruses) but human immune cells fail to do so (**Figure 1**) [66]. Myxovirus resistance 1 (Mx1, a GTPase) is another antiviral protein induced in response to the IFNs is evolutionary conserved in vertebrates and can restrict a wide range of viruses in host cells (**Figure 1**) [67]. In bats these Mx1 proteins protect against Ebola and Influenza viruses through reducing the polymerase activity of these viruses along with other circulating viruses [68]. However, bat Mx1 does not inhibit Thogoto virus (enveloped negative sense ssRNA virus of *Orthomyxoviridae* family) as it does not infect them. On the other hand, mice Mx1 in hematopoietic cells inhibits Thogoto virus infection [67]. Hence, Mx1 is another IFN-induced antiviral protein in bats to protect against severe viral infections (**Figure 1**). Also, the production of type 1 IFN inhibits the NLRP1 and NLRP3 inflammasome-induced IL-1β and IL-18 production and induces IL-10 synthesis via STAT1 transcription factor (**Figure 1**) [69]. The IL-10 further activates STAT3 to reduce the IL-1β and IL-1α levels. IFNs also inhibit inflammasome-mediated Caspase 11 (CASP11) to inhibit the pro-inflammatory IL-1β and IL-18 release via activating immunity-related GTPases M clade 2 (Irgm2) and Gate16 (an ATG8 family member), which inhibit CASP11 maturation or activation [70]. Hence, IFN levels control exaggerated inflammation through different mechanisms.

The cGAS-STING signaling-mediated type 1 IFN production against DNA viruses is lost in bats due to the loss of serine AA at 358 (S358) position of the STING (**Figure 1**) [71, 72]. The S358 AA of the STING from other non-bat mammals is conserved and its phosphorylation is crucial for STING-dependent IRF3 activation and type 1 IFN release. For example, in human STING the S3666 and S358 phosphorylation is crucial for IRF3 binding and activation, but not for TBK1 [73]. Also, the TLR9-dependent cytosolic DNA recognition in bats is not as functional as in other mammals, including humans as result to adapt its high metabolic rate that increases the body temperature over 41°C during migratory flight that can induce DNA damage and its migration to the cytosol (**Figure 1**) [49]. Along with, defective cGAS-STING and TLR9 signaling for cytosolic DNA recognition, absent in melanoma 2 (AIM2) and gamma-interferon-inducible protein Ifi-16 (IFI16 or p204 in mouse) or interferon-inducible myeloid differentiation transcriptional activator are the PYRIN and HIN domain containing (PYHIN) proteins also recognizing cytosolic DNA are absent the genome of most bats, including *P. alecto* and *M. davidii* [74–76]. Both, AIM2 and IFI16 are involved in the cytosolic DNA recognition-induced inflammasome activation, and the maturation and release of pro-inflammatory cytokines (IL-1β and IL-18) (**Figure 1**) [75]. Only, a bat called *Pteronotus parnellii* has a truncated AIM2. Hence, the removal of cytosolic DNA sensors or PRRs adds to escape from the inflammatory immune response generated due to DNA damage observed high metabolic rate-induced rise in temperature during long migratory flights and helps in the coexistence of host and pathogens. Also, the killer immunoglobulin-like receptors (KIRs) encoded by genes in the leukocyte receptor complex (LRC), and killer cell lectin-like receptors (KLRs, also called Ly49 receptors), encoded within the natural killer gene complex (NKC) are required for potent antiviral function of NK cells. However, *P. alecto* lacks both KLRs and KIRs and *M. davidii* has only one Ly49 pseudogene [76].

The pteropodidae or cave nectar bat (*Eonycteris spelae*) monocytes, macrophages and granulocytes resemble human counterparts depending on the immune parameters that are divergent between mice and humans [77]. However, mast cells, eosinophils, basophils, platelets or thrombocytes have not been identified and characterized in different bat species [54]. Further studies are required in this direction. Also, the genome-wide comparison of immune-related genes have indicated their much closer phylogenetic relationship with humans than rodents. Also, bats express largest and most diverse array of apolipoprotein B mRNA editing enzyme, catalytic polypeptide-like 3 (APOBEC3) genes (encode antiviral DNA cytosine deaminases), which are potent antiviral proteins and act as antiviral restriction factors for viruses, including hepadnaviruses (hepatitis DNA virus), and parvoviruses [78, 79]. The potent antiviral immune response of APOBEC3 involves its cytosine deaminase activity that deaminates cytosine residues in the nascent retroviral DNA to block retrovirus replication via hypermutation (**Figure 1**) [80]. This hyper-mutated retroviral DNA, then gets degraded or becomes non-functional [81]. In other mammals, including humans and laboratory mice the expression and action of APOBEC3 might threaten the integrity of the host genome triggering the incidence of cancer [82]. For example, a common APOBEC3 overexpression in humans is associated with the incidence of breast cancer in humans and the overexpression of APOBEC1 (A1) in mice is associated with hepatocellular carcinoma [83–85]. However, bats are more resistant to developing cancer despite expressing APOBEC3 as they express a higher quantity of ABC transporter called ABCB1 than humans and efficiently removes cytotoxic agents (doxorubicin) and damaged DNA [86]. Hence, in bats APOBEC exerts its only antiviral action and remains sans to increase susceptibility to cancer. However, further studies are warranted. Of note, even minor levels of IFNs are able to induce APOBEC3 family of proteins (A3A, A3G, and A3F) expression and their antiviral action [87].

Lower NLRP3 inflammasome activation in the cytosol prevents exaggerated inflammatory immune response in immune cells bats due to lower ROS production (crucial for NLRP3 activation) and apoptosis-associated speck-like protein containing a CARD (ASC) speck formation and secretion of interleukin-1β (**Figure 1**) [88]. Also, bats produce less TNF-α due to the interaction of c-Rel (a member NF-κB family) with the promoter sequence of TNF-α [89]. The antiviral innate immune response in bat macrophages in response to the virus-derived PAMPs is also accompanied by sustained production of an increased amount of anti-inflammatory cytokine (IL-10) (**Figure 1**) [90]. These unique anti-inflammatory mechanisms in bats, including greater mouse-eared bats, *Myotis myotis* may have evolved due to their high metabolic rate (but produce low ROS that regulates NLRP3 inflammasome activation) and long distance flights [90]. For example, this bat species along with other long-distance traveling bats exhibit a delayed aging process as indicated by the absence of shortened telomerase and due to strategies to check induction of severe inflammation, but the induction of potent anti-inflammatory mechanisms [91, 92]. Also, the expression of high basal levels of heat shock proteins (HSP70 and HSP90) in bats protects them from increased metabolic stress that further contributes to their longevity and healthy aging [93]. Hence, these processes may contribute to longevity and healthy aging among bats.

Autophagy is an essential cellular process through which cells maintain homeostasis, including immune homeostasis [94–96]. Autophagy involves the breakdown of cellular components and the sequestration of the portion of cytoplasm into the double or multi-membraned vesicle called autophagosomes, which then fuse with cellular suicide or waste bags or lysosomes (contain hydrolases in their lumen and their membranes have permeases) to form autophagolysosomes or autolysosomes [96–98]. Autolysosomes are the junk crashers of the cell, in which luminal materials, including internal membrane, are degraded and exported out of the cell through permeases to recycle in the cytosol [96]. Hence, autophagy is the renewal process for cytosolic components through which cytoplasmic macromolecules mobilize to generate energy-rich compounds to meet cellular energy requirements during conditions with decreased internal and external energy resources. The impaired autophagy predisposes the host towards premature aging and inflammatory and degenerative diseases. Hence, autophagy helps the host to escape from premature aging and different diseases (cancer, neurodegeneration, and other chronic inflammatory conditions) through cellular self-digestion [99].

Autophagy also plays a crucial role in immune response to infections and inflammation that works downstream to different PRRs (TLRs, NLRs, RLRs, and cGAS-STING signaling) discussed earlier (**Figure 1**) [100–102]. The increased autophagy in Australian black fly foxes also dampens the severity of the lyssavirus infection through suppressing the virus replication and increases the tolerance to the prolonged infection with lesser cell death than humans (**Figure 1**) [103]. Autophagy increases with the increases in the viral load in bats. The pharmacological activation of the autophagy decreases the virus replication that shows its antiviral action. Another virus called Nelson Bay Orthoreovirus (NBV that in humans causes severe respiratory tract infection) isolated from the Australian fruit bat increases autophagy in host cells depending on the viral replication without causing severe infection [104]. Hence, increased autophagy along with increasing longevity and suppressing aging mechanisms among bats also increases their antiviral immune response to protect them from severe productive infection.

## 3. Adaptive immune response in bats to make them resistant severe viral infections

We do not have greater immunological data for adaptive immunity in bats as compared to humans due to lack of experimental reagents specific for bats and corresponding appropriate animal models. The genes [MHC-I and II, TCR (TCR-α and –β) and co-receptors, including CD3, CD4, CD8, and CD28 along with B cell-specific markers (CD22, CD19, CD20, CD27, and Igs)] involved in adaptive immunity in other species are conserved in bats [21–23]. The transcripts of both pro- and anti-inflammatory cytokines (IL-2, IL-4, IL-5, IL-6, IL-12a, IL-12b, IL-17a, IL-23, IL-10, TGF $\beta$, TNF, IFN $\gamma$, IL-1 $\beta$, CCL2, CCL5, and CXCL10) are also present [23]. The alpha1 (α1) domain of the H chain of MHC-I of *P. alecto* have three sequential AAs (Met, Asp, and Leu), which are absent in other mammals, including humans [105]. These 3 extra AAs in bat MHC-I help to form an extra salt-bridge chain between the H chain and the N-terminal of aspartic acid (Asp) of the antigenic peptide that promotes peptide presentation to the MHC I with high affinity during antigen presentation process. This study indicates the induction of stronger MHC-1-dependent T cells ($CD8^+$ cytotoxic T cells) immune response against viruses that helps them to survive otherwise lethal viral infections as seen in other mammals.

*P. alecto* has a predominant population of $CD8^+$T cells in their spleen and $CD4^+$T cells are predominantly present in blood, lymph nodes (LNs), and bone marrow [106]. Forty percent of these splenic T cells constitutively express IL-17, IL-22, and TGF-β mRNA, indicating the polarization of these T cells towards, Th17 and regulatory T cells ($T_{regs}$) [106]. Recent identification and development of bat-specific cross-reactive Abs and establishment of captive experimental bat colonies have advanced the field. Immunoglobulins or Abs, including IgG, IgA, IgM, and IgE have been detected in bats (*P. alecto*) [107, 108]. However, IgA in secretion is lesser than expected but that is compensated by increased presence of IgG in the mucosal surfaces [108]. IgM is the second most abundant Ab in the serum after IgG in *P. alecto*. Of note, bats have a bigger repertoire of germline genes encoding Ig variable (V), diversity (D), and joining (J) segments than humans, indicating a provision of a larger number of antigen (Ag) specificities in their naïve B cell receptor (BCR) repertoire [54]. For example, little brown bats (*Myotis lucifugus*) rely more on the germline encoded repertoire to fight against infections than somatic hypermutation (SHM) [109]. On the other hand, SHM in humans increase the affinities of Abs for diverse antigens [110]. Thus, human Ab response generates more diverse Abs in humans than bats.

The maternal Abs transferred to Egyptian Rousette bats against the Marburg virus last for their first five months after birth and Abs last for approximately 1 year in these bats infected naturally [111]. However, the reinfection of bats with the same virus induces anamnestic immune or Ab response within 5 days of the post viral infection clearing the virus systemically as well as from major organs (salivary glands, intestine, urinary bladder, and the reproductive tract). Hence, reinfection with the virus to bats in the natural environment is not sufficient to induce the productive infection. Another study indicates that the maternally-derived Abs (MDAs) in seasonally breeding bats (African fruit bats) do not last long for other viruses, including Lagos bat lyssavirus (LBV, a member of genus lyssavirus and gamily *rhadoviridae*) [112]. Also, the Abs developed in captive bats decay more slowly than these MDAs, indicating the fast decay of these MDAs. However, Abs produced in captive bats decay faster than seasonally breeding bats living in their natural environment, indicating the Ab may persist for life in natural environment harboring bats.

The Abs-mediated virus neutralization is not a universal mechanism for protection against Ebola, Marburg, and Sosuga (a recently discovered pathogenic Paramyxovirus in Uganda) viruses in the Egyptian Rousette bats [113, 114]. Similarly, maternal Abs to the Henipavirus become undetectable between 4 and 12 months after birth [115]. The seasonal horizontal transmission of the virus makes seronegative bats seropositive for Abs and seasons of late pregnancy/lactation in bats may increase the risk of zoonotic diseases. Further studies have shown that in the straw colored fruit bats (*Eidolon helvum*) fruit bats maternal Abs provide protection against Lagos bat lyssavirus and African Henipavirus for 6 months and acquired immunity in developed adult bats against them lasts for 12 years (Lagos bat virus) and 4 years (Henipavirus) [116]. However, the disturbed pregnancy and lactation (seasonal birth pulse) impacts the maternal Ab-based immunity on persisting virus that depends on the transmission characteristics (prolonged infection period or within host latency). It is interesting to note that despite the diminished Abs level the Egyptian Rousette bats exert a protective immune response against severe Marburg infection that may be due to the anamnestic response generating Abs and type 1 IFNs [117].

Abs specific to the glycoprotein GP2 to another *Filoviridae* family member called Lloviu virus (LLOV) have been detected in insectivorous Schreiber's Bent-winged bats in the caves of Northern Spain [118]. A study has shown that the reinfection with the particular virus is essential to explain the shortness (hours to days) of acute infections and development of immunity lasting for another 1–2 years [119]. Hence, recurring latent infections are warranted for immunoprotection in bats to severe viral infections. The migrating status of the bats or other migratory animals//birds also determine the reactivation or suppression of the latent infection depending on the immune status [120, 121]. For example, the relapse at either the start or end of migration may increase the prevalence across the year and may maintain pathogens with low transmissibility and short infectious periods in the migratory population [120]. For example, relapse at the beginning of the migration may reduce the prevalence of highly virulent or infectious viruses by amplifying death of infected hosts during migration, especially for highly transmissible viruses and those transmitted during migration or breeding season. The long-distance migratory Nathusius' pipistrelles (*Pipistrellus nathusii*) show difference in the immune status, for example, during migration they have increased number of lymphocytes with decreased neutrophils as compared to the non or pre-migratory period [38]. The oxidative stress is higher during migration period without any association between blood oxidative status and immunological impact. Of note, the immune challenge does not induce any changes in the oxidative stress irrespective of the migratory or pre-migratory season.

## 4. Future perspectives and conclusion

Bats always remain the source of attraction and fascinate humans. Even in Hollywood movies the character of the Dracula has been inspired from bats living on blood and coming out for the prey in night time. However, they became important to the medical community upon the first recognition of transfer of rabies virus to the animals serving as their prey for blood in 1959 in Trinidad. Since, then different have been suggested as the career for many viral pathogens that are responsible for different endemics, epidemics, and pandemics, including Nipah virus infection, Hendra virus infection, Ebola virus infection, SARS, MERS, and the current COVID-19 or SARS-CoV-2 infection. However, the direct causal virus for COVID-19, called SARS-CoV-2 has not been directly isolated from them, but genetically related or more close viruses have been identified in them [9, 10]. Hence, understanding the factors responsible for no severe pathogenic outcomes in the bats as compared to other mammals, including humans becomes crucial by keeping in mind the damages (both, life and economical) associated with current COVID-19 pandemic. The bat immune system has evolved in such a way to guard itself through the damages associated with high speed flight for long migration. For example, low ROS production to protect from DNA damage and inflammation. However, to keep a check on invading pathogens, especially viruses it has evolved the potent IFN-dependent antiviral immune response without inducing severe pro-inflammatory immune response as seen in other mammals, including humans during Ebola virus and severe COVID-19 infection. A recent study has shown that the Ebola virus in humans and fruit bats (*Epomops buettikoferi*) evolves differently by undergoing short term evolution as studied through circular sequencing [122]. For example, the Ebola virus (EBOV) passaged in fruit bat (*E. buettikoferi*) cells shows a sequence markers specific for host RNA editing enzyme activity, including evidence for adenosine deaminase acting on RNA (ADAR) editing of the EBOV glycoprotein (GP), show increased G to A transitions depending on the EBOV genome strand, and increased average genomic Shannon entropy compared to Ebola virus passaged in human 293 T cells. The bat EpoNi/22.1 cells express approximately 12-fold more ADAR1 mRNA than 293 T cells due to unique features of bat cells or bats. Hence, host-specific factors, including ADAR impact mutation/evolution of the virus. Of note, the mutation rate for Ebola virus is same for both bat and human cell lines. Hence, studying and identifying bat-specific factors have a potential to answer the unknowns associated with mild or no infection with the same pathogen that proves lethal to humans. For example, the evolution of the pathogen in the reservoir host is drift-driven, but in the incidental host it favors positive selection to adapt and reduces the tropism for primary host (bats) [123]. Hence, the pathogen becomes severe in the incidental host and transmits among human hosts as seen in Ebola virus infection and COVID-19. Also, the virus related to the Rubella called Ruhugu virus (RuhV shares identical genomic structure with the Rubella virus) has also been isolated from cyclops leaf-nosed bats (*Hipposideros cyclops*) sampled in Uganda [124]. This indicates that Rubella virus may have evolved from bat virus or in future Rubella-like infection may affect humans and other mammals as zoonotic disease from bats. Thus the future zoonotic (bats-specific) infections-associated endemics, epidemics, and pandemics, including vampire bat (*D. rotundus*) rabies caused by vampire bat rabies virus (VBRV, Lyssavirus of Rhabdoviridae family) will depend on the host-pathogen evolutionary signatures or relationships [125].

## 5. Conclusion

Bats are unique mammals with a potential to have true flight, harboring different viral pathogens that have caused or may cause severe infections to humans and other mammals. Understanding their immune system associated uniqueness may open avenues to deal effectively with zoonotic diseases coming from them.

## Author contribution

The author developed the idea, wrote and compiled the manuscript, and developed the figure.

## Funding

The author has not received any funding for this work.

## Conflict of interest

The author declares no conflict of interest.

## Author details

Vijay Kumar[1,2,3]

1 Children's Health Queensland Clinical Unit, School of Clinical Medicine, Mater Research, University of Queensland, St Lucia, Brisbane, Queensland, Australia

2 School of Biomedical Sciences, University of Queensland, St Lucia, Brisbane, Queensland, Australia

3 Department of Pharmaceutical Sciences, College of Pharmacy, The University of Tennessee Health Science Center (UTHSC), Madison Avenue, Memphis, Tennessee, USA

*Address all correspondence to: vij_tox@yahoo.com

## References


[1] T.H. Kunz, E.B. de Torrez, D. Bauer, T. Lobova, T.H. Fleming, Ecosystem services provided by bats, Europe 31 (2011) 32.

[2] M. Kasso, M. Balakrishnan, Ecological and Economic Importance of Bats (Order Chiroptera), ISRN Biodiversity 2013 (2013) 187415.

[3] D.T.S. Hayman, Bats as Viral Reservoirs, Annual Review of Virology 3(1) (2016) 77-99.

[4] G.F. McCracken, K. Safi, T.H. Kunz, D.K.N. Dechmann, S.M. Swartz, M. Wikelski, Airplane tracking documents the fastest flight speeds recorded for bats, Royal Society Open Science 3(11) (2016) 160398.

[5] I. Galván, J. Garrido-Fernández, J. Ríos, A. Pérez-Gálvez, B. Rodríguez-Herrera, J.J. Negro, Tropical bat as mammalian model for skin carotenoid metabolism, Proceedings of the National Academy of Sciences 113(39) (2016) 10932-10937.

[6] C.H. Calisher, J.E. Childs, H.E. Field, K.V. Holmes, T. Schountz, Bats: important reservoir hosts of emerging viruses, Clin Microbiol Rev 19(3) (2006) 531-545.

[7] A.D. Luis, D.T.S. Hayman, T.J. O'Shea, P.M. Cryan, A.T. Gilbert, J.R.C. Pulliam, J.N. Mills, M.E. Timonin, C.K.R. Willis, A.A. Cunningham, A.R. Fooks, C.E. Rupprecht, J.L.N. Wood, C.T. Webb, A comparison of bats and rodents as reservoirs of zoonotic viruses: are bats special?, Proc Biol Sci 280(1756) (2013) 20122753-20122753.

[8] F.L. Roes, On the Evolution of Virulent Zoonotic Viruses in Bats, Biol Theory (2020) 1-3.

[9] V. Kumar, Understanding the complexities of SARS-CoV-2 infection and its immunology: A road to immune-based therapeutics, International Immunopharmacology 88 (2020) 106980.

[10] V. Kumar, Emerging human Coronavirus infections (SARS, MERS, and COVID-19): Where they are leading us, International Reviews of Immunology (2020).

[11] A. Caron, M. Bourgarel, J. Cappelle, F. Liégeois, H.M. De Nys, F. Roger, Ebola Virus Maintenance: If Not (Only) Bats, What Else?, Viruses 10(10) (2018) 549.

[12] E.M. Leroy, B. Kumulungui, X. Pourrut, P. Rouquet, A. Hassanin, P. Yaba, A. Délicat, J.T. Paweska, J.P. Gonzalez, R. Swanepoel, Fruit bats as reservoirs of Ebola virus, Nature 438(7068) (2005) 575-576.

[13] J.L. Pawan, Rabies in the vampire bat of Trinidad, with special reference to the clinical course and the latency of infection, Caribb Med J 21 (1959) 137-156.

[14] J.L. Pawan, The transmission of paralytic rabies in Trinidad by the vampire bat (Desmodus rotundus murinus Wagner, Caribb Med J 21 (1959) 110-136.

[15] N. Johnson, N. Aréchiga-Ceballos, A. Aguilar-Setien, Vampire bat rabies: ecology, epidemiology and control, Viruses 6(5) (2014) 1911-1928.

[16] E. De Verteuil, F.W. Urich, The study and control of paralytic rabies transmitted by bats in Trinidad, British West Indies, Caribb Med J 21 (1959) 85-109.

[17] L.K. Koch, S. Cunze, J. Kochmann, S. Klimpel, Bats as putative Zaire ebolavirus reservoir hosts and their habitat suitability in Africa, Scientific Reports 10(1) (2020) 14268.

[18] L. Chen, B. Liu, J. Yang, Q. Jin, DBatVir: the database of bat-associated viruses, Database (Oxford) 2014 (2014) bau021.

[19] T.J. O'Shea, P.M. Cryan, D.T.S. Hayman, R.K. Plowright, D.G. Streicker, Multiple mortality events in bats: a global review, Mammal Review 46(3) (2016) 175-190.

[20] J. Kelley, B. de Bono, J. Trowsdale, IRIS: a database surveying known human immune system genes, Genomics 85(4) (2005) 503-511.

[21] A.T. Papenfuss, M.L. Baker, Z.P. Feng, M. Tachedjian, G. Crameri, C. Cowled, J. Ng, V. Janardhana, H.E. Field, L.F. Wang, The immune gene repertoire of an important viral reservoir, the Australian black flying fox, BMC Genomics 13 (2012) 261.

[22] T.I. Shaw, A. Srivastava, W.C. Chou, L. Liu, A. Hawkinson, T.C. Glenn, R. Adams, T. Schountz, Transcriptome sequencing and annotation for the Jamaican fruit bat (Artibeus jamaicensis), PLoS One 7(11) (2012) e48472.

[23] A.K. Lee, K.A. Kulcsar, O. Elliott, H. Khiabanian, E.R. Nagle, M.E. Jones, B.R. Amman, M. Sanchez-Lockhart, J.S. Towner, G. Palacios, R. Rabadan, De novo transcriptome reconstruction and annotation of the Egyptian rousette bat, BMC Genomics 16 (2015) 1033.

[24] T. Qurkhuli, N. Schwensow, S.D. Brändel, M. Tschapka, S. Sommer, Can extreme MHC class I diversity be a feature of a wide geographic range? The example of Seba's short-tailed bat (Carollia perspicillata), Immunogenetics 71(8-9) (2019) 575-587.

[25] A. Salmier, B. de Thoisy, B. Crouau-Roy, V. Lacoste, A. Lavergne, Spatial pattern of genetic diversity and selection in the MHC class II DRB of three Neotropical bat species, BMC Evol Biol 16(1) (2016) 229.

[26] S.N. Seifert, M.C. Letko, T. Bushmaker, E.D. Laing, G. Saturday, K. Meade-White, N. van Doremalen, C.C. Broder, V.J. Munster, *Rousettus aegyptiacus* Bats Do Not Support Productive Nipah Virus Replication, J Infect Dis 221(Supplement_4) (2020) S407-s413.

[27] C.E. Brook, M. Boots, K. Chandran, A.P. Dobson, C. Drosten, A.L. Graham, B.T. Grenfell, M.A. Müller, M. Ng, L.F. Wang, A. van Leeuwen, Accelerated viral dynamics in bat cell lines, with implications for zoonotic emergence, Elife 9 (2020).

[28] J.M. Emeny, M.J. Morgan, Regulation of the interferon system: evidence that Vero cells have a genetic defect in interferon production, J Gen Virol 43(1) (1979) 247-252.

[29] G.D. Brown, J.A. Willment, L. Whitehead, C-type lectins in immunity and homeostasis, Nature Reviews Immunology 18(6) (2018) 374-389.

[30] V. Kumar, A STING to inflammation and autoimmunity, Journal of Leukocyte Biology 106(1) (2019) 171-185.

[31] K. V, Toll-like receptors in immunity and inflammatory diseases: Past, present, and future, International immunopharmacology 59 (2018) 391-412.

[32] V. Kumar, Toll-like receptors in sepsis-associated cytokine storm and their endogenous negative regulators as future immunomodulatory targets, International immunopharmacology 89(Pt B) (2020) 107087-107087.

[33] J. Rehwinkel, M.U. Gack, RIG-I-like receptors: their regulation and roles in RNA sensing, Nature Reviews Immunology 20(9) (2020) 537-551.

[34] V. Kumar, Inflammasomes: Pandora's box for sepsis, J Inflamm Res 11 (2018) 477-502.

[35] S. Stockmaier, D.K.N. Dechmann, R.A. Page, M.T. O'Mara, No fever and leucocytosis in response to a lipopolysaccharide challenge in an insectivorous bat, Biology Letters 11(9) (2015) 20150576.

[36] A.K. Brunet-Rossinni, Reduced free-radical production and extreme longevity in the little brown bat (Myotis lucifugus) versus two non-flying mammals, Mech Ageing Dev 125(1) (2004) 11-20.

[37] M.Y. Vyssokikh, S. Holtze, O.A. Averina, K.G. Lyamzaev, A.A. Panteleeva, M.V. Marey, R.A. Zinovkin, F.F. Severin, M.V. Skulachev, N. Fasel, T.B. Hildebrandt, V.P. Skulachev, Mild depolarization of the inner mitochondrial membrane is a crucial component of an anti-aging program, Proceedings of the National Academy of Sciences 117(12) (2020) 6491-6501.

[38] C.C. Voigt, M. Fritze, O. Lindecke, D. Costantini, G. Pētersons, G. Czirják, The immune response of bats differs between pre-migration and migration seasons, Sci Rep 10(1) (2020) 17384.

[39] Z. Huang, C.V. Whelan, N.M. Foley, D. Jebb, F. Touzalin, E.J. Petit, S.J. Puechmaille, E.C. Teeling, Longitudinal comparative transcriptomics reveals unique mechanisms underlying extended healthspan in bats, Nature Ecology & Evolution 3(7) (2019) 1110-1120.

[40] D.L. Sun, Y.Z. Gao, X.Y. Ge, Z.L. Shi, N.Y. Zhou, Special Features of Bat Microbiota Differ From Those of Terrestrial Mammals, Front Microbiol 11 (2020) 1040.

[41] G.M. Hughes, J. Leech, S.J. Puechmaille, J.V. Lopez, E.C. Teeling, Is there a link between aging and microbiome diversity in exceptional mammalian longevity?, PeerJ 6 (2018) e4174.

[42] S. Kim, S.M. Jazwinski, The Gut Microbiota and Healthy Aging: A Mini-Review, Gerontology 64(6) (2018) 513-520.

[43] F. Kong, F. Deng, Y. Li, J. Zhao, Identification of gut microbiome signatures associated with longevity provides a promising modulation target for healthy aging, Gut Microbes 10(2) (2019) 210-215.

[44] C. Maynard, D. Weinkove, The Gut Microbiota and Ageing, Subcell Biochem 90 (2018) 351-371.

[45] K. Iha, T. Omatsu, S. Watanabe, N. Ueda, S. Taniguchi, H. Fujii, Y. Ishii, S. Kyuwa, H. Akashi, Y. Yoshikawa, Molecular cloning and expression analysis of bat toll-like receptors 3, 7 and 9, J Vet Med Sci 72(2) (2010) 217-220.

[46] C. Cowled, M. Baker, M. Tachedjian, P. Zhou, D. Bulach, L.F. Wang, Molecular characterisation of Toll-like receptors in the black flying fox Pteropus alecto, Dev Comp Immunol 35(1) (2011) 7-18.

[47] H. Jiang, J. Li, L. Li, X. Zhang, L. Yuan, J. Chen, Selective evolution of Toll-like receptors 3, 7, 8, and 9 in bats, Immunogenetics 69(4) (2017) 271-285.

[48] J. Schad, C.C. Voigt, Adaptive evolution of virus-sensing toll-like receptor 8 in bats, Immunogenetics 68(10) (2016) 783-795.

[49] M. Escalera-Zamudio, M.L. Zepeda-Mendoza, E. Loza-Rubio, E. Rojas-Anaya, M.L. Méndez-Ojeda, C.F. Arias, A.D. Greenwood, The evolution of bat nucleic acid-sensing Toll-like receptors, Mol Ecol 24(23) (2015) 5899-5909.

[50] C. Cowled, M.L. Baker, P. Zhou, M. Tachedjian, L.F. Wang, Molecular

characterisation of RIG-I-like helicases in the black flying fox, *Pteropus alecto*, Dev Comp Immunol 36(4) (2012) 657-664.

[51] A.M. Bruns, C.M. Horvath, LGP2 synergy with MDA5 in RLR-mediated RNA recognition and antiviral signaling, Cytokine 74(2) (2015) 198-206.

[52] R.Y. Sanchez David, C. Combredet, V. Najburg, G.A. Millot, G. Beauclair, B. Schwikowski, T. Léger, J.-M. Camadro, Y. Jacob, J. Bellalou, N. Jouvenet, F. Tangy, A.V. Komarova, LGP2 binds to PACT to regulate RIG-I– and MDA5-mediated antiviral responses, Science Signaling 12(601) (2019) eaar3993.

[53] R. Tarigan, H. Shimoda, K.C.C. Doysabas, M. Ken, A. Iida, E. Hondo, Role of pattern recognition receptors and interferon-beta in protecting bat cell lines from encephalomyocarditis virus and Japanese encephalitis virus infection, Biochem Biophys Res Commun 527(1) (2020) 1-7.

[54] A. Banerjee, M.L. Baker, K. Kulcsar, V. Misra, R. Plowright, K. Mossman, Novel Insights Into Immune Systems of Bats, Front Immunol 11 (2020) 26.

[55] H. Feng, A.-L. Sander, A. Moreira-Soto, D. Yamane, J.F. Drexler, S.M. Lemon, Hepatovirus 3ABC proteases and evolution of mitochondrial antiviral signaling protein (MAVS), Journal of Hepatology 71(1) (2019) 25-34.

[56] S.P. John, J. Sun, R.J. Carlson, B. Cao, C.J. Bradfield, J. Song, M. Smelkinson, I.D.C. Fraser, IFIT1 Exerts Opposing Regulatory Effects on the Inflammatory and Interferon Gene Programs in LPS-Activated Human Macrophages, Cell Reports 25(1) (2018) 95-106.e6.

[57] B. Wu, S. Hur, How RIG-I like receptors activate MAVS, Current opinion in virology 12 (2015) 91-98.

[58] V.J. Munster, D.R. Adney, N. van Doremalen, V.R. Brown, K.L. Miazgowicz, S. Milne-Price, T. Bushmaker, R. Rosenke, D. Scott, A. Hawkinson, E. de Wit, T. Schountz, R.A. Bowen, Replication and shedding of MERS-CoV in Jamaican fruit bats (Artibeus jamaicensis), Sci Rep 6 (2016) 21878.

[59] A. Banerjee, D. Falzarano, N. Rapin, J. Lew, V. Misra, Interferon Regulatory Factor 3-Mediated Signaling Limits Middle-East Respiratory Syndrome (MERS) Coronavirus Propagation in Cells from an Insectivorous Bat, Viruses 11(2) (2019).

[60] A. Banerjee, X. Zhang, A. Yip, K.S. Schulz, A.T. Irving, D. Bowdish, B. Golding, L.-F. Wang, K. Mossman, Positive Selection of a Serine Residue in Bat IRF3 Confers Enhanced Antiviral Protection, iScience 23(3) (2020).

[61] A. Banerjee, S. Subudhi, N. Rapin, J. Lew, R. Jain, D. Falzarano, V. Misra, Selection of viral variants during persistent infection of insectivorous bat cells with Middle East respiratory syndrome coronavirus, Sci Rep 10(1) (2020) 7257.

[62] P. Zhou, C. Cowled, A. Mansell, P. Monaghan, D. Green, L. Wu, Z. Shi, L.F. Wang, M.L. Baker, IRF7 in the Australian black flying fox, Pteropus alecto: evidence for a unique expression pattern and functional conservation, PLoS One 9(8) (2014) e103875.

[63] P. Zhou, C. Cowled, S. Todd, G. Crameri, E.R. Virtue, G.A. Marsh, R. Klein, Z. Shi, L.F. Wang, M.L. Baker, Type III IFNs in pteropid bats: differential expression patterns provide evidence for distinct roles in antiviral immunity, J Immunol 186(5) (2011) 3138-3147.

[64] S.S. Pavlovich, T. Darling, A.J. Hume, R.A. Davey, F. Feng, E. Mühlberger, T.B. Kepler, Egyptian

Rousette IFN-ω Subtypes Elicit Distinct Antiviral Effects and Transcriptional Responses in Conspecific Cells, Front Immunol 11 (2020) 435.

[65] J. Prescott, J.C. Guito, J.R. Spengler, C.E. Arnold, A.J. Schuh, B.R. Amman, T.K. Sealy, L.W. Guerrero, G.F. Palacios, M. Sanchez-Lockhart, C.G. Albariño, J.S. Towner, Rousette Bat Dendritic Cells Overcome Marburg Virus-Mediated Antiviral Responses by Upregulation of Interferon-Related Genes While Downregulating Proinflammatory Disease Mediators, mSphere 4(6) (2019).

[66] I.V. Kuzmin, T.M. Schwarz, P.A. Ilinykh, I. Jordan, T.G. Ksiazek, R. Sachidanandam, C.F. Basler, A. Bukreyev, Innate Immune Responses of Bat and Human Cells to Filoviruses: Commonalities and Distinctions, J Virol 91(8) (2017).

[67] J. Spitaels, L. Van Hoecke, K. Roose, G. Kochs, X. Saelens, Mx1 in Hematopoietic Cells Protects against Thogoto Virus Infection, J Virol 93(15) (2019).

[68] J. Fuchs, M. Hölzer, M. Schilling, C. Patzina, A. Schoen, T. Hoenen, G. Zimmer, M. Marz, F. Weber, M.A. Müller, G. Kochs, Evolution and Antiviral Specificities of Interferon-Induced Mx Proteins of Bats against Ebola, Influenza, and Other RNA Viruses, J Virol 91(15) (2017).

[69] G. Guarda, M. Braun, F. Staehli, A. Tardivel, C. Mattmann, I. Förster, M. Farlik, T. Decker, Renaud A. Du Pasquier, P. Romero, J. Tschopp, Type I Interferon Inhibits Interleukin-1 Production and Inflammasome Activation, Immunity 34(2) (2011) 213-223.

[70] E. Eren, R. Planès, S. Bagayoko, P.-J. Bordignon, K. Chaoui, A. Hessel, K. Santoni, M. Pinilla, B. Lagrange, O. Burlet-Schiltz, J.C. Howard, T. Henry, M. Yamamoto, E. Meunier, Irgm2 and Gate-16 cooperatively dampen Gram-negative bacteria-induced caspase-11 response, EMBO reports 21(11) (2020) e50829.

[71] G. Ni, Z. Ma, B. Damania, cGAS and STING: At the intersection of DNA and RNA virus-sensing networks, PLoS Pathog 14(8) (2018) e1007148.

[72] J. Xie, Y. Li, X. Shen, G. Goh, Y. Zhu, J. Cui, L.-F. Wang, Z.-L. Shi, P. Zhou, Dampened STING-Dependent Interferon Activation in Bats, Cell Host & Microbe 23(3) (2018) 297-301.e4.

[73] Y. Tanaka, Z.J. Chen, STING specifies IRF3 phosphorylation by TBK1 in the cytosolic DNA signaling pathway, Sci Signal 5(214) (2012) ra20.

[74] M. Ahn, J. Cui, A.T. Irving, L.-F. Wang, Unique Loss of the PYHIN Gene Family in Bats Amongst Mammals: Implications for Inflammasome Sensing, Scientific Reports 6(1) (2016) 21722.

[75] L. Unterholzner, S.E. Keating, M. Baran, K.A. Horan, S.B. Jensen, S. Sharma, C.M. Sirois, T. Jin, E. Latz, T.S. Xiao, K.A. Fitzgerald, S.R. Paludan, A.G. Bowie, IFI16 is an innate immune sensor for intracellular DNA, Nature Immunology 11(11) (2010) 997-1004.

[76] G. Zhang, C. Cowled, Z. Shi, Z. Huang, K.A. Bishop-Lilly, X. Fang, J.W. Wynne, Z. Xiong, M.L. Baker, W. Zhao, M. Tachedjian, Y. Zhu, P. Zhou, X. Jiang, J. Ng, L. Yang, L. Wu, J. Xiao, Y. Feng, Y. Chen, X. Sun, Y. Zhang, G.A. Marsh, G. Crameri, C.C. Broder, K.G. Frey, L.-F. Wang, J. Wang, Comparative Analysis of Bat Genomes Provides Insight into the Evolution of Flight and Immunity, Science 339(6118) (2013) 456-460.

[77] A.M. Gamage, F. Zhu, M. Ahn, R.J.H. Foo, Y.Y. Hey, D.H.W. Low, I.H. Mendenhall, C.-A. Dutertre, L.-F. Wang, Immunophenotyping monocytes, macrophages and

granulocytes in the Pteropodid bat Eonycteris spelaea, Scientific Reports 10(1) (2020) 309.

[78] J.A. Hayward, M. Tachedjian, J. Cui, A.Z. Cheng, A. Johnson, M.L. Baker, R.S. Harris, L.F. Wang, G. Tachedjian, Differential Evolution of Antiretroviral Restriction Factors in Pteropid Bats as Revealed by APOBEC3 Gene Complexity, Mol Biol Evol 35(7) (2018) 1626-1637.

[79] M. Renard, M. Henry, D. Guétard, J.P. Vartanian, S. Wain-Hobson, APOBEC1 and APOBEC3 cytidine deaminases as restriction factors for hepadnaviral genomes in non-humans in vivo, J Mol Biol 400(3) (2010) 323-334.

[80] J.N. Mandl, C. Schneider, D.S. Schneider, M.L. Baker, Going to Bat(s) for Studies of Disease Tolerance, Frontiers in Immunology 9(2112) (2018).

[81] E.W. Refsland, R.S. Harris, The APOBEC3 family of retroelement restriction factors, Curr Top Microbiol Immunol 371 (2013) 1-27.

[82] I. Narvaiza, S. Landry, M.D. Weitzman, APOBEC3 proteins and genomic stability: the high cost of a good defense, Cell Cycle 11(1) (2012) 33-38.

[83] S. Yamanaka, M.E. Balestra, L.D. Ferrell, J. Fan, K.S. Arnold, S. Taylor, J.M. Taylor, T.L. Innerarity, Apolipoprotein B mRNA-editing protein induces hepatocellular carcinoma and dysplasia in transgenic animals, Proc Natl Acad Sci U S A 92(18) (1995) 8483-8487.

[84] S. Henderson, T. Fenton, APOBEC3 genes: retroviral restriction factors to cancer drivers, Trends in Molecular Medicine 21(5) (2015) 274-284.

[85] M. Petljak, J. Maciejowski, Molecular origins of APOBEC-associated mutations in cancer, DNA Repair (Amst) 94 (2020) 102905.

[86] J. Koh, Y. Itahana, I.H. Mendenhall, D. Low, E.X.Y. Soh, A.K. Guo, Y.T. Chionh, L.-F. Wang, K. Itahana, ABCB1 protects bat cells from DNA damage induced by genotoxic compounds, Nature Communications 10(1) (2019) 2820.

[87] V. Mohanram, A.E. Sköld, S.M. Bächle, S.K. Pathak, A.L. Spetz, IFN-α induces APOBEC3G, F, and A in immature dendritic cells and limits HIV-1 spread to CD4+ T cells, J Immunol 190(7) (2013) 3346-3353.

[88] M. Ahn, D.E. Anderson, Q. Zhang, C.W. Tan, B.L. Lim, K. Luko, M. Wen, W.N. Chia, S. Mani, L.C. Wang, J.H.J. Ng, R.M. Sobota, C.-A. Dutertre, F. Ginhoux, Z.-L. Shi, A.T. Irving, L.-F. Wang, Dampened NLRP3-mediated inflammation in bats and implications for a special viral reservoir host, Nat Microbiol 4(5) (2019) 789-799.

[89] A. Banerjee, N. Rapin, T. Bollinger, V. Misra, Lack of inflammatory gene expression in bats: a unique role for a transcription repressor, Scientific Reports 7(1) (2017) 2232.

[90] J. Kacprzyk, G.M. Hughes, E.M. Palsson-McDermott, S.R. Quinn, S.J. Puechmaille, L.A.J. O'Neill, E.C. Teeling, A Potent Anti-Inflammatory Response in Bat Macrophages May Be Linked to Extended Longevity and Viral Tolerance, Acta Chiropterologica 19(2) (2017) 219-228, 10.

[91] N.M. Foley, G.M. Hughes, Z. Huang, M. Clarke, D. Jebb, C.V. Whelan, E.J. Petit, F. Touzalin, O. Farcy, G. Jones, R.D. Ransome, J. Kacprzyk, M.J. O'Connell, G. Kerth, H. Rebelo, L. Rodrigues, S.J. Puechmaille, E.C. Teeling, Growing old, yet staying young: The role of telomeres in bats' exceptional longevity, Sci Adv 4(2) (2018) eaao0926.

[92] J. Munshi-South, G.S. Wilkinson, Bats and birds: Exceptional longevity despite high metabolic rates, Ageing Res Rev 9(1) (2010) 12-19.

[93] Y.T. Chionh, J. Cui, J. Koh, I.H. Mendenhall, J.H.J. Ng, D. Low, K. Itahana, A.T. Irving, L.F. Wang, High basal heat-shock protein expression in bats confers resistance to cellular heat/oxidative stress, Cell Stress Chaperones 24(4) (2019) 835-849.

[94] B. Levine, N. Mizushima, H.W. Virgin, Autophagy in immunity and inflammation, Nature 469(7330) (2011) 323-335.

[95] X.-J. Zhou, H. Zhang, Autophagy in immunity: implications in etiology of autoimmune/autoinflammatory diseases, Autophagy 8(9) (2012) 1286-1299.

[96] B. Ravikumar, S. Sarkar, J.E. Davies, M. Futter, M. Garcia-Arencibia, Z.W. Green-Thompson, M. Jimenez-Sanchez, V.I. Korolchuk, M. Lichtenberg, S. Luo, D.C. Massey, F.M. Menzies, K. Moreau, U. Narayanan, M. Renna, F.H. Siddiqi, B.R. Underwood, A.R. Winslow, D.C. Rubinsztein, Regulation of mammalian autophagy in physiology and pathophysiology, Physiol Rev 90(4) (2010) 1383-1435.

[97] David C. Rubinsztein, G. Mariño, G. Kroemer, Autophagy and Aging, Cell 146(5) (2011) 682-695.

[98] H. Appelqvist, P. Wäster, K. Kågedal, K. Öllinger, The lysosome: from waste bag to potential therapeutic target, J Mol Cell Biol 5(4) (2013) 214-226.

[99] N. Mizushima, B. Levine, A.M. Cuervo, D.J. Klionsky, Autophagy fights disease through cellular self-digestion, Nature 451(7182) (2008) 1069-1075.

[100] V. Deretic, Autophagy in immunity and cell-autonomous defense against intracellular microbes, Immunological reviews 240(1) (2011) 92-104.

[101] X. Gui, H. Yang, T. Li, X. Tan, P. Shi, M. Li, F. Du, Z.J. Chen, Autophagy induction via STING trafficking is a primordial function of the cGAS pathway, Nature 567(7747) (2019) 262-266.

[102] V. Deretic, T. Saitoh, S. Akira, Autophagy in infection, inflammation and immunity, Nature Reviews Immunology 13(10) (2013) 722-737.

[103] E.D. Laing, S.L. Sterling, D.L. Weir, C.R. Beauregard, I.L. Smith, S.E. Larsen, L.F. Wang, A.L. Snow, B.C. Schaefer, C.C. Broder, Enhanced Autophagy Contributes to Reduced Viral Infection in Black Flying Fox Cells, Viruses 11(3) (2019).

[104] X.-L. Tao, W. Zhao, W. Tong, X.-F. Wang, L.-L. Dou, J.-M. Chen, N. Liu, Y. Lu, Y.-B. Zhang, X.-P. Jin, Y.-F. Shen, H.-Y. Zhao, H. Jin, Y.-G. Li, The effects of autophagy on the replication of Nelson Bay orthoreovirus, Virology Journal 16(1) (2019) 90.

[105] Z. Qu, Z. Li, L. Ma, X. Wei, L. Zhang, R. Liang, G. Meng, N. Zhang, C. Xia, Structure and Peptidome of the Bat MHC Class I Molecule Reveal a Novel Mechanism Leading to High-Affinity Peptide Binding, J Immunol 202(12) (2019) 3493-3506.

[106] J.M. Martínez Gómez, P. Periasamy, C.-A. Dutertre, A.T. Irving, J.H.J. Ng, G. Crameri, M.L. Baker, F. Ginhoux, L.-F. Wang, S. Alonso, Phenotypic and functional characterization of the major lymphocyte populations in the fruit-eating bat Pteropus alecto, Scientific Reports 6(1) (2016) 37796.

[107] M.L. Baker, M. Tachedjian, L.F. Wang, Immunoglobulin heavy chain diversity in Pteropid bats: evidence for a diverse and highly specific antigen

binding repertoire, Immunogenetics 62(3) (2010) 173-184.

[108] J.W. Wynne, A. Di Rubbo, B.J. Shiell, G. Beddome, C. Cowled, G.R. Peck, J. Huang, S.L. Grimley, M.L. Baker, W.P. Michalski, Purification and characterisation of immunoglobulins from the Australian black flying fox (Pteropus alecto) using anti-fab affinity chromatography reveals the low abundance of IgA, PLoS One 8(1) (2013) e52930.

[109] S. Bratsch, N. Wertz, K. Chaloner, T.H. Kunz, J.E. Butler, The little brown bat, *M. lucifugus*, displays a highly diverse V H, D H and J H repertoire but little evidence of somatic hypermutation, Dev Comp Immunol 35(4) (2011) 421-30.

[110] I.M. Tomlinson, G. Walter, P.T. Jones, P.H. Dear, E.L. Sonnhammer, G. Winter, The imprint of somatic hypermutation on the repertoire of human germline V genes, J Mol Biol 256(5) (1996) 813-817.

[111] Kaposi's sarcoma and Pneumocystis pneumonia among homosexual men--New York City and California, MMWR Morb Mortal Wkly Rep 30(25) (1981) 305-8.

[112] D.T.S. Hayman, A.D. Luis, O. Restif, K.S. Baker, A.R. Fooks, C. Leach, D.L. Horton, R. Suu-Ire, A.A. Cunningham, J.L.N. Wood, C.T. Webb, Maternal antibody and the maintenance of a lyssavirus in populations of seasonally breeding African bats, PLoS One 13(6) (2018) e0198563.

[113] A.J. Schuh, B.R. Amman, T.K. Sealy, M.H. Kainulainen, A.K. Chakrabarti, L.W. Guerrero, S.T. Nichol, C.G. Albarino, J.S. Towner, Antibody-Mediated Virus Neutralization Is Not a Universal Mechanism of Marburg, Ebola, or Sosuga Virus Clearance in Egyptian Rousette Bats, J Infect Dis 219(11) (2019) 1716-1721.

[114] B.R. Amman, C.G. Albariño, B.H. Bird, L. Nyakarahuka, T.K. Sealy, S. Balinandi, A.J. Schuh, S.M. Campbell, U. Ströher, M.E. Jones, M.E. Vodzack, D.M. Reeder, W. Kaboyo, S.T. Nichol, J.S. Towner, A Recently Discovered Pathogenic Paramyxovirus, Sosuga Virus, is Present in *Rousettus aegyptiacus* Fruit Bats at Multiple Locations in Uganda, J Wildl Dis 51(3) (2015) 774-779.

[115] K.S. Baker, R. Suu-Ire, J. Barr, D.T.S. Hayman, C.C. Broder, D.L. Horton, C. Durrant, P.R. Murcia, A.A. Cunningham, J.L.N. Wood, Viral antibody dynamics in a chiropteran host, J Anim Ecol 83(2) (2014) 415-428.

[116] A.J. Peel, K.S. Baker, D.T.S. Hayman, C.C. Broder, A.A. Cunningham, A.R. Fooks, R. Garnier, J.L.N. Wood, O. Restif, Support for viral persistence in bats from age-specific serology and models of maternal immunity, Sci Rep 8(1) (2018) 3859.

[117] A.J. Schuh, B.R. Amman, T.K. Sealy, J.R. Spengler, S.T. Nichol, J.S. Towner, Egyptian rousette bats maintain long-term protective immunity against Marburg virus infection despite diminished antibody levels, Sci Rep 7(1) (2017) 8763.

[118] E. Ramírez de Arellano, M. Sanchez-Lockhart, M.J. Perteguer, M. Bartlett, M. Ortiz, P. Campioli, A. Hernández, J. Gonzalez, K. Garcia, M. Ramos, M.Á. Jiménez-Clavero, A. Tenorio, M.P. Sánchez-Seco, F. González, J.E. Echevarría, G. Palacios, A. Negredo, First Evidence of Antibodies Against Lloviu Virus in Schreiber's Bent-Winged Insectivorous Bats Demonstrate a Wide Circulation of the Virus in Spain, Viruses 11(4) (2019) 360.

[119] E.E. Glennon, D.J. Becker, A.J. Peel, R. Garnier, R.D. Suu-Ire, L. Gibson, D.T.S. Hayman, J.L.N. Wood, A.A. Cunningham, R.K. Plowright, O. Restif,

What is stirring in the reservoir? Modelling mechanisms of henipavirus circulation in fruit bat hosts, Philos Trans R Soc Lond B Biol Sci 374(1782) (2019) 20190021.

[120] D.J. Becker, E.D. Ketterson, R.J. Hall, Reactivation of latent infections with migration shapes population-level disease dynamics, Proc Biol Sci 287(1935) (2020) 20201829.

[121] S. Altizer, R. Bartel, B.A. Han, Animal migration and infectious disease risk, Science 331(6015) (2011) 296-302.

[122] Z.J. Whitfield, A.N. Prasad, A.J. Ronk, I.V. Kuzmin, P.A. Ilinykh, R. Andino, A. Bukreyev, Species-Specific Evolution of Ebola Virus during Replication in Human and Bat Cells, Cell Reports 32(7) (2020) 108028.

[123] R.A. Urbanowicz, C.P. McClure, A. Sakuntabhai, A.A. Sall, G. Kobinger, M.A. Müller, E.C. Holmes, F.A. Rey, E. Simon-Loriere, J.K. Ball, Human Adaptation of Ebola Virus during the West African Outbreak, Cell 167(4) (2016) 1079-1087.e5.

[124] A.J. Bennett, A.C. Paskey, A. Ebinger, F. Pfaff, G. Priemer, D. Höper, A. Breithaupt, E. Heuser, R.G. Ulrich, J.H. Kuhn, K.A. Bishop-Lilly, M. Beer, T.L. Goldberg, Relatives of rubella virus in diverse mammals, Nature 586(7829) (2020) 424-428.

[125] D.G. Streicker, J.C. Winternitz, D.A. Satterfield, R.E. Condori-Condori, A. Broos, C. Tello, S. Recuenco, A. Velasco-Villa, S. Altizer, W. Valderrama, Host–pathogen evolutionary signatures reveal dynamics and future invasions of vampire bat rabies, Proceedings of the National Academy of Sciences 113(39) (2016) 10926-10931.

Section 2

# COVID-19 Origin, Epidemiology, Evolution, and Tools for Drug Development

Chapter 2

# Epidemiology, Zoonotic and Reverse Zoonotic Potential of COVID-19

*Sadia Muneer, Tean Zaheer, Aqsa Ahmad, Muhammad Imran, Amjad Islam Aqib, Iqra Zaheer and Muhammad Imran Arshad*

## Abstract

The demographic patterns of COVID-19 spread can provide clues to develop roadmaps for devising better prevention and control. It is high time to analyze and re-evaluate the zoonotic/reverse zoonotic spread of SARS-CoV-2 globally. To this end, lessons from epidemiology and associated determinants from previous outbreaks of SARS-CoV-1 and MERS need to be cultured and re-visited. Ways to minimize the rates of infection and promote the well-being of the masses need urgent attention owing to the subsequent waves of the global pandemic in most countries. Efforts are being directed for the provision of efficient and cost-effective diagnostics, prophylaxis and therapeutic options for COVID-19. The chapter provides insights, suggesting a potential roadmap for efficiently preventing the future outbreaks of COVID-19, based on the tools of epidemiology, transmission probabilities and public health safety concerns.

**Keywords:** COVID-19, Zoonotic, reverse zoonotic, Epidemiological tools, public health

## 1. Introduction

An outbreak with the name of CoVID-19 was reported from Wuhan, China on December 29, 2019. Initially, it was treated as pneumonia of unknown origin and reported to the local office of the World Health Organization (WHO) in China on December 31, 2019 [1]. The most recent outbreak owing to the probable zoonotic and human-human transmission of coronavirus disease virus, 2019 (COVID-19) has entrapped 220 countries and territories with 162, 773, 940 confirmed cases reported by WHO as of 17 May 2021 more than One Hundred Fifty-eight million people (WHO) affected. The host, agent and environmental factors are crucially involved in the chain of infection following the entry of the 2019 novel Coronavirus (2019-nCoV or SARS-CoV-2) in a susceptible host. The progression of the virus within the host may be as quick as 5–6 days (average), leading to severe clinical symptoms that warrant intensive care. The virus later on named severe acute respiratory syndrome coronavirus 2 (SARS-CoV-2) by the international committee on taxonomy of viruses on February 11, 2020 [2]. Bats and Pangolins were considered the reservoir host and initially blowout through the exposure of human beings to the seafood market in Wuhan, China [3]. The worldwide distribution of the virus was attributed to commercial air travels from epidemic countries to non-epidemic countries including, Taiwan, Japan, Korea, Malaysia, Russia, America, Saudi Arabia, United Arab Emirates, Germany, France, Spain, Italy and Iran etc. [4]. To date, the number of highest positive cases has been encountered by the USA followed by India, Brazil, Europe, UK, Africa and Middle East [5]. In order to respond to the outbreak swiftly and accurately, the public health authorities and policy makers direly need to know the epidemiology and associated risk factors [6]. The risk factors may include; how much time it takes to show the symptoms and which specific individuals having specific characteristics are more prone to infection.

According to CDC, currently several registered vaccines are available in United States to provide protection against CoVID-19. These vaccines are named as Pfizer-BioNTech, Moderna and Johnson & Johnson's Janssen. Other two vaccines Novavax and AstraZeneca are in phase 3 clinical trials.

It is necessary to strictly follow the precautionary measures i.e. wearing mask, social distancing, avoid arranging events and frequently hand washing along with the vaccination because vaccines alone will not prevent the transmission or end the pandemic. Until high level of global vaccine mediated defense is attained throughout the world.

As documented by the WHO, mathematical models specifically designed in a timely fashion may play an important role in providing evidence-based knowledge to public health authorities and policy makers. Moreover, modeling can help in understanding different aspects of the outbreak including (i) the ability of transmission of disease, (ii) prediction of peaks of infections during the progression of the disease, (iii) severity of infection and (iv) the effectiveness of preventive strategies for the intervention of disease. The modelers of infectious diseases worldwide had accepted the challenge of developing simulation models for transmission and dynamics of the disease and promptly reacted to the emerging outbreak of CoVID-19. Various epidemiological models that have been developed by modelers worldwide included: In China, Susceptible-Exposed-Infected-Resistant (SEIR) Model [7–9], Bats-Host-Reservoir-People (BHRP) transmission network model [10], Markov Chain Monte Carlo (MCMC) methods [11], Susceptible individuals (S)-Asymptomatic individuals (E)- Infectious individuals with symptoms(I)- Isolated individuals with treatment (J)- Recovered individual (R) (SEIJR) dynamic compartmental model [12], Exponential growth (EG) and Maximum Likelihood (ML) estimation method [13–15], Incidence Decay and Exponential Adjustment (IDEA) model [16], Susceptible-Exposed-Infected-Recovered-Death-Cumulative (SEIRDC) model [17], Computational modeling of potential epidemic trajectories [18], Simulation of early outbreak trajectories [19], Traveling network based modeling [20], Susceptible-Infected-Recovered (SIR) model and Quarantine model [5] in Italy, Susceptible-Exposed-Infected-Recovered (SEIR) model, Exponential growth (EG), Maximum Likelihood (ML) estimation, Sequential Bayesian (SB) method and Estimation of Time Dependent (TD) reproduction numbers in India [21, 22].

All of these simulation models estimated the Basic Reproduction Number (R0) of the virus. The R0 indicates the transmissibility of the virus from an infected person to a naïve or unexposed population. A value $R0 > 1$ represents that the number of cases will increase in the future while $R0 < 1$ represents that the disease will diminish in the near future. The reason for higher R0 estimates may be attributed to lower numbers of cases and minimum onset time of infection. However, the estimation error will start to decrease as the number of cases increased and real-time pictures of the cases will be available for accurate estimates [13]. In this scenario, statistical models are primarily used to determine the basic viral replication number, the serial interval between primary and secondary cases and virus doubling time which are important epidemic parameters [23, 24]. Additionally, some other approaches may also be required to include mild or asymptomatic cases which may be missed due to limitations of diagnostic methods applied [25]. With time, treatment options of clinical patients were improved and the spread of disease is being controlled through more strict methods like the restricted movement of individuals. The effects of such measures may be measured through statistical reasoning [26, 27]. On the other hand, mathematical models are based on dynamical Equations [28] can give more details related to epidemic characteristics as compared to statistical methods [29].

## 2. Reverse zoonotic potential of coronaviruses

Sporadic detection of natural SARS-CoV-2 infections together with successful experimental infections of certain animals raises concerns about reverse zoonosis (also termed as zooanthroposis: transmission of the infection from humans to animals. As a result of close contact with infected humans, several cats, dogs and zoo animals tested positive for SARS-CoV-2 [30, 31]. However, the incidence of natural infections in these animals has not been ruled out due to limited information on clinical features of the infections in animals. The existing data suggest that clinical features may range from asymptomatic infections to symptomatic disorders with signs that may include sneezing, coughing, nasal discharge, respiratory distress, vomiting, diarrhea, ocular discharge, lethargy and fever etc. [32]. A study from Hong Kong in February 2020 confirmed the transmission of SARS-CoV-2 infection to asymptomatic dogs from their previously diagnosed COVID-19 positive owner. A 17-year-old Pomeranian breed dog and a 2-year-old German shepherd were tested positive for SARS-CoV-2 RNA by RT-PCR on multiple oral and nasal swabs. However, virus isolation and serological testing could not be executed [33]. A summary of potential zoonotic relations of some coronaviruses has been given in **Figure 1**.

As a result of the death of a geriatric dog; presumably due to other underlying health issues, it was concluded that the dog either was contaminated by close contact with an infected individual or had a low level of infection. Similarly, a six-year male German shepherd tested positive for SARS-CoV-2 RNA in the USA in mid-April 2020, who contracted the infection from his COVID-19 positive owner. After five days of infection, he developed active infection followed by nasal discharge, lethargy and difficulty in breathing, blood in urine and vomit, weight loss and difficulty in walking, along with heart murmurs and lymphoma [34]. A case report in March 2020 revealed a cat belonging to a COVID-19 positive owner, tested

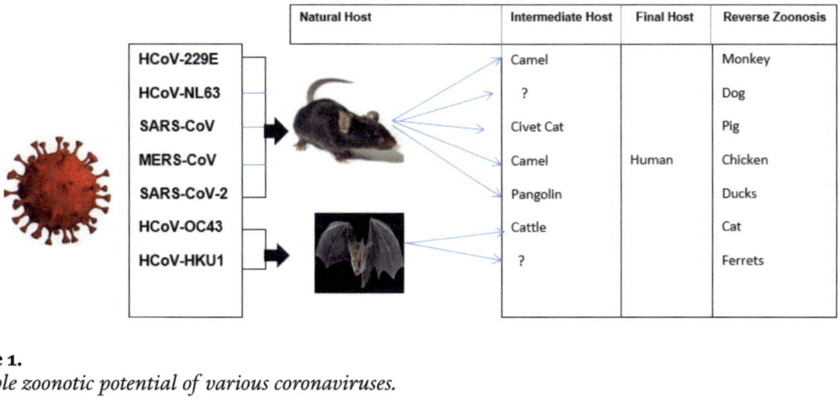


**Figure 1.**
*Probable zoonotic potential of various coronaviruses.*

positive for SARS-CoV-2 RNA by RT-PCR in Belgium, presenting gastrointestinal disease and transient respiratory disorders. While in another report on April 01, 2020, a pet cat belonging to a COVID-19 positive owner was tested positive for SARS-CoV-2 without showing disease symptoms [35]. A report on April 05, 2020, showed transmission of SARS-CoV-2 from a zoo employer who was an asymptomatic carrier of SARS-CoV-2 to one tigress, five tigers and lions at Bronx zoo in New York [35].

In the USA on August 14, 2020, 13 cases of pet cats and 14 cases of dogs were tested positive for SARS-CoV-2 by virus neutralization antibody tests or RT-PCR having close contact history with infected humans [31]. It has also been proven experimentally that susceptible pet cats can also transfer this virus to other healthy cats via short-distance aerosols or droplets due to greater similarity between ACE-2 receptors of feline and humans [36]. In a study, two dogs, two cats, three lions and four tigers were tested positive for the presence of SARS-CoV-2 due to close contact with their COVID-19 positive caretakers [37]. It also provides important information about animal management for COVID-19 control, animal models for SARS-CoV-2 and significant replication of this virus in both lower and upper respiratory tracts of ferrets and cats. Transmission of this virus can occur in ferrets through direct contact and in cats through droplets or aerosols. The presence of this virus in cats from Wuhan, China showed that cats may get infected by this virus by the environment or humans [38]. In a study, 15% of cats were tested positive for the presence of SARS-CoV-2 using an Indirect Enzyme-Linked Immunosorbent Assay while cats tested before the outbreak showed negative results [39]. A study provides important insight about the high susceptibility risk of animals having close contact with humans especially cats and ferrets while poor susceptibility risk in animals like pigs, dogs, ducks and chickens [40].

Based on these findings we may conclude that SARS-CoV-2 has the potential of reverse zoonosis as well. Although the risk of disease transmission from humans to animals and companion or zoo animals to humans or other animals is much less and it depends upon how this virus spreads in various animal species. Therefore, planned investigations, targeted surveillance and continuous monitoring of specific animal species having close contact with their COVID-19 positive or suspected owners or caretakers are mandatory at local or national levels. Although, currently there is no specific testing facility available for SARS-CoV-2 infections in animals. But the situation may change in the future to control and management of COVID-19 infections. To test samples for companion animals, a laboratory in the USA known as IDEXX Laboratories has started a test under the commercial name of SARS-CoV-2 (COVID-19) [41]. Several private and government veterinary laboratories are now trying to develop and use nucleic acid-based tests and serological assays to diagnose SARS-CoV-2 transmission in zoo and pet animals [42].

## 3. Reverse zoonosis in other coronaviruses

### 3.1 SARS-CoV

To probe into the proximal origin of SARS-CoV from china in 2002–2003, an epidemiological surveillance survey was conducted in the animal market of china and adjoining areas during the outbreak from wild, companion and livestock animals to check out their susceptibility for this virus and more importantly to devise means for the management and control of this first documented outbreak [43]. In this report, dogs and goats were tested negative while wild boars and cats were found to be positive for the presence of SARS-CoV using viral detection assays [43]. Chen et al. conducted a field-based surveillance study on different animals through antibody and antigen-based tests. In this study, two pigs were tested positive for SARS-CoV antibodies while cats, dogs and cattle were tested negative. Based on sequence data analysis this study also suggests that transmission is from human-related SARS-CoV [44].

### 3.2 MERS-CoV

During the MERS-CoV outbreak very few reports appeared regarding the chances of human-animal transmission of this virus [45]. Kasem et al. conducted a study to check out the incidence of MERS-CoV infections in goat, sheep and cattle samples due to close contact with MERS-CoV positive individuals. In this study, all the tested samples were negative for MERS-CoV suggesting that no cross-species transmission was occurred [46]. El-Duah et al., conducted a field-based surveillance study on MERS-CoV by taking samples from sheep, pigs, goats, donkeys and cattle of the Ghana area. This study showed that none of the samples were found to be positive for the presence of MERS-CoV [47]. Kandeli et al. conducted an epidemiological surveillance study in Tunisia, Egypt and Senegal area from the field samples received from buffaloes, sheep, cattle, goats, mules, horses and donkeys using PCR and antibody detection kit. The results of this study revealed that both antibody detection tests and PCR were found to be positive for MERS-CoV in goats, sheep, cattle and donkeys. While PCR was negative in horses [48]. These reported studies suggest that transmission of MERS and SARS-CoVs occurred in humans-wild, domestic and companion animals making the possibility of reverse zoonosis [49]. However, still it is not clear whether infected animals shed the virus and are involved in the disease transmission cycle.

## 4. Promoting public health

There are at least 360,497 research studies worldwide, on diagnosis, treatment and prophylaxis of coronavirus that are being supported by NIH [50]. Combined efforts of global health organizations including the World Health Organization (WHO), Centers for Disease Control and Prevention (CDC) and many International, Regional and National NGOs, Government and private bodies are funding, supporting and helping approaches for public health. Food and Drug Administration (FDA) on the other hand, is rapidly analyzing and approving medicines and diagnostics for public use. Some major areas to be considered for tackling the current situation and developing roadmaps for future pandemics have been given in this section.

### 4.1 Elucidating the concept of quarantine and isolation

The COVID-19 crisis is continuously becoming a grave threat to the world and the number of cases is escalating globally. The present pandemic has redefined the human strategies against the control and prevention of this contagious agent responsible for disease outspread [4]. This virus is very lethal and contagious, and the WHO devised measures to control the infectivity and spread of the virus through quarantine and isolation. Some major myths and their busters associated with COVID-19 have been re-developed using WHO research-supported guidelines in **Figure 2**.

| MYTHS | FACTS |
|---|---|
| Elderly people get the virus | All age groups are equally susceptible, co-morbid are more prone |
| Summers/winters kill the virus | No correlation of environment conditions with virus survival |
| Poultry meat has the virus | No scientific evidence supports this myth |
| 5G network spreads virus | Virus need air to travel, not mobile/network signals |
| Recovery rate is poor | More than 95% of cases recover, showing high recovery rates |
| Eating garlic/onion saves against virus | No scientific study proved this |
| Drinking alcohol/bleach save | These are surface disinfectants, unsuitable for drinking |
| Antibiotics/ pneumonia vaccines can save | Only CoVID-19 virus specific vaccines can prevent infection |
| Don't wear mask unless sick | All people having <6ft intra-personal distance should wear masks |
| I don't have certain symptoms, no need to test | Refer to WHO criteria for symptoms scoring |
| Mosquito can get you virus | No link established yet. However, mosquito can transmit other diseases |
| Its only in the air, no need to change/wash clothes or shoes | Virus is of micron meter size, it can stay on fabric, surfaces and shoes for hours |
| Salt water rinsing in nose kills the virus | No scientific evidence supports this myth |

**Figure 2.**
*Major myths and their busters associated with COVID-19.*

Quarantine is separation and restricting the movement of people who have been exposed to a SARS-CoV-2 disease to see if they become sick, according to the CDC. Generally, this quarantine practice takes place at home or generalized facility or restricted movement areas specified for this practice. It can be imposed on individuals or communities constituting exposed individuals. Contact surveillance is required either passively or actively to monitor the individual if they develop the symptoms of the disease. Duration of the quarantine is based on a person's test results for disease or having experienced disease symptoms. If individual tests positive so after that, they are separated or isolated for treatment and monitoring purposes and if the individual is negative for diagnostic test and not showing any disease symptoms, then discharge from the quarantine center [8]. Monitoring must be done in case of quarantined person shows any of the disease symptoms. Government and other global authorities must implement border restriction if necessary, to overcome the spread of disease. The efficacy of this approach allows us to overcome the spread of disease with the early detection of diseased individuals.

Here the question arises after or during this "Quarantine session" what would be our approach if a person is positive for SARS-CoV-2. This question leads us to the term 'isolation'. The Center for Disease Control (CDC) has defined "Isolation" as the separation of sick people with any contagious disease from others who are not sick or at-risk population. This is important to flatten the disease curve so that fewer people become infected over a while. It can be explained as separation and restriction of movement of sick individuals who have a contagious disease, to prevent it from being transmitted to others. These measures are implemented to ensure the close monitoring of individuals with proper treatment and release after full recovery into the community or population to minimize or eliminate the risk of spread of this contagion. However, these individuals can still be monitored for weeks or two, to ensure they do not re-infect or develop severe symptoms after discharge from medical facilities.

### 4.2 Measures for cleaning and disinfection

From the sanitation/disinfection point of view, the Environment Protection Agency (EPA) recommends the use of List N disinfectants for use against COVID-19.

Cleaning the surfaces before applying disinfectants and observing the appropriate contact time are important considerations for efficient utilization. Among the most accessible ones are sodium hypochlorite, hydrogen peroxide, and quaternary ammonium compounds with or without alcohol or phenols. The forms of these disinfectants may be solid, vapor, wipe, dilute-able, which could be easily used to disinfect surfaces. These compounds in their commercial preparations could be safely applied to disinfect keys, doorknobs/handles, slabs, floors, switchboards, equipment, keyboards, tables, cell phones, remote controls, cars, bikes, etc.

Case definitions and their importance to the general public may be well-communicated. Also, smart solutions for handling a large number of outdoor patients may be sought. Un-necessary exposure and increase in case of loads at emergency and intensive care units could be minimized using efficient telemedicine and consultation services. For laboratory testing facilities, it is important to consider biosafety guidelines of level-3 or above, owing to the transmissibility of the virus. Also, solid waste management should be very well planned and executed to spare the risk of dissemination to the general public [51].

### 4.3 Management of COVID-19 patients

It is important to consider the difference of COVID-19 with other prevailing respiratory viral infections e.g. influenza that involves nasopharyngeal or lower respiratory tract infections. Polymerase chain reaction (PCR) is necessary to confirm COVID-19. Further hospitalization of patients involves various factors inclusive of which are the age of patients ($\approx$60 years old); patient having 40% allied morbid conditions like diabetes and cardiac diseases; children exposed, pregnant women with severe illness although there are mild symptoms so far in majority cases and the onset of symptoms and admission to ICU (9–10 days critical) as two-third of patients met criteria of acute respiratory distress syndrome (https://www.ecdc.europ a.eu/en/geographical-distribution-2019-ncov-cases).

The patient's care should be divided into four categories (1) Usual critical care, (2) Modification to usual critical care, (3) Facility planning, (4) COVID-19 specific consideration. Usual critical care will include: Conservative intravenous fluid strategies; Empirical early antibiotics for bacterial pneumonia; Consideration for early invasive ventilation; Lung protective ventilation strategies; Periodic prone position during mechanical ventilation; Consideration of extracorporeal membrane oxygenation. Modification to usual critical care involves: Admission of patients with the suspected disease to private rooms when possible; Use of medical face masks for symptomatic patients during assessment and transfer; Maintain a distance of at least 2-meter distance between patients; Caution when using high-flow nasal oxygen or non-invasive ventilation due to the risk of dispersion of aerosolized virus in the health care setup with poorly fitting masks; Clinicians involved with aerosol-generating procedures should use addition airborne precautions including N95 respirators and eye protection. COVID-19 Specific consideration; Ensure staff updated training in infection prevention and control including PPE; planning at local and regional levels for a potential surge in the need for critical care resources. The facility planning involves: Antiviral or immunomodulatory therapies are yet to be approved, so patients should be left on supportive or targeted therapies.

Three lines of treatments are generally followed (a) COVID-19 with mild acute respiratory distress syndrome (ARDS), (b) COVID-19 with mild ARDS, (c) Adjunct therapies. In the first case ventilator, supply while conservative fluid therapy, and empiric antibiotics are considered. Systematic corticosteroids are uncertain to be used on this occasion. In the second phase, short courses of systemic corticosteroids are considered. In adjunct/rescue therapy (3rd phase), antiviral, chloroquine, and anti-interleukin 6 are uncertain to be used. The hypoxic conditions will be dealt with differently. It is important not to delay intubation if the situation is worsening. COVID-19 hypoxia travels to endotracheal intubation, then it is important to: follow endotracheal intubation, an expert should do intubation in the airway, N95/FFP-2 or equivalent personal protection equipment is necessary, infection control is followed, and staff in the room is minimally kept. In case if the situation is not getting better, endotracheal intubation should immediately be done.

### 4.4 Ensuring mental well-being

Due to social distancing and remote working, maintenance of psychological well-being is pivotal. Social, electronic, print media could play a significant positive role in effectively communicating the risks while assuring mental health. Non-professional people who have a lot of apprehensions about the current pandemic may be discussing their concerns through telecommunication [52, 53]. Another important aspect of lockdown amidst outbreaks worldwide is the less privileged or daily wager community, migrants and internally displaced persons (IDPs). The anxiety due to uncertainty of fiscal matters may affect the mental health of the masses. Also, patients with other diseases, particularly those with chronic diseases may suffer a psychological breakdown. Apart from mental health issues, India has reported suicide due to fear of contracting COVID-19 [54]. It is, therefore, high time to spread hope, offer support and positivity all around.

Studies from one highly infected country *i.e.* Iran have revealed moderate to severe anxiety symptoms in apparently healthy citizens [55]. Suspected patients and cases, belonging to different age groups, may also require support for mental well-being amidst strict isolation. The healthcare workers in the frontline of combating the pandemic may need psychological/moral support, medical insurance and proper PPE. Government, NGOs, private stakeholders, media persons, celebrities, doctors and allied healthcare staff, scientists need to develop stronger communication with the public. These people can motivate people to adopt safety measures and promote public health safety.

## 5. Conclusions and future outlook

The detailed understanding of epidemiological patterns and probable modeling of COVID-19 are highly important. Moreover, there's a need to disseminate the research-based findings to public health. This could be made possible by the thorough collaboration of the National and International organizations that may fetch research-supported data for prevention and ways to control or contain the pandemic at all levels.

## Author details

Sadia Muneer[1], Tean Zaheer[2*], Aqsa Ahmad[1], Muhammad Imran[2], Amjad Islam Aqib[3], Iqra Zaheer[4] and Muhammad Imran Arshad[1]

1 Institute of Microbiology, University of Agriculture, Faisalabad, Pakistan

2 Department of Parasitology, University of Agriculture, Faisalabad, Pakistan

3 Department of Medicine, Cholistan University of Veterinary and Animal Sciences, Bahawalpur, Pakistan

4 Department of Pathology, University of Agriculture, Faisalabad, Pakistan

*Address all correspondence to: teanzaheer942@gmail.com

## References

[1] Zhu, N., Zhang, D., Wang, W., Li, X., Yang, B., Song, J., Zhao, X., Huang, B., Shi, W., Lu, R. and Niu, P., 2020. A novel1. coronavirus from patients with pneumonia in China, 2019. *New England Journal of Medicine*.

[2] Zu, Z.Y., Jiang, M.D., Xu, P.P., Chen, W., Ni, Q.Q., Lu, G.M. and Zhang, L.J., 2020. Coronavirus disease 2019 (COVID-19): a perspective from China. *Radiology*, p.200490.

[3] Huang Chaolin, Wang Yeming, Li Xingwang, Ren Lili, Zhao Jianping, Hu Yi, Zhang Li, Fan Guohui, Xu Jiuyang, Gu Xiaoying, Cheng Zhenshun, Yu Ting, Xia Jiaan, Wei Yuan, Wu Wenjuan, Xie Xuelei, Yin Wen, Li Hui, Liu Min, Xiao Yan, Gao Hong, Guo Li, Xie Jungang, Wang Guangfa, Jiang Rongmeng, Gao Zhancheng, Jin Qi, Wang Jianwei, Cao Bin. Clinical features of patients infected with 2019 novel coronavirus in Wuhan, China. The Lancet. 2020;395(10223):497-506.

[4] National Health Commission of the People's Republic of China Available at: http://www.nhc.gov.cn/

[5] Musa, S.S., Qureshi, S., Zhao, S., Yusuf, A., Mustapha, U.T. and He, D., 2021. Mathematical modeling of COVID-19 epidemic with effect of awareness programs. *Infectious Disease Modelling*, 6, pp.448-460.

[6] Jabeen, K., Haider, M.B.H., Haider, Z., Hassan, A., Ali, S. and Niazi, A.K., 2021. Coronavirus (COVID-19) pandemic: Outbreak, current scenario and impact on human physiology in Pakistan. *Global Journal of Clinical Virology*, 6(1), pp.021-029.

[7] Tang, B., Wang, X., Li, Q., Bragazzi, N. L., Tang, S., Xiao, Y., & Wu, J. (2020). Estimation of the transmission risk of the 2019-nCoV and its implication for public health interventions. *Journal of Clinical Medicine*, *9*(2), 462.

[8] Lin, Q., Zhao, S., Gao, D., Lou, Y., Yang, S., Musa, S.S., Wang, M.H., Cai, Y., Wang, W., Yang, L. and He, D., 2020. A conceptual model for the coronavirus disease 2019 (COVID-19) outbreak in Wuhan, China with individual reaction and governmental action. *International journal of infectious diseases*, *93*, pp.211-216.

[9] Read, J. M., Bridgen, J. R., Cummings, D. A., Ho, A., & Jewell, C. P. (2020). Novel coronavirus 2019-nCoV: early estimation of epidemiological parameters and epidemic predictions. *MedRxiv*.

[10] Chen, T., Rui, J., Wang, Q. *et al.* A mathematical model for simulating the phase-based transmissibility of a novel coronavirus. *Infect Dis Poverty* **9**, 24 (2020).

[11] Wu, J. T., Leung, K., & Leung, G. M. (2020). Nowcasting and forecasting the potential domestic and international spread of the 2019-nCoV outbreak originating in Wuhan, China: a modelling study. *The Lancet*, *395*(10225), 689-697.

[12] Shen, M., Peng, Z., Xiao, Y. and Zhang, L., 2020. Modelling the epidemic trend of the 2019 novel coronavirus outbreak in China. *bioRxiv*.

[13] Liu, T., Hu, J., Kang, M., Lin, L., Zhong, H., Xiao, J., He, G., Song, T., Huang, Q., Rong, Z. and Deng, A., 2020. Transmission dynamics of 2019 novel coronavirus (2019-nCoV).

[14] Zhao, S., Lin, Q., Ran, J., Musa, S.S., Yang, G., Wang, W., Lou, Y., Gao, D., Yang, L., He, D. and Wang, M.H., 2020. Preliminary estimation of the basic reproduction number of novel coronavirus (2019-nCoV) in China,

from 2019 to 2020: A data-driven analysis in the early phase of the outbreak. *International journal of infectious diseases*, *92*, pp.214-217.

[15] Li, Q., Guan, X., Wu, P., Wang, X., Zhou, L., Tong, Y., Ren, R., Leung, K.S., Lau, E.H., Wong, J.Y. and Xing, X., 2020. Early transmission dynamics in Wuhan, China, of novel coronavirus–infected pneumonia. *New England Journal of Medicine*.

[16] Majumder, M. and Mandl, K.D., 2020. Early transmissibility assessment of a novel coronavirus in Wuhan, China. *China (January 23, 2020)*.

[17] Cao, Z., Zhang, Q., Lu, X., Pfeiffer, D., Jia, Z., Song, H. and Zeng, D.D., 2020. Estimating the effective reproduction number of the 2019-nCoV in China. *medRxiv*.

[18] Imai, N., Cori, A., Dorigatti, I., Baguelin, M., Donnelly, C.A., Riley, S. and Ferguson, N.M., 2020. Report 3: transmissibility of 2019-nCoV. WHO Collaborating Centre for Infectious Disease Modelling, MRC Centre for Global Infectious Disease Analysis, J-IDEA, Imperial College London, UK.

[19] Riou, J. and Althaus, C.L., 2020. Pattern of early human-to-human transmission of Wuhan 2019 novel coronavirus (2019-nCoV), December 2019 to January 2020. Eurosurveillance, 25(4), p.2000058.

[20] Lai, S., Bogoch, I.I., Ruktanonchai, N., Watts, A.G., Li, Y., Yu, J., Lv, X., Yang, W., Hongjie, Y., Khan, K. and Li, Z., 2020. Assessing spread risk of Wuhan novel coronavirus within and beyond China, January-April 2020: a travel network-based modelling study.

[21] Mandal, S., Bhatnagar, T., Arinaminpathy, N., Agarwal, A., Chowdhury, A., Murhekar, M., Gangakhedkar, R.R. and Sarkar, S., 2020. Prudent public health intervention strategies to control the coronavirus disease 2019 transmission in India: A mathematical model-based approach. *Indian J Med Res*, *151*.

[22] Rajendrakumar, A.L., Nair, A.T.N., Nangia, C., Chourasia, P.K., Chourasia, M.K., Syed, M.G., Nair, A.S., Nair, A.B. and Koya, M.S.F., 2020. Epidemic Landscape and Forecasting of SARS-CoV-2 in India. *medRxiv*.

[23] Kamalich Muniz-Rodriguez, Gerardo Chowell, Chi-Hin Cheung, Dongyu Jia, Po-Ying Lai, Yiseul Lee, Manyun Liu, Sylvia K. Ofori, Kimberlyn M. Roosa, Lone Simonsen, and Isaac Chun-Hai Fung. Epidemic doubling time of the 2019 novel coronavirus outbreak by rovince in mainland china. medRxiv, 2020.

[24] Shengjie Lai, Isaac Bogoch, Nick Ruktanonchai, Alexander Watts, Yu Li, Jianzing Yu, Xin Lv, Weizhong Yang, Hongjie Yu, Kamran Khan, Zhongjie Li, and Andrew J Tatem. Assessing spread risk of wuhan novel coronavirus within and beyond china, January April 2020: a travel network-based modelling study. medRxiv, 2020.

[25] 10Hiroshi Nishiura, Sung-mok Jung, Natalie M. Linton, Ryo Kinoshita, Yichi Yang, KatsumaHayashi, Tetsuro Kobayashi, Baoyin Yuan, and Andrei R. Akhmetzhanov. The extent of transmission of novel coronavirus in wuhan, china, 2020. Journal of Clinical Medicine, 9(2), 2020.

[26] Matteo Chinazzi, Jessica T. Davis, Marco Ajelli, Corrado Gioannini, Maria Litvinova, Stefano Merler, Ana Pastore y Piontti, Luca Rossi, Kaiyuan Sun, Cecile Viboud, Xinyue Xiong, Hongjie Yu, M. Elizabeth Halloran, Ira M. Longini, and Alessandro Vespignani. The effect of travel restrictions on the spread of the 2019 novel coronavirus (2019-ncov) outbreak. medRxiv, 2020.

[27] Gehui Jin, Jiayu Yu, Liyuan Han, and Shiwei Duan. The impact of tracffic isolation in wuhan on the spread of 2019-ncov. medRxiv, 2020.

[28] Adam J Kucharski, Timothy W Russell, Charlie Diamond, , Sebastian Funk, and Rosalind M Eggo. Early dynamics of transmission and control of 2019-ncov: a mathematical modelling study. medRxiv, 2020.

[29] Tianyu Zeng, Yunong Zhang, Zhenyu Li, Xiao Liu, and Binbin Qiu. Predictions of 2019-ncov transmission ending via comprehensive methods, 2020.

[30] CDC. Coronavirus Disease 2019 (COVID-19) – pets & other animals. 2020. https://www.cdc.gov/coronavirus/2019-ncov/daily-life-coping/positive-pet.html

[31] USDA. Confirmed cases of SARS-CoV-2 in Animals in the United States. 2020. https://www.aphis.usda.gov/aphis/ourfocus/animalhealth/sa_one_health/sars-cov-2-animals-us

[32] AVMA. In-depth summary of reports of naturally acquired SARS-CoV-2 infections in domestic animals and farmed or captive wildlife 2020. https://www.avma.org/resourcestools/animal-health-and-welfare/covid-19/depth-summary-reports-naturally-acquired-sars-cov-2- infections-domestic-animals-and-farmed-or

[33] Sit THC, Brackman CJ, Ip SM, et al. Infection of dogs with SARS-CoV-2. Nature. 2020. DOI. 10.1038/s41586-020-2334-5.

[34] ABC. 1st pet dog in US with COVID-19 dies in NYC, family details his last days. 2020. https://abc13.com/first-dog-with-covid-pets-coronavirus-buddy-german-shepherd/6341676/

[35] Tiwari R, Dhama K, Sharun K. et al. COVID-19: animals, veterinary and zoonotic links. Vet Q. 2020;40(1):169-82.

[36] Guo H, Guo A, Wang C, et al. Expression of feline angiotensin converting enzyme 2 and its interaction with SARS-CoV S1 protein. Res Vet Sci. 2008 Jun;84(3):494-6

[37] Konda, M., Dodda, B., Konala, V. M., Naramala, S., & Adapa, S. (2020). Potential Zoonotic Origins of SARS-CoV-2 and insights for preventing future pandemics through one health approach. *Cureus*, *12*(6).

[38] Zhang Q, Zhang H, Huang K, Yang Y, Hui X, Gao J, He X, Li C, Gong W, Zhang Y, Peng C, Gao X, Chen H, Zou Z, Shi Z, Jin M. SARS-CoV-2 Neutralizing Serum Antibodies in Cats: a Serological Investigation [Internet]. Cold Spring Harbor: bioRxiv; https://www.biorxiv.org/content/10.1101/2020.04.01.021196v1. Updated 2020

[39] Zhang, Q., Zhang, H., Huang, K., Yang, Y., Hui, X., Gao, J., ... & Peng, C. (2020). SARS-CoV-2 neutralizing serum antibodies in cats: a serological investigation. *BioRxiv*.

[40] Shi, J., Wen, Z., Zhong, G., Yang, H., Wang, C., Huang, B., ... & Zhao, Y. (2020). Susceptibility of ferrets, cats, dogs, and other domesticated animals to SARS–coronavirus 2. *Science*, *368*(6494), 1016-1020.

[41] IDEXX SARS-CoV-2 (COVID-19) RealPCR Test 2020. https://www.idexx.com/en/veterinary/reference-laboratories/idexx-realpcr-tests/idexx-sars-cov2-covid-19-realpcr-test/

[42] Munir, K., Ashraf, S., Munir, I., Khalid, H., Muneer, M. A., Mukhtar, N., ... & Zaheer, M. U. (2020). Zoonotic and reverse zoonotic events of SARS-CoV-2 and their impact on global health. *Emerging microbes & infections*, *9*(1), 2222-2235.

[43] Wang, M., Jing, H.Q., Xu, H.F., Jiang, X.G., Kan, B., Liu, Q.Y., Wan, K.L., Cui, B.Y., Zheng, H., Cui, Z.G., Yan, M.Y. (2005). Surveillance on severe acute respiratory syndrome associated coronavirus in animals at a live animal market of Guangzhou in 2004. Zhonghua liu xing bing xue za zhi= Zhonghua liuxingbingxue zazhi. 26(2): 84-87 (In Chinese). DOI: https://pubmed.ncbi.nlm.nih.gov/1592 1605.

[44] Chen, W., Yan, M., Yang, L., Ding, B., He, B., Wang, Y., Liu, X., Liu, C., Zhu, H., You, B., Huang, S. (2005). SARSassociated coronavirus transmitted from human to pig. Emerging Infectious Diseases. 11(3): 446-448. DOI: 10.3201/eid1103.040824

[45] Naveenkumar, V., Nag, B. S., Vijayaraghavan, R., & Porteen, K. (2020). The possible risk of reverse zoonosis in Covid-19: An epidemiological driving approach for the one health future challenges: A review. *Asian Journal of Dairy and Food Research*, *39*(3), 173-179.

[46] Kasem, S., Qasim, I., Al-Hufofi, A., Hashim, O., Alkarar, A., AbuObeida, A., Gaafer, A., Elfadil, A., Zaki, A., Al-Romaihi, A., Babekr, N. (2018). Cross-sectional study of MERSCoV-specific RNA and antibodies in animals that have had contact with MERS patients in Saudi Arabia. Journal of Infection and Public Health. 11(3): 331-338. DOI: 10.1016/j.jiph.2017.09.022

[47] El-Duah, P., Sylverken, A., Owusu, M., Yeboah, R., Lamptey, J., Oppong Frimpong, Y., Burimuah, V., Antwi, C., Folitse, R., Agbenyega, O., Oppong, S. (2019). Potential intermediate hosts for coronavirus transmission: No evidence of Clade 2c coronaviruses in domestic livestock from Ghana. Tropical Medicine and Infectious Disease. 4(1): 34. DOI: 10.3390/tropicalmed4010034.

[48] Kandeil, A., Gomaa, M., Shehata, M., El-Taweel, A., Kayed, A.E., Abiadh, A., Jrijer, J., Moatasim, Y., Kutkat, O., Bagato, O., Mahmoud, S. (2019). Middle East respiratory syndrome coronavirus infection in non-camelid domestic mammals. Emerging Microbes and Infections. 8(1): 103-108. DOI: 10.1080/22221751.2018.1560235.

[49] Chen, W., Yan, M., Yang, L., Ding, B., He, B., Wang, Y., Liu, X., Liu, C., Zhu, H., You, B., Huang, S. (2005). SARSassociated coronavirus transmitted from human to pig. Emerging Infectious Diseases. 11(3): 446-448. DOI: 10.3201/eid1103.040824.

[50] NIH, US national Library of Medicine. 2020. https://clinicaltrials.gov/ct2/results?cond=%22Coronavirus+Infections%22. Last accessed: 12-12-2020.

[51] Chiodini J. (2020). Maps, masks and media - Traveller and practitioner resources for 2019 novel coronavirus (2019-nCoV) acute respiratory virus. Travel medicine and infectious disease, 33, 101574.

[52] Banerjee, D. 2020. The COVID-19 outbreak: Crucial role the psychiatrists can play, Asian Journal of Psychiatry, Volume 50, 2020, 102014.

[53] Javadi, S.M.H., M. Arian, M. Qorbani-Vanajemi. The need for psychosocial interventions to manage the coronavirus crisis. Iran. J. Psychiatry Behav. Sci., 14 (1) (2020), Article e102546.

[54] Goyal, K., Chauhan, P., Chhikara, K., Gupta, P., Singh, M.P. 2020. Fear of COVID 2019: First suicidal case in India!, Asian Journal of Psychiatry, Volume 49, 2020, 101989.

[55] Moghanibashi-Mansourieh, A. 2020. Assessing the anxiety level of Iranian general population during COVID-19 outbreak, Asian Journal of Psychiatry, Volume 51, 2020, 102076.

Chapter 3

# Coronavirus Disease 2019 (COVID-19): Origin, Impact, and Drug Development

*Amaresh Mishra, Nisha Nair, Amit K. Yadav, Pratima Solanki, Jaseela Majeed and Vishwas Tripathi*

## Abstract

At the end of December 2019, in Wuhan, China, a rapidly spreading unknown virus was reported to have caused coronavirus disease of 2019 (COVID-19). Origin linked to Wuhan's wholesale food market where live animals are sold. This disease is caused by SARS Coronavirus-2 (SARS-CoV-2), which is closely related to the Severe Acute Respiratory Coronavirus (SARS-CoV) and the Middle East Respiratory Syndrome Coronavirus (MERS-CoV). This virus shares a high sequence identity with bat-derived SARS-like Coronavirus, which indicating its zoonotic origin. The virus spread globally, provoking widespread attention and panic. This Coronavirus is highly pathogenic and causes mild to severe respiratory disorders. Later, it was declared a global pandemic by the World Health Organization (WHO) due to its highly infectious nature and worldwide mortality rate. This virus is a single-stranded, positive-sense RNA genome, and its genome length about 26 to 32 kb that infects a broad range of vertebrates. The researchers worldwide focus on establishing treatment strategies on drug and vaccine development to prevent this COVID-19 pandemic. A drug repurposing approach has been used to identify a rapid treatment for the people affected by COVID-19, which could be cost-effective and bypass some Food and Drug Association (FDA) regulations to move quickly in phase-3 trials. However, there is no promising therapeutic option available yet. This book chapter addresses current information about the COVID-19 disease, including its origins, impacts, and the novel potential drug candidates that can help treat the COVID-19.

**Keywords:** COVID-19, Zoonotic virus, SARS-CoV-2, Epidemiology, Drug discovery, Therapeutics

## 1. Introduction

Nowadays, there is growing concern and perceived threat due to the outbreak of the novel coronavirus disease, COVID-19, as named by the World Health Organization (WHO), which poses a peril of pandemic to the global public health. The epicenter of the novel Coronavirus was located in Wuhan province of China, where the outbreak originated in December 2019 due to Severe Acute Respiratory Syndrome coronavirus 2 (SARS-CoV-2) [1]. This disease has spread to 220 countries, with over 158 million confirmed coronavirus cases of 3.3 million confirmed deaths with 136 million recoveries worldwide as of May 10, 2021 [2]. Also, millions of people's lives have been affected as mandatory isolations/quarantines instructed. The adverse effect of the COVID-19 outbreak could bring significant challenges to the health system globally and could have far-reaching consequences on the global economy if the virus's spread is not effectively curtailed [3, 4].

Coronaviruses (CoVs) are encapsulated within a membrane envelope containing a single-stranded positive-sense RNA genome. Spikes of glycoprotein that give coronaviruses their crown-like appearance are studded with the viral membrane. Coronaviruses infect humans as well as animals such as bats that host the widest range of coronaviruses [5]. There are four types of alpha, beta, gamma, and delta-designated coronaviruses. Extreme acute respiratory syndrome virus (SARS-CoV), Middle East respiratory syndrome (MERS-CoV), and SARS-CoV-2 are included in the beta coronavirus class [6, 7]. SARS-CoV-2 targets the lower respiratory system to induce viral pneumonia, similar to SARS-CoV and MERS-CoV, but may also affect the heart, kidney, liver, and central nervous system, resulting in multiple organ failure [8]. New evidence suggests that SARS-CoV-2 is more contagious/transmissible than SARS-CoV and MERS-CoV [9]. Glycosylated spike (S) protein acts as a significant inducer of host immune responses, which mediates both SARS-CoV and SARS-CoV-2 host cell invasion by binding with angiotensin-converting enzyme 2 (ACE2) located on the host cells of the surface membrane [1].

With the onset of the second wave of COVID-19 infection, developing countries like India seem to be reeling in the most catastrophic damages. Since late March of 2021, the emergence of COVID-19 infected patience has skyrocketed to more than 22 million people and have touched a record number of 4000 death per day in the first week of May 2021. The outbreak has left the country struggling hard to cope with the healthcare needs of patients. This silent killer disease creates havoc on earth, yet the upcoming course of this virus is unpredictable. Therefore, necessary measures are needed to control and eradicate this alarming problem to save the people's precious life and the country's economy [4, 10]. However, significant steps have been taken by the government of different countries. Many countries such as Italy, Germany, and India have "lockdown" the whole country to break the chain by quarantine and confinement of people to the homes. To date, there is no clinically approved antiviral drug or vaccine available to be used against COVID-19; therefore, it has posed a public health emergency and a global threat to the entire world. Repurposing existing medications is an affordable and effective therapeutic technique. The scientific community reacted quickly with a suggested list of current drugs with therapeutic potential for COVID-19, based on genomic sequence knowledge. This chapter examines the source of infection, the SARS-CoV-2 transmission pathway, and the medications currently being clinically tested for COVID-19 management to include references for follow-up research, prevention, and treatment that may help readers gain the latest understanding of this emerging infectious disease.

## 2. History

The first case of Coronavirus infection was detected in 1960. Twice in the past two decades, history has seen incidences where β-coronavirus has cross over from animal to humans in severe infectious diseases. Till 2003, coronavirus infection was considered to be a non-fatal disease. However, with many mortally affecting cases of severe acute respiratory syndrome cropping up in Hong Kong, the United States of America, Vietnam, Taiwan, and Thailand culminated in the deciphering of the deadly pathogenesis of this disease and led to the declaration of disease as a state emergency by World health organization (WHO) in 2004 [10–13]. In 2012, almost a decade later, the Middle East respiratory syndrome coronavirus, also known as MERS-CoV, arose in Saudi Arabia, killing 858 and affecting 2494 people. This virus also originated from bats, and dromedary camels were possibly its intermediate host [14].

## 3. Origin and prevalence of COVID-19

It all started in the Hubei province's capital city, Wuhan, in December 2019, when several adults with severe pneumonia were admitted to the nearby hospitals. The surveillance team was triggered and collected the samples of respiratory patients for the etiologic study. It was investigated that numerous patients had contact with the Huanan wholesale seafood, where dead and live animals were sold and traded. At the end of December 2019, China declared the outbreak of this disease to the WHO. This virus had more than 95% homology with bat coronavirus (SARS-like bat CoVs) and more than 70% resemblance with SARS-CoV, and hence the virus was recognized as Coronavirus on January 7, 2020. The environmental samples obtained from the Huanan seafood market were also tested positive, which indicated that the virus took origin from the Huanan seafood market [15]. Though the Coronavirus originated from bats, the existing possibility of an intermediary animal that gets transferred to humans may be snakes or pangolins. Xu. Et al. have isolated SARS-CoV-2 from pangolin and found pangolin to be the potential intermediate host of the SARS-CoV-2 as it shows high similarity (99%) between the coronaviruses affecting the humans [16]. However, these current results are not sufficient to prove the potential host and intermediate of COVID-19. **Figure 1** shows a schematic view of crucial reservoirs and the mode of transmission of COVID-19.

According to Wu, JT, Leung et al. of York University, the estimated Basic Reproduction Number ($R_0$), which means the average amount of secondary infection that patients may develop without intervention in a completely susceptible population, varies with several research groups [17]. Utilizing the Susceptible-Exposed-Infectious-Recovered (SEIR) model and Incidence Decay with Exponential Adjustment (IDEA) model, the estimated $R_0$ value of novel COVID-19 was found to be 2.47–2.86 [18] and 2.0–3.3 [19] respectively, which is higher than other viruses of β–coronaviruses such as MERS-CoV (2.0–6.7) [20] and SARS-CoV (2.2–3.6) [21]. This elevated value of $R_0$ points towards the fact that COVID-19 has a comparatively high transmission rate. It is also indicated from the overall case-fatality rate (CFR) that elderly male citizens are more prone to this Coronavirus, especially those with chronic health issues (heart disease, diabetes, hypertension) than other groups of the viruses. Thus, SARS-CoV-2 shows a high prevalence, and the population is easily susceptible to this virus. Among the RNA viruses, Coronavirus contains the most extensive genome sequence of about 26 to 32 Kilobases with 14 Open Reading Frames (ORFs). These ORFs code for 27 structural and non-structural proteins of the virus [22, 23]. Spike protein, membrane protein, envelope, and nucleocapsid, along with eight accessory proteins, lie in the 3′ end of the SARS-CoV-2 genome. A very high sequence resemblance is shared between structural proteins of SARS-CoV-2 and its predecessor human coronaviruses (hCoVs) (82%) (except in the 8a, 8b, and 3b accessory protein); suggests common molecular pathophysiology and pathogenesis among COVID-19, SARS, and MERS [24]. Genomic analysis has surmised the relevance of the Sans N gene in coronaviruses. Positive selection, mutation, and adaptation affect the pathogenicity and stability of the virus and might play an essential role in widespread infection in a large population [25]. This also poses a threat to the generation of newer strains of the virus that may result from mutation and adaptation, making the threat of transmission even more potent [26].

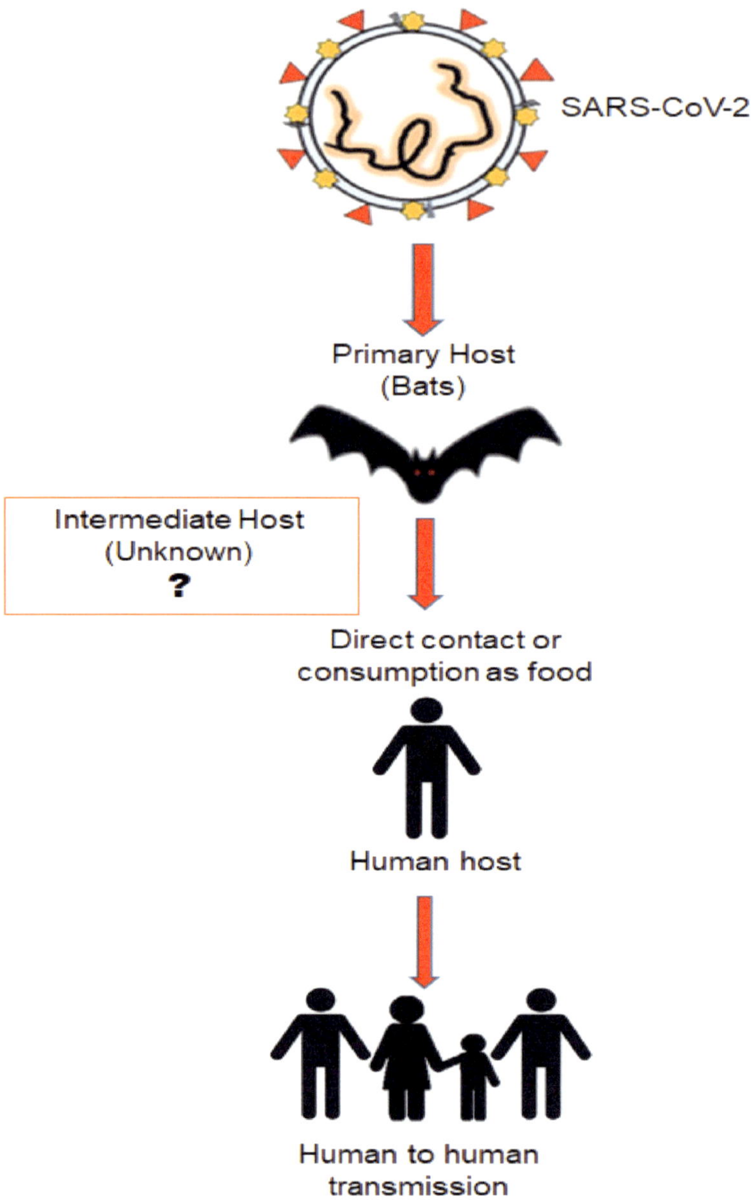


**Figure 1.**
*Schematic view of the critical reservoirs and mode of transmission of coronaviruses.*

## 4. Drug repurposing

Drug repurposing is an old weapon in the arsenal for new drug development strategies. This approach identifies new therapeutic indications for available marketed drugs making it time-efficient in a cost-effective manner [27, 28]. It has been assumed that about 75% of existing drugs could be repurposed for various diseases [29]. Global pandemic like novel coronavirus disease 2019 (COVID-19) has an urgent need to select appropriate therapeutic options with limited time to discover the new drug candidates [30]. It takes 10–15 years to develop a new drug, and the actual cost would be more than a billion dollars, with only 2.01% of its success rate

[31, 32]. Existing drug compounds, including Raltegravir, Paritaprevir, Bictegravir, and Dolutegravir, identify promising inhibitors against 3C-like protease 2′-O-ribose methyltransferase from COVID-19 is cost-effective and a drug repurposing approach [33, 34]. A recent in-silico study suggested that natural compounds like guggulsterone and drug rifampicin can be repurposed for COVID-19, insights from the molecular docking analysis [35, 36]. Thus, the concept of drug repurposing could be utilized as a novel drug discovery process to discover an effective therapeutic option against COVID-19. Recent examples of drug repurposing against COVID-19 are given in **Table 1**.

Based on previous experiences in the treatment of previous coronavirus diseases like SARS-CoV and MERS-CoV, drugs currently being implemented in the management of this disease are entry or inhibitors of SARS-CoV-2, RNA mutagens that stop replication, host inflammatory response inhibitors, viral protease inhibitors, monoclonal antibodies (mAbs), and convalescent plasma-based immunogenicity, blockers of the release of mature virion and glucocorticoids based cell tissue and organ injury management apart from necessary ventilation for support [54]. It is an urgent need to perform more prospective, rigorous population studies and further preclinical and clinical trials to gain a perspective on the safety and therapeutic effect of new and potential therapeutic agents that may help contain the spread and enhance recovery from SARS-CoV-2 infection.

| S.No. | Drug name | Primary use | Description | Ref. |
|---|---|---|---|---|
| 1. | Remdesivir | Ebola Virus Disease | Viral RNA polymerase inhibitor | [37, 38] |
| 2. | Chloroquine & Hydroxychloroquine | Malaria | Antimalarial; interferent with protein post-translational processes; Mitogen-activated protein kinase (MAPK) inhibitor; pro-inflammatory cytokines inhibitor | [39–41] |
| 3. | Arbidol and Oseltamivir | Treatment of influenza virus infections | Blocks virus entry into the cell | [40, 42–45] |
| 4. | Danoprevir | Hepatitis C virus (HCV) | Nonstructural protein 3 (NSP3) inhibitor | [46] |
| 5. | Xiyanping | Antibacterial and antiviral | Blocks virus entry into the cell | [47] |
| 6. | Darunavir | HIV protease inhibitor | Using among the COVID-19 pneumonia patients | [48] |
| 7. | Thalidomide | Anti-inflammatory action | Reduce tumor necrosis factor-α (TNFα), increase interleukins secretion, and activate natural killer cells | [49, 50] |
| 8. | Methylprednisolone | Corticosteroid therapy | Prolongs the survival time among the severe stage COVID-19 patients | [51, 52] |
| 9. | Lopinavir-Ritonavir | HIV treatment | Viral Protease inhibitors | [40, 43] |
| 10. | Ribavirin | Viral RNA synthesis inhibitor | Viral RNA-dependent RNA polymerase (RdRp) inhibitor | [53] |

**Table 1.**
*Recent examples of drug repurposing against COVID-19.*

## 5. Drugs under clinical trials for COVID-19

As the epidemic spreads more and more, scientists worldwide are in a quest to explore drugs that may be potentially effective in combating COVID-19. During a pandemic that causes morbidity and mortality to grow exponentially, well-structured, randomized, controlled trials are necessary to evaluate new or repurposed drugs' safety and efficacy to protect the community from ineffective, unnecessary, or unsafe drugs [55]. World Health Organization and partners have launched an international clinical trial – Solidarity trial, to assist in the accelerated search for a therapeutic regimen for COVID-19. Solidarity trail is one of the most extensive international randomized trials for COVID-19 to evaluate drugs on three essential outcomes that were needed for assisted ventilation, mortality, and duration of hospital stay. Solidarity Trial also aims to assess the chances of drugs improving survival or reducing the need for ventilation or hospital stay duration [56]. Currently, repurposed antiviral therapies are under significant scrutiny in clinical trials as disease-specific and designated antiviral therapy may have a maximum impact on disease progression and optimized treatment of COVID-19 [57].

### 5.1 RNA mutagens

RNA and DNA viruses encode RNA-dependent RNA polymerase (RdRp) core, which is requisite for RdRP catalytic function and viral replication. Hence, it is one of the prime targets for intervention infection. RdRp facilitates the elongation of the RNA strand and genome replication [7, 58]. RNA mutagens are nucleotide analogs that halt RNA elongation by RdRp by inserting themselves into the RNA chain. RdRp has no host cell homolog making this antiviral drug development superior as it reduces the risk of affecting human cells or protein. Thus, mutagenic nucleoside analog inhibitors like remdesivir, favipiravir, and ribavirin targeting RdRp are explored for their function to block viral RNA synthesis against human coronaviruses [7].

Remdesivir is a known antiviral against SARS-CoV and the MERS-CoV and has been a drug choice for SARS-CoV-2 due to its proven activity to inhibit SARS-CoV-2 in vitro [59]. A randomized, placebo-controlled, double-blind trial of intravenous remdesivir in hospitalized adults suffering from lower respiratory tract infection due to COVID-19 shows an average recovery day of 14 days and clinical improvement at day 15, emphasizing that remdesivir abbreviate time to recovery among COVID-19 patients. The trial also suggested that a remdesivir treatment regimen may prevent disease progression to more severity and a lower incidence of respiratory support requirement [60]. Another randomized, open-label trial among patients with severe COVID-19 who required oxygen support showed recovery among patients with both 5- and 10-day courses of remdesivir [61]. In another randomized phase 3 clinical trial, compared to standard of care treatment, the period of 5 days of remdesivir had significant improvement in patient's clinical status [62]. Prompted by such conclusive evidence, the US Food and Drug Administration has granted remdesivir a status of Emergency Use Authorization for SARS-CoV-2 infected patients of about 12 years of age and with pneumonia [57].

Favipiravir is a broad-spectrum oral RNA-dependent RNA polymerase (RdRp) currently under study in numerous clinical and preclinical trials for its Role in inhibiting the viral replication phase of SARS-CoV-2. Glenmark Pharmaceuticals evaluates Favipiravir in Phase 3 clinical trial for COVID-19 among mild to moderately infected patients of COVID-19 and has observed a marked 40% faster recovery of patients by day 4 [63].

In another prospective, randomized, controlled, open-label multicentered trial involving adult patients with COVID-19 in china, Favipiravir, compared to Arbidol, significantly improved the viral clearance, relief for pyrexia and cough with mild and manageable adverse effects [64]. Such promising results have cast the attention of healthcare providers to use RNA mutagens in treatments for SARS-CoV-2 infection [65].

### 5.2 Protease inhibitors

Lopinavir/Ritonavir is a combination therapy used as a potent inhibitor of the human immunodeficiency virus protease. Lopinavir is a protease inhibitor that inhibits the protease enzyme necessary for the virus to catalyze the cleavage of polyprotein essential for completing the viral infectious cycle. In contrast, ritonavir is used in combination with Lopinavir to inhibit cytochrome P450 and increase its half-life for a longer duration of action [66]. Lopinavir/ritonavir was also employed in the treatment of MERS. In vitro experiments have shown lopinavir/ritonavir potential in limiting replication of Coronavirus. 400 mg Lopinavir with 50 mg Ritonavir (Kaletra) is an efficacious oral anti-HIV drug [67]. A study on SARS-CoV demonstrates the inhibitory activity of Lopinavir (4 μg/mL) in plaque reduction assay.

In contrast, combination therapy of Lopinavir (400 mg) and Ritonavir (100 mg) two times a day for 14 days in SARS-CoV infected patients exhibited lessening of viral load in patients [68]. Subsequently, a randomized control trial known as the MIRACLE trial (MERS-CoV Infection Treated With A Combination of Lopinavir/Ritonavir and Interferon Beta-1b) was started to establish the therapeutic efficacy of combination therapy of interferon β-1b along with lopinavir/ritonavir among MERS-CoV infected patients [69]. Whereas in a retrospective case–control study, treatment by a combination of Lopinavir/Ritonavir (LPV/r) and Ribavirin yielded depreciated Acute Respiratory Distress Syndrome (ARDS) as well as mortality in SARS patients [70].

Darunavir (DRV), another protease inhibitor that shares a similar mechanism for inhibiting HIV replication, like Lopinavir, is in phase III studies. In combination with Cobicistat, Darunavir showed better efficacy and tolerability among Covid-19 patients with less diarrhea and dyslipidemia and fewer adverse reaction compared with LPV/r [71].

### 5.3 Virus entry and fusion blockers

S proteins of Coronavirus interact with angiotensin-converting enzyme 2 (ACE2) to initiate entry into the host cell, and hence ACE2 is a critical molecular target for drugs aiming to inhibit cellular access of SARS-CoV-2 [72]. Several drugs have been known to inhibit ACE2, and they are under significant scrutiny for clinical studies.

Chloroquine and Hydroxychloroquine are the drugs from natural sources being employed as the first line of drugs, potential broad-spectrum antiviral drugs. Both are also being used to treat infection by SARS-CoV [73–75]. In Simian Vero cells, both chloroquine phosphate and Hydroxychloroquine have shown inhibition of replication of SARS-CoV-2, and in a physiologically-based pharmacokinetic model, 400 mg twice daily was established as the necessary dose [76, 77]. A pilot trial in about ten hospitals from Wuhan, Guangzhou, Jinzhou, Shanghai, Beijing, Chongqing, and Ningbo emphasizes Chloroquine phosphate's superior ability to inhibit pneumonia, reduce viral load, and improving pulmonary findings, and reducing the duration of COVID-19 disease [77]. An open-label non-randomized clinical trial demonstrated that in 57% of patients, COVID-19 patients who underwent treatment with a daily dose of 600 mg Hydroxychloroquine for six days showed virological clearance. In contrast, in another randomized clinical trial in Wuhan, sixty-two COVID-19 patients showed improvement in 5 days of treatment by a daily dose of 400 mg hydroxychloroquine [39, 78]. This confirmation from the above smaller studies has propelled many prospective studies to investigate Chloroquine and Hydroxychloroquine efficiency in patients of SARS-CoV-2 infection [79, 80].

Umifenovir (Arbidol) is a drug that blocks virus entry inside the host cell by inhibiting endocytosis. It halts viral membrane from fusing into the host cell and subsequent viral entry and has been used in prophylaxis of influenza A and B viruses and inhibits numerous viruses, including Ebola virus, Hepatitis C virus, Lassa virus making it a critical antiviral [81–83]. Arbidol has been tested for its efficiency against COVID-19 conducted in Wuhan, China, where patients receiving 400 mg Umifenovir showed reduced viral load and decreased mortality [84]. A retrospective cohort study among Umifenovir-treated patients showed malicious SARS–COV-2 detection by RT-PCR was, and 69% of patients had improved chest computed tomography scans [85]. These promising results have led to the clinical trial investigation of Umifenovir to be recently initiated [85–88].

Immunotherapy has proven to be effective against infectious diseases such as influenza, SARS, MERS, and Ebola, using monoclonal antibodies (mAbs) to mitigate contagious diseases [89]. Monoclonal antibodies bind to a specific target in the body, enabling it to mimic, block, or cause changes and provide a therapeutic effect for the particular diseases [90]. SARS-CoV-2 and SARS-CoV show many similarities among them, and this suggests the use of SARS antiviral monoclonal antibodies that can identify Receptor Binding Domain (RBD) in subunit S1 in SARS-CoV-2. mAbs can block RBD interaction and its ACE2 receptor, making it anti-spike protein therapy [91, 92]. A cocktail of monoclonal antibodies that can target S-proteins in SARS-CoV and detect different epitopes can potentially destroy viral cells. For example, a cocktail of monoclonal antibodies (MAB)- CR3022 show CR3022, and CR3014 showed neutralization in laboratory setup [92, 93]. Combination of Casirivimab and Imdevimab, popularly known as REGN-COV2 is a monoclonal antibody that can bind to SARS-CoV-2 spike protein and prevent it from entering healthy cells and is under scrutiny for the same. LY3819253- a mAb isolated from a recovered COVID-19 patient, is also under evaluation that has been sponsored by Eli Lilly and Company of Indianapolis, Indiana [94].

### 5.4 Virus-release blockers

Oseltamivir, branded as Tamiflu, is Food and Drug Admission (FDA) approved drug that acts as a neuraminidase inhibitor and has since been used popularly in treating influenza A and B [95]. Oseltamivir is being tried as a first-line antiviral drug in symptomatic patients with COVID-19 posts its successful use in SARS-CoV in 2003. A study by Zhang et al. brings light to the fact that that the active site of the Spike (S) 1 Protein of SARS shows a striking similarity to neuraminidase, making use of neuraminidase inhibitors useful to treat SARS-CoV [96]. Clinical trials are currently evaluating Oseltamivir in combination with favipiravir and Chloroquine in treating SARS-CoV-2 infection [97].

### 5.5 Non-virus-targeting treatments

Tocilizumab is a humanized mAb employed in Rheumatoid Arthritis treatment, and numerous studies have included tocilizumab for consideration as anti-SARS-CoV-2 therapy. A larger multicentred clinical trial of tocilizumab has been launched in China and had about 500 patients treated already enrolled [98, 99]. Anakinra is an FDA-approved modified human IL-1 receptor antagonist (IL-1RA) for RA treatment, which blocks innate immune response associated with cytokine storm resultant inflammation [100, 101].

Dexamethasone is a glucocorticoid that curbs lung injury resultant from inflammation, respiratory failure, and death in ARDS by decreasing ventilator days and mortality. World Health Organization has put Dexamethasone on the list of essential medicines. National Institutes of Health has recommended glucocorticoids in patients hospitalized with Covid-19 in the United States [102]. Randomized Evaluation of COVID-19 Therapy (RECOVERY Trial) - a large human study was initiated in the United Kingdom by Oxford University in March 2020 to test the utility of several previously known drugs against the COVID-19 trial. The initial report announced that Dexamethasone at a dose of 6 mg once daily for up to 10 days could bring down mortality significantly in critically ill COVID-19 patients validating the use of Dexamethasone for COVID-19 patients [103]. In another recent trial, dexamethasone therapy given to patients showed 15% lower mortality in ARDS patients [104].

CD24Fc, also known as Cluster of differentiation 24, is a recombinant fusion protein and a biological immunomodulator comprising the Fc region of human Immunoglobin G1 (IgG1) attached to the nonpolymorphic areas of CD24, making it an innate checkpoint against the inflammatory responses against tissue injuries associated with cytokine storm. The protection and biological activity of CD24Fc in suppressing the expression of multiple inflammatory cytokines have been demonstrated in preclinical and clinical studies carried out. A Phase II clinical trial in patients with leukemia indicates that three doses of CD24Fc effectively eliminated the appearance of extreme acute Graft vs. Host Diseases (GVHD) due to overreacting immune system and recipient target attacking transplanted T cells. CD24Fc may therefore be investigated as a prime candidate for non-antiviral COVID-19 therapy intervention for the control of cytokine storms in affected cells [105].

Dapagliflozin (Farxiga), a sodium-glucose co-transporter-2 (SGLT-2) inhibitor, has currently been assessed under "Dapagliflozin in Respiratory Failure in Patients with COVID-19" or DARE-19 in a phase-3 randomized trial designed to evaluate its efficacy as a treatment option for COVID-19 at risk of developing comorbidity such as organ failure [106]. SGLT-2 inhibitors play a role in instigating the renin-angiotensin-aldosterone pathway through the expression of angiotensin-converting enzyme type-2 (ACE2). Renin-angiotensin-aldosterone system (RAAS) pathway is essential in the pathophysiology of SARS-CoV-2. Organ-protective effects are provided by SGLT-2 inhibitors complementary to its glycaemic benefits and hence may afford additional vital organ protection to the patients [107, 108]. Patients in DARE-19 are to be treated with a daily dose of 10 mg Dapagliflozin once a day.

## 6. Future prospective

The evolution of Zoonotic Chinese Coronavirus SARS-CoV-2 needs to be better monitored through implementing better surveillance and precautionary steps. Due to this COVID-19 pandemic, scientists worldwide were encouraged to search for novel therapeutic options, including vaccines, drugs, and diagnostics. However, until now, there is no effective treatment approved and recommended for COVID-19 globally. Utilization of such computer-aided-drug design (CADD) and bioinformatics tools such as Immune Epitope Database (IEDB) software to predict a computational vaccine and target drug compounds for COVID-19 is also encouraging [109]. In this way, drug repurposing emerged as a promising therapeutic approach in a time-saving and cost-effective manner. There are many drugs repurposed in the case of COVID-19 treatment. Drugs like Remdesivir, Dexamethasone, and a combination of Lopinavir-Ritonavir, reported positive outcomes to treat COVID-19.

Similarly, there are currently more than 100 vaccine candidates under development for the COVID-19, and it will likely be ready by early/late 2021. 38 Vaccines are in the first stage for the testing safety and dosage, 17 Vaccines are in their second phase and expanded safety trials, 12 Vaccines are in the third phase comes in large-scale efficacy tests, and 6 Vaccines approved for first or limited use. None of the vaccines are approved for full use. The safety issue is concerning and the most significant challenge when tested in diverse populations, especially in countries like India and China. Large-scale production, storage, and distribution of vaccines are also another challenge. However, further investigations and experiments are needed to discover an effective treatment option.

## 7. Conclusion

The Zoonotic Chinese Coronavirus SARS-CoV-2 outbreak likely started in the seafood market in Wuhan, China, where live animals are sold. The spread of this disease has been declared a global pandemic by WHO as it rapidly expanded worldwide and still infecting people exponentially. However, it is suggested that bats are the natural hosts for SARS-CoV-2. Bat-derived coronavirus identified from a sequence analysis shares 93.3% nucleotide identity with SARS-CoV-2 complete virus genome and 97.2% identity in the 1ab gene. However, the origins of the virus remain unclear. There is no effective therapeutic option available against human coronaviruses. This pandemic may get worsened soon if no effective therapeutics or vaccine is developed to combat COVID-19.

Nevertheless, researchers and scientists are searching for the vaccines or/ and drugs used against this deadly virus. Different broad-spectrum medications, including repurposed antiviral drugs, either alone or in combinations, are evaluated for their efficacy to treat COVID-19 patients. Few drugs give positive results to block the COVID-19 infection, including Remdesivir, Oseltamivir, Lopinavir, and Ritonavir. A predictive analysis says that more such viral pandemic could emerge shortly and cause deadly outbreaks. Therefore, to prevent the emergence of a new viral pandemic, strategies should be developed to minimize its consequences.

*DOI: http://dx.doi.org/10.5772/intechopen.98358*

## Author details

Amaresh Mishra[1], Nisha Nair[2], Amit K. Yadav[3], Pratima Solanki[3], Jaseela Majeed[4] and Vishwas Tripathi[1*]

1 School of Biotechnology, Gautam Buddha University, Greater Noida, India

2 Department of Pharmaceutical Chemistry, Delhi Pharmaceutical Education and Research University, Government of NCT of Delhi, New Delhi, India

3 Special Centre for Nanoscience, Jawaharlal Nehru University, New Delhi, India

4 School of Allied Health Sciences, Delhi Pharmaceutical Sciences and Research University, Government of NCT of Delhi, New Delhi, India

*Address all correspondence to: drvishwastripathi@gmail.com; vishwas@gbu.ac.in

## References

[1] Jalandra, R., et al., Strategies and perspectives to develop SARS-CoV-2 detection methods and diagnostics. Biomedicine & Pharmacotherapy 2020; 110446.

[2] Organization, W.H., Novel Coronavirus ( 2019-nCoV): situation report, 3. 2020.

[3] of the International, C.S.G., The species Severe acute respiratory syndrome-related Coronavirus: classifying 2019-nCoV and naming it SARS-CoV-2. Nature Microbiology 2020; 5(4) 536.

[4] Kupferschmidt, K. and J. Cohen, *Will novel virus go pandemic or be contained?* 2020, American Association for the Advancement of Science.

[5] Anthony, S.J., et al., Global patterns in coronavirus diversity. Virus evolution 2017; 3(1).

[6] Chan, J.F.-W., et al., Interspecies transmission and emergence of novel viruses: lessons from bats and birds. Trends in microbiology 2013; 21(10) 544-555.

[7] Zhu, N., et al., A novel coronavirus from patients with pneumonia in China, 2019. New England Journal of Medicine 2020.

[8] Zhang, Y., et al., New understanding of the damage of SARS-CoV-2 infection outside the respiratory system. Biomedicine & Pharmacotherapy 2020; 110195.

[9] Tang, B., et al., An updated estimation of the risk of transmission of the novel Coronavirus (2019-nCov). Infectious disease modelling 2020; 5 248-255.

[10] Tsang, T., et al., Update: outbreak of severe acute respiratory syndrome-worldwide, 2003. MMWR: Morbidity & Mortality Weekly Report 2003; 52(12) 241-241.

[11] Update, W., 31-Coronavirus never before seen in humans is the cause of SARS. Unprecedented Collaboration Identifies New Pathogen in Record Time 2003; 16.

[12] Organization, W.H., Summary of probable SARS cases with onset of illness from 1 November 2002 to 31 July 2003. http://www. who. int/csr/sars/country/table2004_04_21/en/index.html 2003.

[13] Peiris, J., et al., Coronavirus as a possible cause of severe acute respiratory syndrome. The Lancet 2003; 361(9366) 1319-1325.

[14] Memish, Z.A., et al., Middle East respiratory syndrome. The Lancet 2020.

[15] Singhal, T., A review of coronavirus disease-2019 (COVID-19). The Indian Journal of Pediatrics 2020; 1-6.

[16] Xu, X., et al., Evolution of the novel Coronavirus from the ongoing Wuhan outbreak and modeling of its spike protein for risk of human transmission. Science China Life Sciences 2020; 63(3) 457-460.

[17] Remais, J., *Modelling environmentally-mediated infectious diseases of humans: transmission dynamics of schistosomiasis in China*, in *Modelling parasite transmission and control*. 2010, Springer. p. 79-98.

[18] Wu, J.T., K. Leung, and G.M. Leung, Nowcasting and forecasting the potential domestic and international spread of the 2019-nCoV outbreak originating in Wuhan, China: a modelling study. The Lancet 2020; 395(10225) 689-697.

[19] Majumder, M. and K.D. Mandl, Early transmissibility assessment of a novel coronavirus in Wuhan, China. China (January 23, 2020) 2020.

[20] Lipsitch, M., et al., Transmission dynamics and control of severe acute respiratory syndrome. Science 2003; 300(5627) 1966-1970.

[21] Majumder, M.S., et al., Estimation of MERS-coronavirus reproductive number and case fatality rate for the spring 2014 Saudi Arabia outbreak: insights from publicly available data. PLoS currents 2014; 6.

[22] Wu, A., et al., Genome composition and divergence of the novel Coronavirus (2019-nCoV) originating in China. Cell host & microbe 2020.

[23] Lu, R., et al., Genomic characterisation and epidemiology of 2019 novel Coronavirus: implications for virus origins and receptor binding. The Lancet 2020; 395(10224) 565-574.

[24] Lau, Y.L. and J.M. Peiris, Pathogenesis of severe acute respiratory syndrome. Current opinion in immunology 2005; 17(4) 404-410.

[25] Chen, N., et al., Epidemiological and clinical characteristics of 99 cases of 2019 novel coronavirus pneumonia in Wuhan, China: a descriptive study. The Lancet 2020; 395(10223) 507-513.

[26] Liu, S., et al., Genetic spectrum and distinct evolution patterns of SARS-CoV-2. Frontiers in Microbiology 2020; 11 2390.

[27] Ahn, D.-G., et al., Current status of epidemiology, diagnosis, therapeutics, and vaccines for novel coronavirus disease 2019 (COVID-19). 2020.

[28] Ke, Y.-Y., et al., Artificial intelligence approach fighting COVID-19 with repurposing drugs. Biomedical Journal 2020.

[29] Huang, F., et al., Identification of amitriptyline HCl, flavin adenine dinucleotide, azacitidine and calcitriol as repurposing drugs for influenza A H5N1 virus-induced lung injury. PLoS Pathogens 2020; 16(3) e1008341.

[30] Dyall, J., et al., Repurposing of clinically developed drugs for Treatment of Middle East respiratory syndrome coronavirus infection. Antimicrobial agents and chemotherapy 2014; 58(8) 4885-4893.

[31] Wong, H.-H., et al., Examination of clinical trial costs and barriers for drug development final. 2014.

[32] Yeu, Y., Y. Yoon, and S. Park, Protein localization vector propagation: a method for improving the accuracy of drug repositioning. Molecular BioSystems 2015; 11(7) 2096-2102.

[33] Khan, R.J., et al., Targeting SARS-CoV-2: a systematic drug repurposing approach to identify promising inhibitors against 3C-like proteinase and 2′-O-ribose methyltransferase. Journal of Biomolecular Structure and Dynamics 2020; 1-14.

[34] Harrison, C., Coronavirus puts drug repurposing on the fast track. Nature biotechnology 2020; 38(4) 379-381.

[35] Mishra, A., et al., Natural compounds as potential inhibitors of novel coronavirus (COVID-19) main protease: An in silico study. 2020.

[36] Pathak, Y., A. Mishra, and V. Tripathi, Rifampicin may be repurposed for COVID-19 Treatment: Insights from an in-silico study. 2020.

[37] ClinicalTrials.gov.A Trial of Remdesivir in Adults With Severe COVID-19. ClinicalTrials.gov Identifier: NCT04257656.National Library of MedicineDate. Published. https://clinicaltrials.gov/ct2/show/NCT04257656

[38] ClinicalTrials.gov.Mild / Moderate 2019-nCoV Remdesivir RCT. NCT04252664.Published. https://clinicaltrials.gov/ct2/show/NCT04252664

[39] Gautret, P., et al., Hydroxychloroquine and azithromycin as a treatment of COVID-19: results of an open-label non-randomized clinical trial. International journal of antimicrobial agents 2020; 105949.

[40] ClinicalTrials.gov.A Prospective/Retrospective,Randomized Controlled Clinical Study of Antiviral Therapy in the 2019-nCoV pneumonia. ClinicalTrials.gov Identifier: NCT04255017.National Library of Medicine (US); Date. Published. https://clinicaltrials.gov/ct2/show/NCT04255017

[41] ClinicalTrials.gov.Chloroquine/Hydroxychloroquine Prevention of Coronavirus Disease (COVID-19) in the Healthcare Setting (COPCOV). ClinicalTrials.gov Identifier: NCT04303507.National Library of Medicine (US).Date. Published. https://clinicaltrials.gov/ct2/show/NCT04303507

[42] ClinicalTrials.gov.Clinical Study of Arbidol Hydrochloride Tablets in the Treatment of Pneumonia Caused by Novel Coronavirus. ClinicalTrials.gov Identifier: NCT04260594.Published. https://clinicaltrials.gov/ct2/show/NCT04260594

[43] ClinicalTrials.gov.The Efficacy of Lopinavir Plus Ritonavir and Arbidol Against Novel Coronavirus Infection (ELACOI). ClinicalTrials.gov Identifier: NCT04252885.National Library of Medicine (US); Date. Published. https://clinicaltrials.gov/ct2/show/NCT04252885

[44] ClinicalTrials.gov.The Clinical Study of Carrimycin on Treatment Patients With COVID-19. ClinicalTrials.gov Identifier: NCT04286503.National Library of Medicine (US)Date. Published. https://clinicaltrials.gov/ct2/show/NCT04286503

[45] ClinicalTrials.gov.Favipiravir, Protease Inhibitors, Oseltamivir -Gpo, Hydroxychloroquine for Treatment of COVID-19 (FIGHT-COVID-19). ClinicalTrials.gov Identifier: NCT04303299.National Library of Medicine (US). Date. Published. https://clinicaltrials.gov/ct2/show/NCT04303299

[46] Markham, A. and S.J. Keam, Danoprevir: first global approval. Drugs 2018; 78(12) 1271-1276.

[47] Tang, T., Application of Xiyanping in Treatment of infantile rotavirus diarrhea. J Hainan Med Univ 2016; 22(13) 113-5.

[48] ClinicalTrials.gov.Efficacy and Safety of Darunavir and Cobicistat for Treatment of COVID-19 (DC-COVID-19). ClinicalTrials.gov Identifier: NCT04252274.National Library of Medicine (US)Date. Published. https://clinicaltrials.gov/ct2/show/NCT04252274

[49] ClinicalTrials.gov.The Efficacy and Safety of Thalidomide Combined With Low-dose Hormones in the Treatment of Severe COVID-19. ClinicalTrials.gov Identifier: NCT04273581.National Library of Medicine (US)Date. Published. https://clinicaltrials.gov/ct2/show/NCT04273581

[50] ClinicalTrials.gov.The Efficacy and Safety of Thalidomide in the Adjuvant Treatment of Moderate New Coronavirus (COVID-19) Pneumonia. ClinicalTrials.gov Identifier: NCT04273529.National Library of Medicine (US)Date. Published. https://clinicaltrials.gov/ct2/show/NCT04273529

[51] ClinicalTrials.gov.Glucocorticoid Therapy for COVID-19 Critically Ill

Patients With Severe Acute Respiratory Failure. ClinicalTrials.gov Identifier: NCT04244591.National Library of Medicine (US)Date. Published. https://clinicaltrials.gov/ct2/show/NCT04244591

[52] Long, Y., et al., Clinical recommendations from an observational study on MERS: Glucocorticoids was benefit in treating SARS patients. International Journal of Clinical and Experimental Medicine 2016; 9(5).

[53] Hung, I.F.-N., et al., Triple combination of interferon beta-1b, Lopinavir–ritonavir, and ribavirin in the treatment of patients admitted to hospital with COVID-19: an open-label, randomised, phase 2 trial. The Lancet 2020; 395(10238) 1695-1704.

[54] Li, H., et al., Updated approaches against SARS-CoV-2. Antimicrobial agents and chemotherapy 2020; 64(6).

[55] Rome, B.N. and J. Avorn, Drug evaluation during the Covid-19 pandemic. New England Journal of Medicine 2020.

[56] Organisation, W.H. *"Solidarity" clinical trial for COVID-19 treatments*. 2020 October 16 2020; Available from: https://www.who.int/emergencies/diseases/novel-coronavirus-2019/global-research-on-novel-coronavirus-2019-ncov/solidarity-clinical-trial-for-covid-19-treatments.

[57] Sanders, J.M., et al., Pharmacologic treatments for coronavirus disease 2019 (COVID-19): a review. Jama 2020; 323(18) 1824-1836.

[58] Gorbalenya, A.E., et al., The palm subdomain-based active site is internally permuted in viral RNA-dependent RNA polymerases of an ancient lineage. Journal of molecular biology 2002; 324(1) 47-62.

[59] Sheahan, T.P., et al., Comparative therapeutic efficacy of remdesivir and combination lopinavir, ritonavir, and interferon beta against MERS-CoV. Nature communications 2020; 11(1) 1-14.

[60] Beigel, J.H., et al., Remdesivir for the treatment of Covid-19. New England Journal of Medicine 2020.

[61] Goldman, J.D., et al., Remdesivir for 5 or 10 days in patients with severe Covid-19. New England Journal of Medicine 2020.

[62] Spinner, C.D., et al., effect of remdesivir vs standard care on clinical status at 11 days in patients with moderate COVID-19: a randomized clinical trial. Jama 2020; 324(11) 1048-1057.

[63] Games, A., et al., Glenmark also continues its Phase 3 clinical trials on antiviral Favipiravir monotherapy for COVID-19 patients in India.

[64] Chen, C., et al., Favipiravir versus Arbidol for COVID-19: a randomized clinical trial. MedRxiv 2020.

[65] Cai, Q., et al., Experimental Treatment with favipiravir for COVID-19: an open-label control study. Engineering 2020.

[66] Benson, C.A., et al., Safety and antiviral activity at 48 weeks of lopinavir/ritonavir plus nevirapine and 2 nucleoside reverse-transcriptase inhibitors in human immunodeficiency virus type 1-infected protease inhibitor-experienced patients. The Journal of infectious diseases 2002; 185(5) 599-607.

[67] Corbett, A.H., M.L. Lim, and A.D. Kashuba, Kaletra (lopinavir/ritonavir). Annals of Pharmacotherapy 2002; 36(7-8) 1193-1203.

[68] Chu, C., et al., Role of lopinavir/ritonavir in the Treatment of SARS:

initial virological and clinical findings. Thorax 2004; 59(3) 252-256.

[69] Arabi, Y.M., et al., Treatment of Middle East respiratory syndrome with a combination of lopinavir-ritonavir and interferon-β1b (MIRACLE trial): study protocol for a randomized controlled trial. Trials 2018; 19(1) 1-13.

[70] Chan, J.F.-W., et al., treatment with lopinavir/ritonavir or interferon-β1b improves outcome of MERS-CoV infection in a nonhuman primate model of common marmoset. The Journal of infectious diseases 2015; 212(12) 1904-1913.

[71] Chen, J., et al. *Antiviral activity and safety of darunavir/cobicistat for the Treatment of COVID-19*. in *Open forum infectious diseases*. 2020. Oxford University Press US.

[72] Li, W., et al., Angiotensin-converting enzyme 2 is a functional receptor for the SARS coronavirus. Nature 2003; 426(6965) 450-454.

[73] Ben-Zvi, I., et al., Hydroxychloroquine: from malaria to autoimmunity. Clinical reviews in allergy & immunology 2012; 42(2) 145-153.

[74] Savarino, A., et al., New insights into the antiviral effects of Chloroquine. The Lancet infectious diseases 2006; 6(2) 67-69.

[75] Vincent, M., et al., *Chloroquine is a potent inhibitor of SARS coronavirus infection and spread. Virol J2: 69*. 2005.

[76] Keyaerts, E., et al., In vitro inhibition of severe acute respiratory syndrome coronavirus by Chloroquine. Biochemical and biophysical research communications 2004; 323(1) 264-268.

[77] Gao, J., Z. Tian, and X. Yang, Breakthrough: Chloroquine phosphate has shown apparent efficacy in Treatment of COVID-19 associated pneumonia in clinical studies. Bioscience trends 2020.

[78] Chen, Z., et al., efficacy of Hydroxychloroquine in patients with COVID-19: results of a randomized clinical trial. MedRxiv 2020.

[79] Zhang, Q., et al., Clinical trial analysis of 2019-nCoV therapy registered in China. Journal of medical virology 2020; 92(6) 540-545.

[80] Cortegiani, A., et al., A systematic review on the efficacy and safety of Chloroquine for the Treatment of COVID-19. Journal of critical care 2020.

[81] Boriskin, Y.S., E.-I. Pécheur, and S.J. Polyak, Arbidol: a broad-spectrum antiviral that inhibits acute and chronic HCV infection. Virology journal 2006; 3(1) 56.

[82] Blaising, J., et al., Arbidol inhibits viral entry by interfering with clathrin-dependent trafficking. Antiviral research 2013; 100(1) 215-219.

[83] Pécheur, E.-I., et al., The synthetic antiviral drug arbidol inhibits globally prevalent pathogenic viruses. Journal of virology 2016; 90(6) 3086-3092.

[84] Wang, Z., et al., Clinical features of 69 cases with coronavirus disease 2019 in Wuhan, China. Clinical infectious diseases 2020.

[85] Deng, L., et al., Arbidol combined with LPV/r versus LPV/r alone against Corona Virus Disease 2019: A retrospective cohort study. Journal of Infection 2020.

[86] Li, Y., et al., An exploratory randomized, controlled study on the efficacy and safety of lopinavir/ritonavir or Arbidol treating adult patients hospitalized with mild/moderate COVID-19 (ELACOI). MedRxiv 2020.

[87] Wen, C., et al., Real-world efficacy and safety of lopinavir/ritonavir and Arbidol in treating with COVID-19: an observational cohort study. Zhonghua nei ke za zhi 2020; 59 E012.

[88] Huang, H., et al., Chloroquine, Arbidol (umifenovir) or lopinavir/ritonavir as the antiviral monotherapy for COVID-19 patients: a retrospective cohort study. 2020.

[89] Cutino-Moguel, M.T., et al., Immunotherapy for infectious diseases in haematological immunocompromise. British journal of haematology 2017; 177(3) 348-356.

[90] Lu, R.-M., et al., development of therapeutic antibodies for the treatment of diseases. Journal of biomedical science 2020; 27(1) 1-30.

[91] Wong, S.K., et al., A 193-amino acid fragment of the SARS coronavirus S protein efficiently binds angiotensin-converting enzyme 2. Journal of Biological Chemistry 2004; 279(5) 3197-3201.

[92] Duan, J., et al., A human SARS-CoV neutralizing antibody against epitope on S2 protein. Biochemical and biophysical research communications 2005; 333(1) 186-193.

[93] Sheikhshahrokh, A., et al., Frontier therapeutics and vaccine strategies for sars-cov-2 (COVID-19): A review. Iranian Journal of Public Health 2020; 49 18-29.

[94] Marovich, M., J.R. Mascola, and M.S. Cohen, Monoclonal antibodies for prevention and Treatment of COVID-19. Jama 2020; 324(2) 131-132.

[95] Hayden, F.G., et al., use of the oral neuraminidase inhibitor oseltamivir in experimental human influenza: randomized controlled trials for prevention and treatment. Jama 1999; 282(13) 1240-1246.

[96] Zhang, X.W. and Y.L. Yap, The 3D structure analysis of SARS-CoV S1 protein reveals a link to influenza virus neuraminidase and implications for drug and antibody discovery. Journal of Molecular Structure: THEOCHEM 2004; 681(1-3) 137-141.

[97] Rosa, S.G.V. and W.C. Santos, Clinical trials on drug repositioning for COVID-19 treatment. Revista Panamericana de Salud Pública 2020; 44 e40.

[98] Fu, B., X. Xu, and H. Wei, Why tocilizumab could be an effective treatment for severe COVID-19? Journal of translational medicine 2020; 18(1) 1-5.

[99] Registry, C.C.T., A multicenter, randomized controlled trial for the efficacy and safety of tocilizumab in the treatment of new coronavirus pneumonia (COVID-19). 2020.

[100] Dinarello, C.A., Overview of the IL-1 family in innate inflammation and acquired immunity. Immunological reviews 2018; 281(1) 8-27.

[101] Wu, R., et al., An update on current therapeutic drugs treating COVID-19. Current Pharmacology Reports 2020; 1.

[102] Moazzam, M., et al., Understanding COVID-19: From Origin to Potential Therapeutics. International Journal of Environmental Research and Public Health 2020; 17(16) 5904.

[103] Juszczak, E. and A. Montgomery, Dexamethasone in Hospitalized Patients with Covid-19—Preliminary Report. New England Journal of Medicine.

[104] Villar, J., et al., Dexamethasone treatment for the acute respiratory distress syndrome: a multicentre, randomised controlled trial. The Lancet Respiratory Medicine 2020; 8(3) 267-276.

[105] ClinicalTrials.gov.CD24Fc as a Non-antiviral Immunomodulator in COVID-19 Treatment (SAC-COVID). ClinicalTrials.gov Identifier: NCT04317040.Published. https://ichgcp.net/clinical-trials-registry/NCT04317040

[106] Bonnet, F. and A. Scheen, Effects of SGLT2 inhibitors on systemic and tissue low-grade inflammation: The potential contribution to diabetes complications and cardiovascular disease. Diabetes & metabolism 2018; 44(6) 457-464.

[107] Kawanami, D., et al., SGLT2 inhibitors as a therapeutic option for diabetic nephropathy. International journal of molecular sciences 2017; 18(5) 1083.

[108] Cheng, H., Y. Wang, and G.Q. Wang, Organ-protective effect of angiotensin-converting enzyme 2 and its effect on the prognosis of COVID-19. Journal of medical virology 2020.

[109] Ibrahim, H.S. and S.K. Kafi, A Computational Vaccine Designing Approach for MERS-CoV Infections. Immunoinformatics 2020; 39-145.

Chapter 4

# Utilization from Computational Methods and Omics Data for Antiviral Drug Discovery to Control of SARS-CoV-2

*Ömür Baysal and Ragıp Soner Silme*

## Abstract

SARS-CoV-2 pandemic issue threatening world health and economy became a major problem with its destructive impact. The researchers have seen that conventional methods related to medicine and immunological background do not resolve this disease by gained knowledge of viruses previously studied. Advances in computational biology comprising bioinformatics, simulation, and yielded databases have accelerated and strengthened our facilities to predict some cases related to the biological complex by comparison with the use of artificial intelligence. Various novel drugs by using *in silico* resources and *in vivo* imaging techniques associated with high-resolution technologies can cause the confidential development of methods for the detection of antiviral drugs and the production of diagnosis kits. In the future, we will start seeing these novel techniques' positive reflection and their advantages in cost/time effective profits. This chapter highlights these approaches and addresses updated knowledge currently used for research and development.

**Keywords:** Computational biology, Drug discovery, Genomics, Omics science, SARS-CoV-2

## 1. Introduction

Coronaviruses (CoVs) are positive-strand RNA viruses belonging to the order of *Nidovirales* including three families *Arteriviridae*, *Coronaviridae*, and *Roniviridae* [1]. Relied on the genetic studies, they classify CoVs into four genera as alpha, beta, gamma, and delta CoVs [2]. The diameter of CoVs is between 80 to 120 nm and their shapes are spherical. The fundamental structural proteins of CoVs are envelope (E), membrane (M), nucleocapsid (N), and spike (S) [1]. Its RNA genome composes of six to ten open reading frames (ORFs) [3].

The new studies will fill the knowledge gaps to reveal how the virus is evolving and adapting to new conditions. In recent years, the advanced findings on nucleic acid amplification technologies have been the reason for improving of automated DNA sequencing with the help of bioinformatics tools to characterize and classification of all kinds of infectious disease agents. One of the single-stranded RNA viruses, the Coronaviruses, has been classified using molecular tools. On sequence analysis, the genomes were identified by direct RNA extraction of the clinical specimens isolated from nasopharyngeal aspirate or stool, as the template, since the viruses are non-cultivable [4–11]. The collection of SARS-CoV-2 sequences has been started in 2020 under the GISAID database. The analysis of viral genomes provided the preventing of possible viral mutations during *in vitro* viral replication. These provided data helped us to understand the virus, threatening the world health, at genomic and *in silico* levels, which gave rise to new experiments carried out in the laboratory. Protein function prediction methods mainly fall into sequence- and structure-based approaches. Using precisely important databases and tools relied on comparison for sequence, structural differentiation, and gene ontology enables us to find exact protein function annotation [12]. Given the destructive effect of the virus SARS-CoV-2 on human health and its contagious virulence, it has attracted the attention of researchers to find its efficiently curative method. We have realized that antiviral chemotherapy with small molecules for their properties as nucleoside analogs can identify new uncharacterized viral genes for producing antiviral drugs related to viral glycoproteins to cellular receptors, viral regulatory proteins. These drugs may block the synthesis and replication of the viral genome that induce the host immune response [13, 14].

These targeted regions can reduce the crucial function required for survival of the virus, by polymerase and/or protease assay enabled us getting of high throughput screening for identification of inhibitor small molecules and enzymes, which can be beneficial for the development of effective antiviral components and synthesized novel molecules [15]. Understanding of viral gene products could overcome the challenge of the development of antiviral drugs contributing to essential functions on the virus, with assays carried out *in vitro* considering molecular mechanisms involved in gene products and biochemical processes. New technology related to omics science is suggesting novel possibilities to find the right answers to inquiries resulting from unexplored pathogenic behavior of the virus. Bioinformatics promises to generate new knowledge on virus and host interaction that can help drive the efforts in more detail to the discovery and development of antiviral therapies [16]. Genomics, proteomics, and related technologies will also be beneficial in molecular virology as suited techniques and approaches for big data.

## 2. Bioinformatics and computational tools

The progress in the fields of genomics and proteomics are encouraging biological studies on the virus. Genomic sequences and bioinformatics are also major tools in this field and quantities of raw data which has tremendously increased besides their complexity. Therefore, significant computational resources required to manage the volumes of data and their manipulation, researchers studying in these fields for any future drug discovery projects are using these new technologies. Bioinformatics resources (GISAID; NCBI) required to analyze the data, identify patterns and display the patterns help to investigators for understanding the problem, testing, and confirmation of their hypothesis in the laboratory to focus on prioritized compounds or genes [17]. Computational methods applied in the study of SARS-CoV-2 could be paved for the characterization of the virus collected from unique specimens and comparison with similar genomes resulted from sequence similarity. Comprehensively studied investigations on the characterization of the viruses to set a unique set of well-described genomes compared within each other have been reported [18]. Bioinformatics workflows and tools related to SARS-CoV-2 to the detection of potential drug targets and providing beneficial knowledge on therapeutic strategies have also been recently acknowledged [19]. New bioinformatics tools applied to these genomes to test their ability and to predict the organization of viral genes involving coding capacity and the function of the viral proteins are commonly used [20]. These tools are assisting for the confirmation of transcriptional patterns, gene expression, and gene function which are essential studies earlier than *in vitro* studies not to lose time and labor cost [21].

Data relevant to the discovery of new drugs contain information related to biological function, chemical structure, and the biologic activity of small molecules that all findings can help for the searching for new compounds. Even the nature of this problem is inherently complex, bioinformatics is a useful tool to handle the volumes of data required with databases. Small molecule inhibitors could target the computational methods, suggesting aspects of the viral genomic property. Then they may be the reason for identification of the small molecules well-described with their biological effects, which could be used to probe for following of the cellular functions related to chemical structure, protein structure, biochemical activity, and biologic activity of the virus. As another branch of data mining on whole existing data shows a way for screening on inhibitory chemicals with known biochemical activities according to their chemical classes.

## 3. Impact of omics science and related fields on SARS-CoV-2 research

With advanced techniques and bioinformatics tools, the scientific landscape has dramatically changed in recent years. The huge data yielding on omics science plays an important role in the steps related to the biology of SARS-CoV-2 infections towards understanding more [22]. These resources are tremendously necessary to scientists studying SARS-CoV-2 infections and provide a map and common reference points to reach the data for describing precisely viral transcripts and ORFs. Comparison of different genomic organizations among all the SARS-CoV-2 isolates forms a starting point to determine the evolutionary relationships in this virus family. The most important point that should not be missed is the instability of the nucleotide sequences in the virus genome, which causes high ratio mutations. Viral genomes data inherently in GenBank involves missing annotated parts that sequence needs to be corrected. Annotations of viral genomes conducted with the best tools are available to test gene prediction with precise algorithms to identify new genes [23]. The annotation process may cause inconsistent findings for different genomes as the terminology used to describe gene function [24]. Viral genomes need to be updated and re-annotated as additional strains are of importance for comparing sequences for the continual annotation process considering analogous by released versions in NCBI [25].

The RNA sequence and structure of the genomes could be easily sequenced, but to predict their role in infection with any certainty seems difficult at the course of an infection. *In vitro* experimentation results should prove the different ORFs identified through algorithms such as codon/pair usage, dinucleotide/junction usage, RNA structure differentiation which are detected by bioinformatics tools on a viral infection [26]. Even microarray using oligonucleotide probes to hybridize with putative exons and splice junctions could be beneficial for following the expression of predicted transcripts and splice variants in virus genome [27], single-cell RNA sequencing analysis of SARS-CoV-2 will help define how the virus integrates into a human as use host cell organization to regulate and code for all the required biologic process [28]. As this knowledge with different biological assays increasingly supports findings on SARS-CoV-2 and its pathogenic behavior, the proteomics data obtained on up/down-regulated expression levels expressed by the virus reflects ongoing RNA transcripts that can be evaluated as biological cases related to post-translational processing playing role in protein formation complexity. Proteomics methods have also the potential to follow the modification of viral gene products during viral infection, which will help to characterize how post-translation modification that affects viral replication. Since omics technology maybe not sufficient alone to find effective compounds inhibiting viral replication and invasive negative effects that occurred on the human body, we should consider the detection of the genomic parts showing stability without a high mutation ratio to design targeted molecules with inhibitory potential [13]. Genomic screening using specific algorithms to identify conserved motifs and to predict protein structure could be an efficient way to understand protein functions [29]. In immunological studies, model organism, yeast, thanks to its two-hybrid (Bait and Prey) system that can be suggested to prove the protein–protein interactions among viral-cellular proteins and potential gene products cooperating in biological processes can be clarified by the construction of protein–protein interaction maps [30].

## 4. Drug discovery by means of omics data on SARS-CoV-2

Genomics and proteomics are promising new areas affecting apparently whole biological fields with widespread data and tools provided by databases.

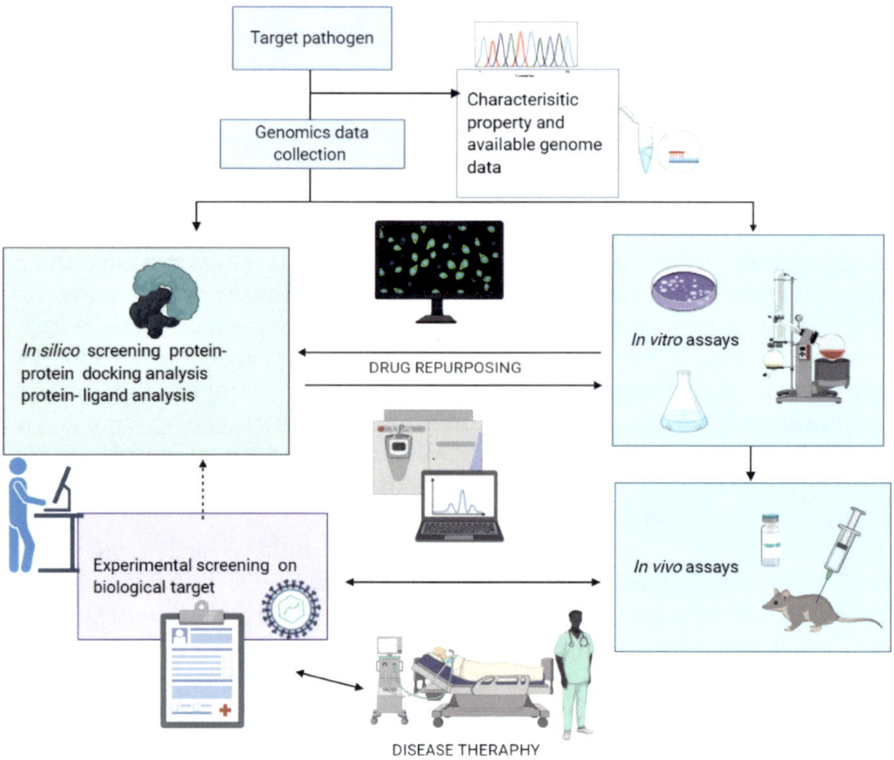


**Figure 1.**
*The experiment-based approach is activity-based repositioning of original drugs for new pharmacological indications based on experimental assays, which involves protein target-based and cell/organism-based screening* in vitro *and/or* in vivo *assays. These studies are followed with cell assay, animal model approach and clinical approach. Illustration was created with BioRender.com by the authors of this chapter.*

The DNA Data Bank of Japan (DDBJ) (https://www.ddbj.nig.ac.jp/), GISAID initiative (https://www.gisaid.org/), National Center for Biotechnology Information (The GenBank) (http://www.ncbi.nlm.nih.gov/) and The European Bioinformatics Institute (EMBL-EBI) (http://www.ebi.ac.uk/) are important resources to researchers as nucleotide databases provided on the web. Most functions in micro/ macro organism are directed by interactions of proteins and ligands. Hence, computational techniques comprising *in silico* techniques to predict the protein complex formed can be remarkably cheaper and quicker than experimental methods. They are being a guide for subsequent targeted experiments before initiating *in vitro* studies cause of their predictive capability. Predicting the binding possibilities of multiple proteins is critical for understanding their biological function in any target organism to design of drugs addressing the impairment of biological processes (**Figure 1**). Many solutions generated from a pair of static molecular structures with scoring function comprise the specific position of each atom, giving rise to the simulation of modeling that is seriously sensitive to the specific packing of atoms at the interface [31–33]. For modeling the protein, dynamics and correct protein arrangement are required, considering scoring functions related to the feature of docking poses using techniques such as molecular dynamics (MD) [34, 35].

## 5. Importance of drug discovery and molecular docking

The docking method relies on steric complementarity at the protein–protein interface level. These interfaces are observed in co-crystallized complexes available in the Protein Data Bank (PDB). They have been the major driving force in the development of docking with the addition of physicochemical and statistics-based properties [36, 37].

Homology modeling and protein prediction analysis enables us to test different proteins on SARS-CoV-2 with various ligands. Analysis by protein-ligand docking servers (**Table 1**) is available for geometric shape complementarity score (GSC score) and approximate interface area (AI area). Additionally, different software-based tools for molecular dynamic analysis could be used. The interaction analysis of protein-ligand complexes and their amino acid position with bond distances calculated and visualized through the software provides an opportunity for molecular docking simulations. Protein docking servers can confirm the results within the protein and ligand [44]. They can get an insight into their all binding preferences within the active site of the protein and ligand (**Figure 2**).

| Program | Country | Year | Reference |
|---|---|---|---|
| AADS | India | 2011 | [38] |
| AutoDock Vin | USA | 2010 | [39] |
| BetaDock | South Korea | 2011 | [40] |
| LigDockCSA | South Korea | 2011 | [41] |
| PythDock | South Korea | 2011 | [42] |
| VoteDock | Poland | 2011 | [43] |

**Table 1.**
*List of most commonly used protein-ligand softwares, comprising the updated ones.*

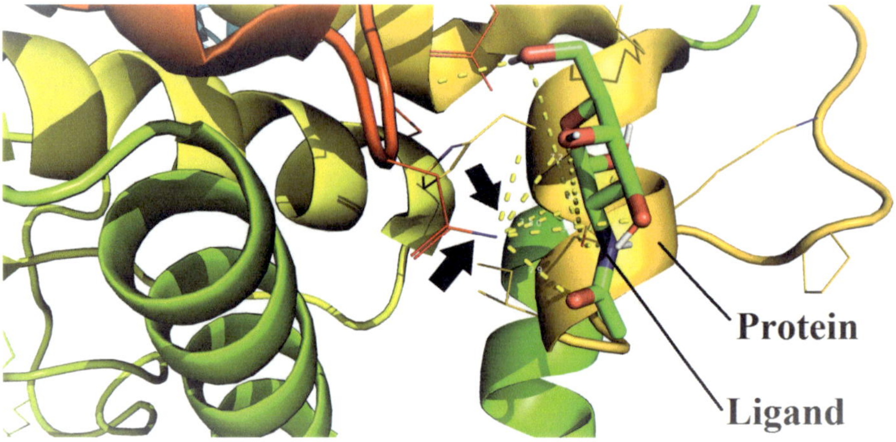


**Figure 2.**
*Protein- ligand interaction illustration from Baysal et al. [13]. Arrows indicate the binding possibilities.*

## 6. The effect of circadian rhythm on SARS-CoV-2-infection and host immune response

Many physiological processes influenced by 24-hour circadian rhythms has been known within individual cells. Even virology and circadian rhythms seem like different fields of biology, studies have suggested a novel interaction between viral infection and the circadian clock [45]. Edgar et al. showed 10 times higher viral replication in the mice infected at the start of their resting phase, likely as late evening for humans [45]. The finding confirmed the relationship between the circadian phase and virus infection. This data shows viral infection can directly affect the advantage of physiological rhythms in combating viruses. Noteworthy, a new study also indicated that the expression of the genes exhibited circadian rhythm in monocytes are shifting between two-time points showing the active and the resting periods in human individuals, which also indirectly affects SARS-CoV-2 replication [46]. The drug intake should also be adjusted considering the circadian rhythm of the body and virus to increase the efficacious of inhibitory compounds (**Figure 3**).

Another study also shows circadian clock has a central role in coordinating daily physiological processes involving immunity and biological process that humans are more susceptible to infections at certain times of the day cause of the function related to defense systems (**Figure 3**) with a daily rhythmic pattern [47]. In viral diseases, deciphering the complex relationships between circadian timekeeping, host immunity, and host-virus interactions has a great potential to unravel the complexity of severe acute respiratory syndrome coronavirus pathogenicity. Infection severity which may be regulated by the circadian clock affecting therapy positively against the novel pathogen may also result in recession of the pathogen. Therefore, circadian nature accounted for responses needs urgent studies on clock–infection biology in SARS-CoV-2. Even the pathophysiology of SARS-CoV-2 infection and its severe complications are not well understood, SARS-CoV-2 severity may also depend on day-night cycle (**Figure 3**). The battle between virus replication and its neutralization by the host immune system could move simultaneously with the circadian activity phase of the host. Accelerating the activity of circadian immunity factors may help to control virus replication, as circadian clocks provide a competitive advantage to the host against SARS-CoV-2.

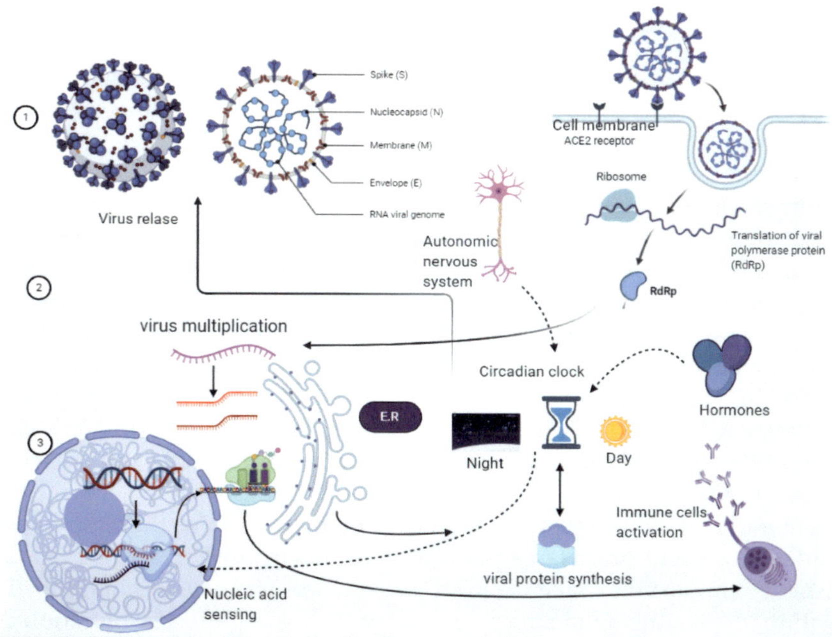


**Figure 3.**
*Cellular clock affects the virus life cycle (1) which directly/ indirectly influenced by circadian clock of the host cell. These cases trigger multiple steps in regulation of different pathways (2) against virus and its replication phases involving particle genesis. In addition, immune responses combating viral infections regulated by circadian clocks could change depending on day and night (3). Illustration was created with BioRender.com by the authors of this chapter.*

As known defect on the circadian clock in hosts causes increasing of pathogen replication and invasion, which indicates that the severity of infection influenced by circadian rhythms. All these cases can be followed by omics technologies comprising genomics, transcriptomics and proteomics data [48, 49]. We stress the combination of the whole omics data to understand all biological cases related to SARS-CoV-2 and host defense mechanism. In consequence, exact treatment times aiming to control of virus will provide higher success in managing the disease. Circadian Expression Profiles Database (CircaDB) (http://circadb.hogeneschlab.org/) could be beneficial for the evaluation of omics data with expression profiles related to the circadian clock [50]. Notably, the expression profiles of potential drug targets considering the circadian rhythm of the host could provide a new strategy for effective compounds depending on application doses, which may affect the efficiency of tested pre-purposed or novel compounds. We need to better understand how the circadian clock affects SARS-CoV-2 infection to optimal clinical management of the virus.

Another highlighted point for drawing the attention of the scientists, virulent agents causing infections could help to shape our genome that is also responsible for various polymorphic structure involving many loci related to MHC antigen processing [51]. There is also strong evidence on the effect of the virus infection depending on HLA allele's expression [52], even their influence is moderate level. Accordingly, the resistance to pathogens comprising viruses conferred by several genes acts at different stages of the host-pathogen interaction. The finding on another virus HIV at least 250 genes affecting the success of the infection has been demonstrated [53]. Consequently, the lack of genes or its impairment could have a negative or less effect on the virus invasion. These cases arise from deficient genes which lead to increased susceptibility to different virus infections [54].

## 7. Mutational changes in virus genome and traceability

As the inherent property of the virus genome, there is a higher mutational tendency compared to other micro/macro-organisms. The RNA virus replication does not comprise proofreading, as in the DNA cycle that this case renders genetic material to convenient for missing in the transcriptional phase [55]. This feature of RNA virus replication gives rise to high mutation possibility and formation of high yields, occurring of replication in a short time. RNA virus replication involves a complex and dynamic mutant formation ratio in certain genomic sites affecting the nucleotide sequence, caused by environmental factors. The model described for the evolution of virus shows comprehensible pathogenic behavior as quasispecies that have special population structure with a huge number of variant genomes relied on mutations [56]. These high mutation rates raised continually are changing in the relative frequency of the replication and selection. This process is the adoption of primitive replicons involving mutant distributions as seen in RNA viruses within their host [56, 57].

This mutational tendency depends on the population size of the virus involved in the infection. Therefore, a large population results in rapid fitness for cellular organisms. An important challenge in studies on RNA virus evolution is the differentiation, depending on phenotypic traits with ongoing specific mutations. They may associate different mutations with the biological behavior of the virus, which may be existence for the expression of phenotypic traits. These cases are the reason for the formation of restricted types. The findings on epidemiological, functional genomics, and structural studies showed the tolerance of the genetic changes on RNA viruses which are indispensable characteristic properties stemming from the virus evolution. However, the extinction of the viral infection cannot be estimated just from the characteristics of the existing sequence that is an unpredictable transitional phase of the genetic information based on lethal mutagenesis. Relied on the genomic data, the mutational ratio on viral sequences can be easily followed, but the effect of the mutation resulted in less epidemical and pathogenic behavior cannot be determined without clinical studies and monitoring on the host. Even the omics science provides predicational data on the virus, this is not enough alone if not supported by filiation studies on epidemic cases. This mutation limiting the pathogenicity of the virus may result in alternative solutions occurring spontaneously in nature for ending the viral infections.

## 8. Future outlook

According to our current knowledge on SARS-CoV-2, our facilities limit to the efficient management of the disease and do not be enough to cut down the severity of the pathogen invasion except for protective methods relied on vaccination. Even it seems a major alternative method within other possibilities we are not sure how long the virus will keep its genetic stability without the mutation, which will not render all developed vaccines possible and effective approach for further infection waves. Particularly, we now need to determine whether SARS-CoV-2 is also more severe at certain times of the day or not, which is directly related with crosstalk between the circadian clocks and viral infections besides immunological strategies based on vaccination. Drug designing or testing of pre-purposed compounds with high potential inhibitory on viral replication should be accelerated without wasting time. We are not sure what will tomorrow bring us and how other biotic and abiotic reasons will affect the pathogenicity and genetically that may change the SARS-CoV-2 and other viruses.

## 9. Conclusions

Given the existing advanced techniques present today for following the genetic structure of the RNA viruses, we are able to find a solution for combating them. But it is possible to face the novel viruses that appeared in further periods in the world cause of shifting in ecological balance and the negative effect of global warming. We should be prepared for the further worst epidemic scenarios resulted from not only due to the virus but also by other microorganisms. It appears this kind of devastating case will be not the last one if the human being continues wasting of the irreversible property of nature and ecological biodiversity. As the genetic material RNA, viruses have their own unique repair process that emerged as early as 3.5 to 2.5 billion years ago in the crust of the world. The uncovered genomic data puts insights on many biological processes for deciphering the dramatic scientific cases threatening world health, environmental issues. We believe that the post-genomic area at which we have completed genomic characterization of whole macro/micro-organisms will serve for the harvesting of the fruits, which will be useful for the scientists. The data on the genome sequences available, already /or will be soon, will offer all the information concerning the threats such as SARS-CoV-2. Bioinformatics will have a dramatic impact on improving our understanding of this kind of unclear cases. Omics science and yielded purified data are expected to be an important contributor to the global issues waiting for outbreaks cause of pandemic cases. Researches in this field will play a major role and will impact drug discovery and pharmaceutical development comprising health care and the environment.

We stress in this chapter; bioinformatics tools will increase the potential of curing the diseases and producing new effective solutions besides accurately correlated clinical parameters of patient responsiveness to therapy. Bioinformatics used in the building of global databases in molecular microbiology to enhance the accumulative knowledge in the purpose of the experimental data and meta-data about microorganisms. Drastically, whole bioinformatics tools and data yielding with omics science involving data mining will establish dynamically updated and flexible portals upon the novel microbial diversity with biotechnological innovations by our efforts aimed to reach end-products.

## Acknowledgements

The authors wish to thank to Prof. Dr. Nazlı Arda for her valuable support on our studies related to SARS-CoV-2. Moreover, the authors dedicate this chapter to scientists who think outside the box.

## Conflict of interest

The authors declare no conflict of interest.

## Author details

Ömür Baysal[1]* and Ragıp Soner Silme[2]

1 Faculty of Science, Molecular Microbiology Unit, Department of Molecular Biology and Genetics, Muğla Sıtkı Koçman University, Muğla, Turkey

2 Center for Research and Practice in Biotechnology and Genetic Engineering, Istanbul University, Istanbul, Turkey

*Address all correspondence to: omurbaysal@mu.edu.tr

## References

[1] Masters PS. The molecular biology of coronaviruses. Advances in Virus Research. 2006;**66**:193-292. DOI: 10.1016/S0065-3527(06)66005-3

[2] de Wilde AH, Snijder EJ, Kikkert M, van Hemert MJ. Host factors in coronavirus replication. Current Topics in Microbiology and Immunology. 2018;**419**:1-42. DOI: 10.1007/82_2017_25

[3] Belouzard S, Millet JK, Licitra BN, Whittaker GR. Mechanisms of coronavirus cell entry mediated by the viral spike protein. Viruses. 2012;**4**(6):1011-1033. DOI: 10.3390/v4061011

[4] Woo PC, Lau SK, Lam CS, Lai KK, Huang Y, Lee P, Luk GS, Dyrting KC, Chan KH, Yuen KY. Comparative analysis of complete genome sequences of three avian coronaviruses reveals a novel group 3c coronavirus. Journal of Virology. 2009;**83**(2):908-917. DOI: 10.1128/JVI.01977-08

[5] Woo PC, Wang M, Lau SK, Xu H, Poon RW, Guo R, Wong BH, Gao K, Tsoi HW, Huang Y, Li KS, Lam CS, Chan KH, Zheng BJ, Yuen KY. Comparative analysis of twelve genomes of three novel group 2c and group 2d coronaviruses reveals unique group and subgroup features. Journal of Virology. 2007;**81**(4):1574-1585. DOI: 10.1128/JVI.02182-06

[6] Tang XC, Zhang JX, Zhang SY, Wang P, Fan XH, Li LF, Li G, Dong BQ, Liu W, Cheung CL, Xu KM, Song WJ, Vijaykrishna D, Poon LL, Peiris JS, Smith GJ, Chen H, Guan Y. Prevalence and genetic diversity of coronaviruses in bats from China. Journal of Virology. 2006;**80**(15):7481-7490. DOI: 10.1128/JVI.00697-06

[7] Lau SK, Woo PC, Li KS, Huang Y, Tsoi HW, Wong BH, Wong SS, Leung SY, Chan KH, Yuen KY. Severe acute respiratory syndrome coronavirus-like virus in Chinese horseshoe bats. Proceedings of the National Academy of Sciences of the United States of America. 2005;**102**(39):14040-14045. DOI: 10.1073/pnas.0506735102

[8] Chu DK, Peiris JS, Chen H, Guan Y, Poon LL. Genomic characterizations of bat coronaviruses (1A, 1B and HKU8) and evidence for co-infections in *Miniopterus* bats. The Journal of General Virology. 2008;**89**(5):1282-1287. DOI: 10.1099/vir.0.83605-0

[9] Mihindukulasuriya KA, Wu G, St Leger J, Nordhausen RW, Wang D. Identification of a novel coronavirus from a beluga whale by using a panviral microarray. Journal of Virology. 2008;**82**(10):5084-5088. DOI: 10.1128/JVI.02722-07

[10] Zhang J, Guy JS, Snijder EJ, Denniston DA, Timoney PJ, Balasuriya UB. Genomic characterization of equine coronavirus. Virology 2007;**369**(1):92-104. DOI: 10.1016/j.virol.2007.06.035

[11] Lau SK, Woo PC, Li KS, Huang Y, Wang M, Lam CS, Xu H, Guo R, Chan KH, Zheng BJ, Yuen KY. Complete genome sequence of bat coronavirus HKU2 from Chinese horseshoe bats revealed a much smaller spike gene with a different evolutionary lineage from the rest of the genome. Virology. 2007;**367**(2):428-439. DOI: 10.1016/j.virol.2007.06.009

[12] Grant MA. Integrating computational protein function prediction into drug discovery initiatives. Drug Development Research, 2011;**72**(1):4-16. DOI: 10.1002/ddr.20397

[13] Baysal O, Silme RS, Karaaslan C, Ignatov A. Genetic uniformity of a specific region in SARS-CoV-2 genome

and repurposing of N-Acetyl-D-Glucosamine. Fresenius Environmental Bulletin. 2021;**30**(3):2848-2857. DOI: 10.5281/zenodo.4621319

[14] Ahmed SF, Quadeer AA, McKay MR. Preliminary identification of potential vaccine targets for the COVID-19 coronavirus (SARS-CoV-2) based on SARS-CoV immunological studies. Viruses. 2020;**12**(3):254. DOI: 10.3390/v12030254

[15] Dooley AJ, Shindo N, Taggart B, Park JG, Pang YP. From genome to drug lead: Identification of a small-molecule inhibitor of the SARS virus. Bioorganic & Medicinal Chemistry Letters. 2006;**16**(4):830-833. DOI: 10.1016/j.bmcl.2005.11.018

[16] Collins FS, Green ED, Guttmacher AE, Guyer MS. A vision for the future of genomics research. Nature. 2003;**422**:835-847. DOI: 10.1038/nature01626

[17] Venter JC, Levy S, Stockwell T, Remington K, Halpern A. Massive parallelism, randomness and genomic advances. Nature Genetics. 2003;**33**:219-227. DOI: 10.1038/ng1114

[18] Chaitanya KV. Structure and organization of virus genomes. In: Genome and Genomics. 1st ed. Singapore: Springer; 2019. p. 1-30. DOI: 10.1007/978-981-15-0702-1_1

[19] Hufsky F, Lamkiewicz K, Almeida A, Aouacheria A, Arighi C, Bateman A, Baumbach J, Beerenwinkel N, Brandt C, Cacciabue M, Chuguransky S, Drechsel O, Finn RD, Fritz A, Fuchs S, Hattab G, Hauschild AC, Heider D, Hoffmann M, Hölzer M, Hoops S, Kaderali L, Kalvari I, von Kleist M, Kmiecinski R, Kühnert D, Lasso G, Libin P, List M, Löchel HF, Martin MJ, Martin R, Matschinske J, McHardy AC, Mendes P, Mistry J, Navratil V, Nawrocki EP, O'Toole ÁN, Ontiveros-Palacios N, Petrov AI, Rangel-Pineros G, Redaschi N, Reimering S, Reinert K, Reyes A, Richardson L, Robertson DL, Sadegh S, Singer JB, Theys K, Upton C, Welzel M, Williams L, Marz M. Computational strategies to combat COVID-19: useful tools to accelerate SARS-CoV-2 and coronavirus research. Briefings in Bioinformatics. 2020;**bbaa232**:1-22. DOI: 10.1093/bib/bbaa232

[20] Pappas N, Roux S, Hölzer M, Lamkiewicz K, Mock F, Marz M, Dutilh BE. Virus bioinformatics. Reference Module in Life Sciences. 2020:1-9. DOI: 10.1016/B978-0-12-814515-9.00034-5

[21] Hölzer M, Marz M. Software dedicated to virus sequence analysis "bioinformatics goes viral". Advances in Virus Research. 2017;**99**:233-257. DOI: 10.1016/bs.aivir.2017.08.004

[22] Shu Y, McCauley J. GISAID: Global initiative on sharing all influenza data – From vision to reality. EuroSurveillance. 2017;**22**(13):30494. DOI: 10.2807/1560-7917.ES.2017.22.13.30494

[23] Mills R, Rozanov M, Lomsadze A, Tatusova T, Borodovsky M. Improving gene annotation of complete viral genomes. Nucleic Acids Research. 2003;**31**(23):7041-7055. DOI: 10.1093/nar/gkg878

[24] Koonin EV, Galperin MY. Genome Annotation and Analysis. Sequence - Evolution - Function: Computational Approaches in Comparative Genomics. Boston: Kluwer Academic; 2003. Chapter 5, Available from: https://www.ncbi.nlm.nih.gov/books/NBK20253/ [Accessed 2020-12-12]

[25] Holmes EC. RNA virus genomics: A world of possibilities. The Journal of Clinical Investigation. 2009;**119**(9):2488-2495. DOI: 10.1172/JCI38050

[26] Kames J, Holcomb DD, Kimchi O, DiCuccio M, Hamasaki-Katagiri N, Wang T, Komar AA, Alexaki A, Kimchi-Sarfaty C. Sequence analysis of SARS-CoV-2 genome reveals features important for vaccine design. Scientific Reports. 2020;**10**:15643. DOI: 10.1038/s41598-020-72533-2

[27] Shoemaker DD, Schadt EE, Armour CD, He YD, Garrett-Engele P, McDonagh PD, Loerch PM, Leonardson A, Lum PY, Cavet G, Wu LF, Altschuler SJ, Edwards S, King J, Tsang JS, Schimmack G, Schelter JM, Koch J, Ziman M, Marton MJ, Li B, Cundiff P, Ward T, Castle J, Krolewski M, Meyer MR, Mao M, Burchard J, Kidd MJ, Dai H, Phillips JW, Linsley PS, Stoughton R, Scherer S, Boguski MS. Experimental annotation of the human genome using microarray technology. Nature. 2001;**409**:922-927. DOI: 10.1038/35057141

[28] Mahalingam R, Dharmalingam P, Santhanam A, Kotla S, Davuluri G, Karmouty-Quintana H, Ashrith G, Thandavarayan RA. Single-cell RNA sequencing analysis of SARS-CoV-2 entry receptors in human organoids. Journal of Cellular Physiology. 2020;1-9. DOI: 10.1002/jcp.30054

[29] Grant MA. Integrating computational protein function prediction into drug discovery initiatives. Drug Development Research. 2011;**72**(1):4-16. DOI: 10.1002/ddr.20397

[30] Brückner A, Polge C, Lentze N, Auerbach D, Schlattner U. Yeast two-hybrid, a powerful tool for systems biology. International Journal of Molecular Sciences. 2009;**10**(6):2763-2788. DOI: 10.3390/ijms10062763

[31] Chen R, Li L, Weng Z. ZDOCK: An initial-stage protein docking algorithm. Proteins. 2003;**52**(1):80-87. DOI: 10.1002/prot.10389

[32] Tovchigrechko A, Vakser IA. GRAMM-X public web server for protein-protein docking. Nucleic Acids Research. 2006;**34**(suppl_2): W310-W314. DOI: 10.1093/nar/gkl206

[33] Kozakov D, Brenke R, Comeau SR, Vajda S. PIPER: An FFT-based protein docking program with pairwise potentials. Proteins. 2006;**65**(2):392-406. DOI: 10.1002/prot.21117

[34] Jackson RM, Gabb HA, Sternberg MJE. Rapid refinement of protein interfaces incorporating solvation: Application to the docking problem. Journal of Molecular Biology. 1998;**276**(1):265-285. DOI: 10.1006/jmbi.1997.1519

[35] Krol M, Tournier AL, Bates PA. Flexible relaxation of rigid-body docking solutions. Proteins. 2007;**68**(1):159-169. DOI: 10.1002/prot.21391

[36] Gray JJ, Moughon S, Wang C, Schueler-Furman O, Kuhlman B, Rohl CA, Baker D. Protein-protein docking with simultaneous optimization of rigid-body displacement and side-chain conformations. Journal of Molecular Biology. 2003;**331**(1):281-299. DOI: 10.1016/s0022-2836(03)00670-3

[37] Zacharias M. Protein-protein docking with a reduced protein model accounting for side-chain flexibility. Protein Science. 2003;**12**(6):1271-1282 DOI: 10.1110/ps.0239303

[38] Singh T, Biswas D, Jayaram B. AADS - an automated active site identification, docking, and scoring protocol for protein targets based on physicochemical descriptors. Journal of Chemical Information and Modeling. 2011;**51**(10):2515-2527. DOI: 10.1021/ci200193z

[39] Trott O, Olson AJ. AutoDock Vina: Improving the speed and accuracy of docking with a new scoring function, efficient optimization, and multithreading. Journal of

Computational Chemistry. 2010;**31**(2):455-461. DOI: 10.1002/jcc.21334

[40] Kim DS, Kim CM, Won CI, Kim JK, Ryu J, Cho Y, Lee C, Bhak J. BetaDock: Shape-priority docking method based on beta-complex. Journal of Biomolecular Structure & Dynamics. 2011;**29**(1):219-242. DOI: 10.1080/07391102.2011.10507384

[41] Shin WH, Heo L, Lee J, Ko J, Seok C, Lee J. LigDockCSA: Protein-ligand docking using conformational space annealing. Journal of Computational Chemistry. 2011;**32**(15):3226-3232. DOI: 10.1002/jcc.21905

[42] Chung JY, Cho SJ, Hah JM. A python-based docking program utilizing a receptor bound ligand shape: PythDock. Archives of Pharmacal Research. 2011;**34**:1451-1458. DOI: 10.1007/s12272-011-0906-5

[43] Plewczynski D, Lazniewski M, Von Grotthuss M, Rychlewski L, Ginalski K. VoteDock: Consensus docking method for prediction of protein-ligand interactions. Journal of Computational Chemistry. 2011;**32**(4):568-581. DOI: 10.1002/jcc.21642

[44] Mashiach E, Schneidman-Duhovny D, Peri A, Shavit Y, Nussinov R, Wolfson HJ. An integrated suite of fast docking algorithms. Proteins. 2010;**78**(15):3197-3204. DOI: 10.1002/prot.22790

[45] Edgar RS, Stangherlin A, Nagy AD, Nicoll MP, Efstathiou S, O'Neill JS, Reddy AB. Cell autonomous regulation of herpes and influenza virus infection by the circadian clock. Proceedings of the National Academy of Sciences of the United States of America. 2016;**113**(36):10085-10090. DOI: 10.1073/pnas.1601895113

[46] Diallo AB, Gay L, Coiffard B, Leone M, Mezouar S, Mege JL. Daytime variation in SARS-CoV-2 infection and cytokine production. bioRxiv. 2020.09.09.290718. DOI: 10.1101/2020.09.09.290718

[47] Man K, Loudon A, Chawla A. Immunity around the clock. Science. 2016;**354**(6315):999-1003. DOI: 10.1126/science.aah4966

[48] Mazzoccoli G, Vinciguerra M, Carbone A, Relógio A. The circadian clock, the immune system, and viral infections: The intricate relationship between biological time and host-virus interaction. Pathogens. 2020;**9**(2):83. DOI: 10.3390/pathogens9020083

[49] Borrmann H, McKeating JA, Zhuang X. The circadian clock and viral infections. Journal of Biological Rhythms. 2020. DOI: 10.1177/0748730420967768

[50] Pizarro A, Hayer K, Lahens NF, Hogenesch JB. CircaDB: A database of mammalian circadian gene expression profiles. Nucleic Acids Research. 2013;**41**(D1):D1009-D1013. DOI: 10.1093/nar/gks1161

[51] Segal S, Hill AV. Genetic susceptibility to infectious disease. Trends in Microbiology. 2003;**11**(9):445-448. DOI: 10.1016/s0966-842x(03)00207-5

[52] Goulder PJ, Watkins DI. Impact of MHC class I diversity on immune control of immunodeficiency virus replication. Nature Reviews Immunology. 2008;**8**:619-630. DOI: 10.1038/nri2357

[53] Brass AL, Dykxhoorn DM, Benita Y, Yan N, Engelman A, Xavier RJ, Lieberman J, Elledge SJ. Identification of host proteins required for HIV infection through a functional genomic screen. Science. 2008;**319**(5865):921-926. DOI: 10.1126/science.1152725

[54] Kenney AD, Dowdle JA, Bozzacco L, McMichael TM, St Gelais C, Panfil AR,

Sun Y, Schlesinger LS, Anderson MZ, Green PL, López CB, Rosenberg BR, Wu L, Yount JS. Human genetic determinants of viral diseases. Annual Review of Genetics. 2017;**51**:241-263. DOI: 10.1146/annurev-genet-120116-023425

[55] Drake JW, Holland JJ. Mutation rates among RNA viruses. Proceedings of the National Academy of Sciences of the United States of America. 1999;**96**(24):13910-13913. DOI: 10.1073/pnas.96.24.13910

[56] Eigen M, McCaskill J, Schuster P. Molecular quasi-species. Journal of Physical Chemistry. 1988;**92**(24):6881-6891. DOI: 10.1021/j100335a010

[57] Nowak MA. What is a quasispecies? Trends in Ecology & Evolution. 1992;**7**(4):118-121. DOI: 10.1016/0169-5347(92)90145-2

Chapter 5

# Organoid Technology and the COVID Pandemic

*Ria Sanyal and Manash K. Paul*

## Abstract

COVID-19 is caused by the Severe Acute Respiratory Syndrome Coronavirus 2 (SARS-CoV-2) and has emerged as a devastating pandemic. SARS-CoV-2 not only causes respiratory illness but also leads to impairment of multi-organ function. Scientists are racing to evaluate a range of experimental therapeutics to target COVID-19 systemically. The World Health Organization (WHO) and the Center for Disease Control and Prevention (CDC) are accelerating global research priorities to mobilize innovation towards diagnostics, treatments, and vaccines against COVID-19. In this scenario, information about appropriate organ-specific physiologically relevant models is critical to generate knowledge about the pathophysiology and therapeutic targeting of COVID-19. Human and animal organoids are providing a unique platform, demonstrating their applicability for experimental virology. This review provides a brief analysis of the available organoid models used to study and device strategies to combat COVID-19.

**Keywords:** COVID-19, Organoids, Infection, ACE2, Challenges, Gut, Lung, Brain

## 1. Introduction

It is quite well-known that classical 2D cell lines and *in vivo* models have been used near universally to investigate biological mechanisms and assess novel therapies across a large range of clinical problems [1]. Nevertheless, the results from these experiments are critically limited by a systemic lack of translational power for the response, efficacy, safety, and toxicity in humans despite its primary benefits in clinical research [2, 3]. Cell lines generically display insufficiency and inaccuracy in modeling the immune system, stromal components, and organ-specific functions after multiple passages [4]. Leaving aside animal welfare arguments, species-specific variations in organ development and pathogenesis are a long-standing bottleneck due to which animal models cannot mimic a given human disease that is polymorphic, to begin with [5]. Therefore, to define and treat disease pathology seamlessly, biologists exploited the critical features of stem-cell and came up with three-dimensional (3-D) or organotypic cultures or organoids from human samples that could successfully phenocopy cell-type composition, architecture, and to some extent, functionality (e.g., contraction, filtration, excretion, neural activity, etc.) of their natural counterparts [6–8].

Organoids, a term coined for referring to 'mini organs', [9] are best described as *in vitro* three dimensional (3D) cellular clusters exclusively derived from healthy cells – like primary tissue, embryonic stem cells, or induced pluripotent stem cells (iPSCs) [10] or even tumor cells [11]. Since these cells are capable of self-renewal and self-organization, organoids portray outstanding similarity to organ functionality as the tissue of origin compared to other conventional routes [2, 12]. The sole purpose of developing organoids is to recreate and miniaturize the multicellular structure of organs while retaining the 3-dimensional construct indefinitely.

It can now be commented that the development of organoid technology has generated a robust new methodology to zoom into the physiological events *ex vivo*, and this fact can be explained. Firstly, scientists have a wider domain of cell types to choose from, some of which were historically hard-to-access; secondly, organoids contain multiple differentiated cell types; and thirdly, organoids are genetically stable [13]. The intrinsic nature of this innovative near-physiological technology has created a paradigm shift in our understanding of basic developmental biology or stem cell research directed to a host-pathogen relationship in infectious diseases, degenerative conditions, genetic disorders, oncology, genome engineering, biobanking, and regenerative and personalized medicine [14, 15]. Through a complete visualization of spatiotemporal cellular interactions, organoid modeling reflects the predominant structural and functional properties of essential organs like kidneys [16], lungs [17–20], gut [21], brain [22], prostate [23], heart [24] and retina [25].

Human organoids are intrinsically human-derived, rapid-to-set-up, robust in scaling up, and ideal for genetic manipulation and personalization [26]. In simple terms, the organoid is an attractive strategy for clinical applications and bridges the gap between basic research and clinical practice. Along these lines, biomedical and pharmaceutical investigations on particularly relevant, rigorously designed, well-characterized, and controlled organotypic models will travel a long way in redefining fundamental discoveries, testing novel hypotheses at the 3D level and for the validation of critical data without sacrificing the integrity of any living being in the name of science. It should also be kept in mind that this technology is still in its infancy; much of the current hype originates from its enormous potential rather than a finite number of real-life scientific advancements. Hence, COVID-19 researchers use bronchial, respiratory, liver, kidney, intestine, and brain organoids to study the pathogenesis of SARS-CoV-2 and virus-specific cellular reaction on various organ systems.

In this chapter, we aim to answer a plethora of scientific questions related to the situation around the SARS-CoV-2 battle in the light of organoid technology, emphasizing key findings in therapeutic interventions meant to prevent and cure the serious medical threats imposed by SARS-CoV-2. We will highlight the state-of-the-art tools and methodologies available for human organoid lines and deep-dive into the case studies of fantastic *in vitro* organ models that well-known research groups have employed for understanding the root cause of COVID-19 devastation.

## 2. Virology and organoid

It is well-known that immortalized cell lines and animal models have paved the way for identifying the pathobiology of obligate intracellular parasites or viruses. Despite their paramount role in this field, none can adequately reproduce human disease pathology or exactly recapitulate the homeostatic functions of a normal cell. Therefore, virologists have moved on from carrying out investigations on non-natural hosts to patient-derived organoid models to address the unmet need for human model systems in studying virology and its therapeutic interventions [27]. Organoid technology, a human-based model technique, has broadened the scope for studying viral infections by enhancing the translatability of results from *in vitro* cell cultures or *ex vivo* animal systems to a more human *in vivo* mimicking condition. Since the route of host-pathogen interactions largely varies based on virus nature and its host type, including age, sex demographic profile, and genetic constitution of the hosts, it is crucial to have an accurate prototype of its natural host to conduct the experiments.

### 2.1 Culturing the unculturable

At almost all stages of replication, viruses associate closely with the host cell, and therefore the cell model used to research virus infection is crucial. Primary cells better represent the phenotype of healthy cells *in vivo* but have a short lifetime, are difficult to culture, and are heterogeneous and thereby renders manipulating them difficult. The widespread use of immortalized cell lines for culturing diverse virus strains is a common practice, but the induction of interferon-stimulated genes and other antiviral defenses is defective in many tumor-derived and artificially immortalized cell lines. These flaws can interfere with virus replication, particularly when cells are infected at lower, more physiologically important multiplicities. Moreover, there are some challenging cases where the virus fails to adapt in man-made culture conditions, like, norovirus or other enteric viruses, which remain unculturable to date in any kind of cell line system. Luckily for us, stem-cell-derived human intestinal organoids have successfully grown and studied these viral cultures up to one round of infection [28]. Similarly, respiratory viruses which are challenging to grow in cell lines like human coronavirus HKU1, human bocavirus, and human rhinovirus C could be successfully isolated from clinical specimens using Human airway epithelial (HAE) cultures [29–31]. These data prove that there is room for discovering unknown viruses and their mechanism of infection, pathogenesis, and immune escape through the fine-tuning of crucial features of the organoid platform [32].

### 2.2 Reproducing the natural virus host environment

Viruses isolated from patient samples like feces, blood, or nasopharyngeal swabs infested with a particular infection, can be grown on organoids without any imposed mutation or adaption. These cultures will now exactly recapitulate the fundamental features and infectivity profiles of the natural host cell [33, 34]. Therefore, conclusions drawn on the various aspects of organotropism, receptor usage, innate immunity induction, etc., is now even more reliable than laboratory-adapted or ATCC strains. The readouts used for post-infection analysis may differ in cell lines vs. organoids based on the culture environment and discussed in the following sections.

### 2.3 Provide new insights

Data from cell lines have earlier shown that the small open reading frame upstream of the main polyprotein ORF which is also present in the 5'UTR genomic region in enteroviruses, cannot be utilized for the initiation of translation [35]. Lulla et al. had reported for the first time that the small protein encoded by this uORF is crucial for virus release in human intestinal organoids [36]. The viruses lacking this uORF are therefore attenuated in this model. Later on, other publications on intestinal organoids have reiterated that different enteroviruses infect different cell types and induce an antiviral response characteristic of a particular cell type [37, 38].

To assess the influence of host conditions such as age and comorbidities on the progress and severity of viral infections, cross-interactions between co-detected pathogens in a single host can be studied closely with organoids. This was never feasible with cell lines because different viruses are often not culturable on the same cell line. For example, respiratory viruses are well-known for causing asthma and pathologies like cystic fibrosis or chronic obstructive pulmonary disease. HAE infection samples collected from healthy and asthmatic donors with rhinovirus have shown a unique airway epithelial structure with inflammatory signaling in asthmatic patients [39, 40].

### 2.4 Utilization in fighting the SARS-CoV-2 pandemic

Multiple types of organoid models were used to study the detrimental effect of SARS-CoV-2 infection on human hosts and its potential therapeutic interventions [41]. To begin with, HAE cultures served as faithful models for the lungs where efficient replication occurred through the infection of ciliated cells in the airway [42]. Therapeutic investigations on organoid models showed the repurposed drug remdesivir and remdesivir–diltiazem to be functional in resisting further SARS-CoV-2 infection [43]. Lamers et al. had proved for the first time that the human gut epithelium is the second major replication site of the virus [44]. Combined with the novel insights from other organoid research groups, it was proved that the SARS-CoV-2 genome is detectable in feces even after the virus is absent from oropharyngeal swabs, which explains the outcome of intestinal infection and potential fecal transmission [45].

These findings were closely followed by the observation of increased efficiency to infect secondary tissue by the virus. In terms of relative importance, the next area of investigation using organoids has been establishing the neuro-invasive aspect of SARS-CoV-2 by using brain organoid models [46]. Epidemiological studies showed the direct contribution of SARS-CoV-2 infection to neurological complications like headaches, ischemic stroke, and encephalitis, including cranial nerve-related complications such as anosmia and hyposmia, and ageusia [47, 48]. Recently, Pellegrini et al. utilized choroid plexus organoids to demonstrate the potential viral tropism for choroid plexus epithelial cells that affect the epithelium [49]. Damage to this barrier is suspected as a possible entry route for the virus into the cerebrospinal fluid and the brain.

### 2.5 Extensive research in Zika virus pandemic

Zika virus, a mosquito-borne flavivirus, is reportedly the causative agent for the infection known as ZIKV. Although adult victims show mild symptoms, newborns are marked with microcephaly, a condition in which infants are born with an abnormally small head. Being spread in over 70 countries and territories globally, [50] ZIKV is declared a global health emergency by WHO whereby microcephalic fetal tissues have shown traces of ZIKV in damaged fetal brains [51]. Due to accessibility challenges with live infected human fetal samples and postmortem tissues showing a diverse range of quality and genetic history, clinical examinations are replaced for good by brain organoid model studies. These focus on cellular tropism and pathogenesis mechanisms of ZIKV in controlled settings [52].

In 2016, the first study on brain organoid models was published by Tang et al., where they used monolayer cultures of forebrain-specific neural progenitor cell (NPCs) to model ZIKV infection during human brain development [53]. These were the initial results towards projecting that ZIKV more efficiently infects NPCs layers over human pluripotent stem cells (hPSCs) or immature neurons. Infection of cerebral organoids and human neurospheres with ZIKV and dengue virus 2 (DENV2) has proved that only ZIKV attenuates NPC growth, suggesting that the extreme aftereffect of ZIKV infection as an exceptional feature of the flavivirus family [54]. Later on, studies using brain organoids derived from hPSCs have also led to a significant understanding of various other aspects of ZIKV infection on fetal brain development [52].

Due to the limited accessibility of organoid methodologies to virology research groups and the delay in the pace of commercialization of this technology, the majority of the published work so far has been a result of cross-functional collaborative efforts [55]. This challenge is closely followed by complications arising from heterogeneity inherent to the structural complexity and cell-type diversity in brain organoid models compared to simpler analogs such as neurospheres [56]. Moreover, the low-throughput nature of culturing and analyzing organoids creates a significant obstacle in drug screening which usually needs a high-throughput styled experimental protocol. We anticipate the evolution of more sophisticated brain organoids in the future that involves the co-culturing of endothelial cells or microglial cells to enhance the physiological relevance of modeling ZIKV infection during fetal human brain development.

### 2.6 Technical challenges

The classical nature of 3D organoid models was closed round structures embedded in Matrigel, challenging to infect with viruses as receptors needed for infection are always located deep inside. This shortcoming was overcome in HAE cultures where cells are grown on a Transwell. Therefore, round gut organoids can be easily transformed into an open organoid model where they are accessible from the upper and lower sides simultaneously to establish the desired infection [28, 57, 58]. This model system is technically advantageous for infectious disease studies and drug-testing in antimicrobial therapy.

The next significant challenge worth consideration is readouts used for analysis after infection. Due to the release of viral particles in a nonlytic manner, virus cultures in primary cellular models do not result in plaque-like cytopathic effect (CPE) most of the time, for example, in the case of enterovirus A71. Huang et al. have shown using human intestinal organoids that are infected with enterovirus A71 that viral release happens through exosomes instead of a lytic process characteristic of a classical RD cell line [59]. This production is quantified through back titration or plaque assays using cell lines. The aforementioned protocol of measurement of the number of viral particles is a matter of concern in the case of primary cultures, which calls for more suitable evaluation methods.

## 3. COVID-19 and organoid

The severe acute respiratory syndrome coronavirus (SARS-CoV) first emerged in the human population in November 2002. Phylogenetic analysis of this viral isolate indicated that it has a zoonotic origin, and horseshoe bats (*R. sinicus*) seem to be its natural reservoir. With local travel restrictions and a wildlife trade ban, there were no further naturally acquired human cases of SARS in Guangdong, China. In late 2019, a novel coronavirus, SARS-CoV-2, again crossed the animal-to-human interspecies barrier to infect humans [60]. Palm civets and other mammals acted as their amplification hosts, which resulted in a super-transmissible form that could effectively spread from human to human at an unprecedented rate. This rapid propagation happened by the deposition of infected droplets or aerosols on the respiratory epithelium. This led to a pneumonia outbreak in Wuhan, China [61] which causes coronavirus disease-19 (COVID-19) marked by symptoms like fever, cough, shortness of breath, myalgia, fatigue, and sometimes gastrointestinal symptoms such as nausea, vomiting, and diarrhea [62]. Viral RNA was detected in patients' respiratory, stool and urine specimens. This condition can extend to severe lung injury and multi-organ failure, eventually leading to death in senile and comorbid patients.

In a few months, the virus had disseminated globally and sustained its pathogenicity irrespective of external factors. After WHO declared this a public health emergency of pandemic proportions, there were several lockdowns, social distancing protocols, hygienic measures, strict travel bans, strategic medical care, and vaccination programs to control the obnoxity of this outbreak. Even after one year of a relentless pandemic situation, the world is trying hard to combat the collateral damage to the global economy, public health, and civil life.

Genomic analyses of SARS-CoV-2 prove ~96% identity to the bat coronavirus BatCoV RaTG13 and 88% identity to two other bats SARSr-CoVs [61, 63, 64]. Sharing multiple similarities with SARS-CoV [65], phylogenetic analysis of SARS-CoV-2 shows that it belongs to lineage B of the beta-coronavirus genus in the family Coronaviridae [63] and has a possible common host cell receptor due to similarity in the receptor-binding domain. Animal model studies further confirmed that Angiotensin-converting enzyme 2 (ACE2)-dependent viral entry into cells is a critical step [66]. The evolution of different mutants is another concern, and quick studies can help understand the infectivity, pathogenesis, and targeting better. The B.1.1.7 variants in England, B.1.351 mutant in South Africa, P.1 in Brazil, B.1.427 in California, and now B.1.617, a "double mutant" common in India, have caused havoc on life and the economy.

Like SARS and MERS, pathobiology of the recently emerged COVID-19 is not limited to the respiratory tract because the damage has been observed and confirmed repeatedly in multiple organs [65], albeit the lungs are the main site of the infection. To investigate the rationale behind the organotropism of SARS-CoV-2, we need 3D model systems that mimic the physiological conditions at their best. Herein, organoid technology comes in as the basic framework of COVID-19 research with a much higher impact than animal models and cellular studies. Fortunately, the past decade has witnessed a revolutionary breakthrough in the generation of organoids for almost every human organ, including intricate systems like the heart, intestine, brain, and lung organoids. In the following sub-sections, we will discuss the constitution, contribution, limitations, and future applications of organoid technology in understanding the mechanism of organotropism by SARS-CoV-2 (Section 3.1-3.4), which influences and, in most cases, aggravates comorbid conditions in COVID-19 patients.

The first step in the pipeline of using 2D and 3D models for COVID-19 studies *in vitro* starts with tissue dissociation from different organs and is followed by stem/progenitor cell isolation using popular sorting methods like fluorescence-activated cell sorting (FACS) and magnetic-activated cell sorting (MACS) (**Figure 1**). Sorted stem/progenitor cells are cultured in a 3D organoid culture system and subjected to SARS-CoV-2, which mimics the organ-specific infection. Different aspects of the post-infection studies like infection rate, gene expression analysis, infection mechanism, immune-response, inflammatory response, and histology can be studied. The 3D-organoid models can then be subjected to drug screening, drug repurposing, and vaccine development-related studies (**Figure 1**). **Figure 1** provides a layout of the COVID-19 research platform.

### 3.1 Lung organoid

Dan et al. described an approach to synthesizing patient-specific lung tissue in a modular method to model relevant human lung disease, as well as for high-throughput drug screening to detect targeted therapies [67]. The first development of long-term differentiated human airway organoid cultures, which can morphologically and functionally simulate human airway epithelium, was done by Z. Zhou

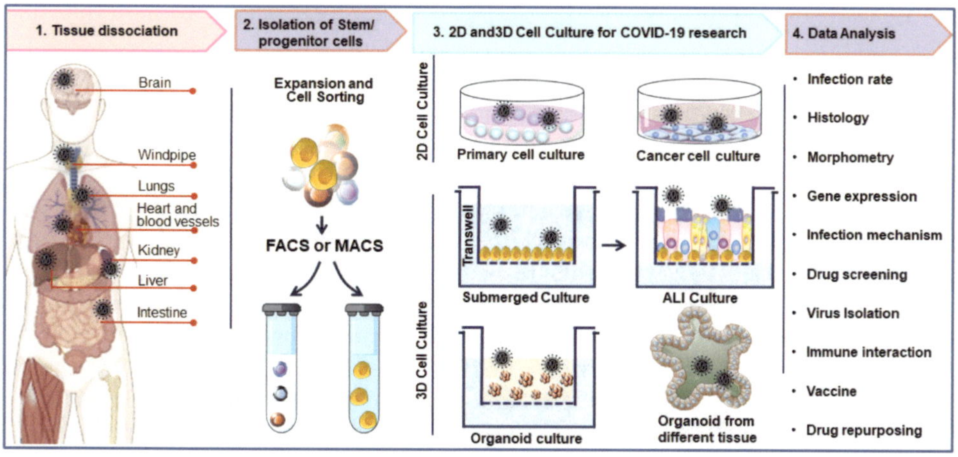


**Figure 1.**
*The COVID-19 research platform's layout using 3D organoids. Tissue dissociation from various organs is the first step in the pipeline for using 2D and 3D models for Covid-19 studies* in vitro. *Isolated stem/progenitor cells by fluorescence-activated cell sorting (FACS) and magnetic-activated cell sorting (MACS) cells are grown in 3D using extracellular matrix mimetics and nourished with niche-specific culture medium. Stem/progenitor cells derived from various tissues self-organize into tissue-specific organoids. 3D organoid cultures are infected with SARS-CoV-2. Various aspects of post-infection studies can be conducted as shown.*

et al. to predict the infectivity of influenza viruses [68]. Optimized to contain the four major airway epithelial cell types- ciliated, goblet, club, and basal cells, these organoids were exposed to two 'pairs' of already studied viruses. Resultantly, the pair of humans-infective virus replicated more robustly than the pair of matched viruses poorly infective in humans.

Several *in vitro* models, such as Vero cells, Huh7 cells, and human airway epithelial cells, have been used early on in the COVID-19 pandemic to isolate and study the SARS-CoV-2 virus. These studies took a notch up when SARS-CoV-2 was isolated and propagated in TMPRSS2-expressing Vero E6 cells, thereby proving the indispensable role of TMPRSS2 serine protease in viral replication. Nevertheless, these models are limited by their poor representation of the histology, physiology, and pathology of the events occurring in our respiratory tract [69]. Y. Han et al. have developed a lung organoid model of alveolar type II cells using human pluripotent stem cells (hPSCs) that could be adapted for drug screens [70]. This organotypic culture was able to express ACE2 and are permissive to SARS-CoV-2 infection. High throughput screening experiments identified FDA-approved drug candidates, ima-tinib and mycophenolic acid, which are efficient inhibitors of SARS-CoV-2 entry. Pre- or post-treatment with these drugs at physiologically relevant levels decreased SARS-CoV-2 infection of hPSC-derived lung organoids.

To test the validation of Remdesivir, a Covid-19 drug candidate, A. Mulay et al. successfully developed and infected differentiated air-liquid interface cultures of proximal airway epithelium and organoid cultures of alveolar epithelium by SARS-CoV-2 [71]. They displayed an epithelial cell-autonomous proinflammatory response that proved the relevance of this platform for studying COVID-19 pathobiology and rapid drug screening against SARS-CoV-2.

### 3.2 Brain organoid

While the Coronavirus disease 2019 manifests clinically acute respiratory symptoms along with fever [72], a large subset of patients, especially younger victims, develop complete or partial olfactory dysfunction (anosmia/hyposmia) during the course of infection [73]. This loss in olfaction occurred without (83%) associated rhinorrhea or nasal congestion at a median of 0.5 days after symptom onset [74]. While the majority of patients recovered within a couple of weeks from the onset of olfactory symptoms, few continued to have refractory and disabling anosmia [75]. Neurological symptoms like headache, dysgeusia, confusion, seizure, and viral encephalitis have been reported in 36.4% of 214 COVID-19 patients in Wuhan, China, where 45.5% of patients had severe SARS-CoV-2 infections [47, 76]. Similarly, France and Germany reported neurologic findings in 84.5% (49/58) and 36.4% (8/22) of COVID-19 patients, respectively, of which the latter studies had detected viral RNA in brain biopsies of patients who succumbed to the disease [77].

In 2016, D. Pamies et al. had put forward human mini-brains or BrainSpheres-an organotypic brain model derived from iPSC for the first time [78], comprising of different types of neurons, astrocytes, and oligodendrocytes. After its application on Zika, Dengue, HIV, and John Cunningham (JC) virus, they used this model to understand the extent of SARS-CoV-2 virus infection in human brain cells. Their results demonstrated that SARS-CoV-2 could infect and replicate in cells of neuronal origin, thereby proving the critically potential neurotropism of SARS-CoV-2. In yet another study, the same group had shown that SARS-CoV-2 could directly infect and effectively damage the olfactory sensory neurons of golden Syrian hamsters [75]. The entry receptor of the spike protein in SARS-CoV-2, ACE2, is widely detected in the brain, especially in the substantia nigra, middle temporal gyrus, and posterior cingulate cortex [79, 80]. Interestingly, serine protease TMPRSS2 expression was undetectable in the BrainSpheres, which suggests an alternative mechanism for spike (S) protein priming during viral entry. Together, these findings indicate that the human brain might be an extra-pulmonary target of SARS-CoV-2 infection.

Initially, it was proposed that anosmia and ageusia happen due to infection of non-neuronal cells in the olfactory system [81], which was busted by reports supporting the presence of viral particles in the CNS biofluid [82] and signs of neural damage biomarkers in the plasma of COVID-19 patients [83]. Taken together, a direct infection rather than a secondary immune response seems more accountable for neurological outcomes and predicted future neurodevelopmental disorders. Given that the human brain is arguably an extra-pulmonary target of SARS-CoV-2 infection, biologists and neuroscientists also need to figure out the impact of SARS-CoV-2 on a prototypical developing brain. Brain organoid research or the BrainSphere model is also limited by the absence of microglia or brain immune cells since they originate from the mesoderm germ layer and invade the developing brain from the blood, unlike neural precursor cells [84].

### 3.3 Gut organoid

While most COVID-19 patients suffer from mild to severe respiratory illnesses, >50% of patients manifest gastrointestinal disorders with prolonged symptoms like diarrhea, nausea, etc., which becomes severe to fatal when left unattended [85]. Although the virus has been detected in the upper respiratory tract of humans, proving the nasopharynx as a prominent site of replication, the highest expression of ACE2 occurs in the brush border of intestinal enterocytes [86]. Interestingly, when 53% of a cohort of 73 hospitalized patients had SARS-CoV-2 RNA in stool specimens, viral RNA was found in rectal swabs of 23% of patients even after negative nasopharyngeal testing, which implied fecal-oral transmission route leading to gastrointestinal infection or vice-versa [87, 88]. Of note, viral nucleoprotein-positive cells were found in the gastrointestinal epithelial cells from biopsy specimens [89] and pediatric patients [90]. Also, the SARS-CoV-2 receptor ACE2 is highly expressed on differentiated enterocytes suggesting that the intestine is a vital target organ for the pathogen. Therefore, models to understand the mechanism of SARS-CoV-2 and validate drug efficiency in the gut for COVID-19 patients are the need of the hour.

Based on the high homology of SARS-CoV-2 to SARS-related coronaviruses isolated from horseshoe bats, J. Zhou et al. established and characterized expandable intestinal organoids derived from Chinese horseshoe bats of the *Rhinolophus sinicus* species that can recapitulate bat intestinal epithelium [41]. These bat enteroids were readily infectable and could sustain SARS-CoV-2 replication. They also demonstrated active replication of SARS-CoV-2 in human intestinal organoids along with isolation of infectious virus from the stool specimen of diarrheal COVID-19 patients [91]. This again confirmed that the established culture conditions for human intestinal organoids could be extended to other members of the mammalian species.

This report, along with the work done by M. M. Lamers et al. [44] and R. Zang et al., unanimously reported that the intestine is a potential site of SARS-CoV-2 replication since enterocytes, the most common cell type of the intestinal epithelium, get readily infected [92]. M. M. Lamers et al. established human small intestinal organoids (hSIOs) from primary gut epithelial stem cells containing all proliferative and differentiated cell types of the *in vivo* epithelium [44]. Of note, hSIOs have been utilized for *in vitro* culturing of norovirus for the first time. The authors used confocal and electron microscopy to show that SARS-CoV and SARS-CoV-2 infect enterocyte lineage cells in an hSIO model. They reported similar infection rates of enterocyte precursors and enterocytes, whereas ACE2 expression increased ~1000-fold upon differentiation at the mRNA level. Therefore, while the infected enterocytes upregulated the viral response genes through cytoplasmic sensing of the viral RNA genome, the host-cell membrane-bound serine proteases TMPRSS2 and TMPRSS4 were found to cleave the SARS-CoV-2 spike protein to facilitate viral entry. They conclude the following facts from this study: (a) intestinal epithelium supports SARS-CoV-2 replication, (b) hSIOs serve as a faithful biological model for coronavirus infection, and (c) viral entry is supported even at low ACE2 concentrations.

Since organotypic cultures are derived from pluripotent or organ restricted stem cells having the ability to mimic a natural 3D environment, they need a cell source with excellent self-renewal ability. The gut is one such source that allows unlimited replenishments of a particular cell type or tissue. Single-layered human intestinal organoids (HIOs) derived from human adult gut stem cells contain only epithelial cell types [93]. Pluripotent stem cells derived from HIOs (PSC-HIOs) made of endodermal/mesodermal progeny [94], resembling epithelium and fibroblasts or gut capillaries, respectively [95]. While PSC-HIOs are not 100% mature, HIOs are architecturally too simple, resulting in lower *in vivo* transplantability and analytical access to intermediate developmental stages. Until further modifications are done on them, both models are comparable and complementary to each other with model-specific pros and cons. As per previous reports, HIOs express ACE2 and are susceptible to SARS-CoV-2 [44, 92].

Inspired by the prior human intestinal organoids derived from pluripotent stem cells (PSC-HIOs) for modeling of gastrointestinal infections, J. Kruger et al. used this organoid model to dissect SARS-CoV-2 pathogenesis and then study its inhibition by remdesivir and famotidine (histamine-2-blocker), a potential drug candidate for COVID-19 treatment [96]. Immunostaining for ACE2 and TMPRSS2 showed large expression in the gastrointestinal tract with maxima in the intestine. This ready infection of organoids with SARS-CoV-2 followed by the viral spread across entire PSC-HIOs subsequently led to organoid deterioration except goblet cells lacking ACE2 expression. The drug testing data showed that remdesivir and EK1 (but not famotidine) effectively inhibited SARS-CoV-2 infection in a dose-dependent manner at a low micromolar concentration which rescued the morphology of PSC-HIOs. This is a benchmark study that has established the applicability of PSC-HIOs in the field of organ-specific drug testing related to gut infection, like SARS-CoV-2, rotavirus, norovirus, enterovirus 71, and human adenovirus.

### 3.4 Human capillary organoids

Since ACE2 is the SARS-Cov-2 receptor, clinical-grade human recombinant soluble ACE2 (hrsACE2) has already undergone clinical phase 1 and phase 2 testing. hrsACE2 slowed or even stopped the virus's systemic dissemination from the lungs to other tissues, including potentially reducing SARS-CoV-2 attacks on the endothelial cells of the blood vessel linings. hrsACE2 has shown promising therapeutic efficacy in treating severe COVID-19 [97]. To this end, V. Monteil et al. pursued the development of engineered human blood vessel organoids and human kidney organoids to get confirmatory evidence on the effect of hrsACE2 on SARS-CoV-2 infection in multiple human organoid models [98].

To begin with, they first isolated the SARS-CoV-2 from a nasopharyngeal sample of a patient in Sweden with confirmed COVID-19, cultured it on Vero E6 cells, and successfully isolated the virus for characterization by next-generation sequencing and electron microscopy. The cellular studies showed that hrsACE2 can reduce viral growth in Vero E6 cells by a factor of 1,000–5,000. Their data demonstrated that hrsACE-2 can inhibit *in vitro* SARS-CoV-2 infection in a dose-dependent manner, unlike mouse rsACE2 highlighting the specificity of hsrACE2 in blocking SARS-CoV-2 entry. With the *in vitro* evidence at hand, they moved on to the organoid model studies.

Before getting into the deeper details, let us have a look at the background for capillary organoid research in the light of SARS-CoV-2. It was already well-known during that time that viremia initiates during the course of COVID-19 despite the irregular observation of viral RNA in blood [88]. However, a viral size of 80–100 nm is suggestive of the fact that local tissue infections can only occur through the viremic invasion into vascular endothelial cells unless there is preexisting tissue damage. This hypothesis was tested by infecting iPSC-derived human capillary organoids, which resemble human capillaries with clear lumen, lined by CD31+ endothelial cells and PDGFR+ pericyte cells and basal membrane [99]. A qRT-PCR analysis of these organoids for the presence of viral RNA indicates a gradual rise in the levels of viral RNA from day 3 to 6 of infection, proving active replication and production of progeny virus. This was followed by a marked decrease in replication without any associated toxicity on adding hrsACE2 to the capillary organoid culture.

SARS-CoV-2 can directly infect blood vessel cells which can also shed progeny viruses. Most importantly, this can be significantly inhibited by hrsACE2 at the early stages of the infection. This is the underlying rationale behind the hope of using soluble ACE2 for protecting the host body from lung injury and block the virus from entering target cells. Having said that, no data on its impact during the advanced stage of COVID-19 is currently accessible [98].

### 3.5 Kidney organoids

Since renal organotropism was becoming increasingly prominent in SARS-CoV-2, M. Glatzel et al. did an *in silico* data analysis of single-cell RNA sequencing that was available in the public datasets. Their calculations revealed that RNA of genes (ACE2, TMPRSS2, CTSL) that help to promote the viral infection is enriched in multiple kidney-cell types from fetal development through adulthood. This corroborates previous reports stating that enrichment may facilitate SARS-CoV-2–associated kidney injury [77]. They also quantified the SARS-CoV-2 viral load in precisely defined kidney compartments obtained with the use of tissue microdissection from the samples of patients who underwent autopsy. The findings revealed that 50 percent of patients had observable SARS-CoV-2 viral loads in all kidney compartments tested, with glomerular cells being the most often infected [100].

V. Monteil et al. adapted their previously published procedure [97] to produce kidney organoids from human embryonic stem cells into 3D suspension culture to assess if SARS-CoV-2 would directly invade human tubular kidney cells [101]. Kidney organoids showed conspicuous tubular-like shapes, as observed by Lotus tetraglobus lectin (LTL), a standard marker of proximal tubular epithelial cells. Similar to their human capillary organoid study, infections of kidney organoids were monitored for at least six days post-infection, and their qRT-PCR data were analyzed for the presence of viral RNA. The team used Vero E6 cells to determine the virus's progeny. SARS-CoV-2 reproduced in kidney organoids, as predicted in cells and tissues that express ACE2. The engineered kidney organoids developed infectious progeny virus, as shown by the ability of supernatant from infected kidney organoids to infect Vero E6 cells on day six post-infection. hrsACE2 significantly decreased SARS-CoV-2 infections in a dose-dependent way in the human kidney organoids, with no evidence of toxicity. In summary, engineered human kidney organoids can also be infected with SARS-CoV-2, and this infection can be inhibited by hrsACE2, similar to blood vessel organoids.

Taken together, renal tropism explains the major clinical signs of kidney injury in patients with COVID-19 having mild or severe symptoms. These studies also predict that SARS-CoV-2 infection can potentially aggravate any preexisting renal conditions. The coronavirus receptor ACE2 is expressed in kidney organoids, which may help researchers further understand the disease's systemic effects, and multiple questions regarding the pathogenesis can be answered. Thus, the development of multi-organ organoids can address the multi-organ dysfunction, a symptom of COVID-19 illness.

## 4. Future directions and conclusion

After SARS-CoV and MERS-CoV, SARS-CoV-2 is the third coronavirus in terms of pathogenicity to jump to humans within two decades. This suggests that similar zoonotic coronavirus spillovers can happen again in the near future. Nevertheless, the events relating to coronavirus pathogenesis and transmission are not completely known yet. There is a lack of efficient *in vitro* systems to accurately model host tissues. As conventional animal models, like mice, are not natural hosts to SARS-CoV-2 infection, there is a surge in the development of alternate pre-clinical models to recapitulate the targeted human organs.

Herein, organoid technology used to model human organ development and various human pathologies in a petri dish has played a significant role in understanding SARS-CoV-2 infection and replication. For drug response studies, drug screening, and repurposing, organoids, especially patient-derived organoids, have become popular. Organoid-based studies are leading to personalizing drugs, formulating regenerative medicine, and establishing gene therapy. In comparison to age-old animal models and cell lines, there has been a noticeable improvement in the reproducibility of results and statistical power of experiments. From all previous data, human organoids of lung, gut, kidney, brain, and blood vessels represent excellent experimental models to study the biology of SARS-CoV-2 [44].

Having said that, researchers working in this field are still trying to identify and troubleshoot the inherent challenges in various aspects of handling organoids, including the maintenance costs, cross-technique artifacts, and interpretation of data [26]. It is now well known that the generation and handling of organoids are way more tedious than two-dimensional cell culture protocols. Moreover, the essential growth factors being more expensive and not explicitly tested for applications in the organoid system, one has to prepare them in-house. With the emergence of various commercial sources for reagents tailored to the organoid culture, there is reason to believe that this problem will be fixed quickly. Moreover, the range of cellular heterogeneity for a particular organoid system needs to be improved. Also, mimicking the native micro-and matrix-environment encountered by cells within organoids remains a challenge. Reverse engineering methodologies are only in their infancy as it comes to developing rigorous protocols for the *in vitro* maturation of organoids that are largely fetal-like in cultures [102]. Advances in stem cell, progenitor cell, and pluripotent stem cell handling and directed differentiation techniques will soon help create more physiologically relevant organoids.

In combination with genome editing techniques for manipulating 3D models, organoid technology will be implemented at a large scale in basic and clinical research in the forthcoming era [14]. Progress with other technologies, such as microRNA switches and potentially CRISPR–Cas9, 3D bioprinting, and 3D organoids, will further advance the fast-developing multi-organ disease modeling COVID-19 and its associated therapeutic build-up. Though organoid technology suffers from multiple lacunae but COVID-19 has shown the feasibility and practicality of the organoid platform, suggesting further investment to create an *in vitro* organ mimicking reliable system for successful and effective discovery of therapeutics.

## Author details

Ria Sanyal[1] and Manash K. Paul[2*]

1 Department of Chemistry, University of Minnesota, Minneapolis, MN, USA

2 Department of Pulmonary and Critical Care Medicine, David Geffen School of Medicine, University of California Los Angeles (UCLA), Los Angeles, CA, USA

*Address all correspondence to: paul_cancerbiotech@yahoo.co.in

## References

[1] Hoarau-Véchot, J., et al., *Halfway between 2D and Animal Models: Are 3D Cultures the Ideal Tool to Study Cancer-Microenvironment Interactions?* International Journal of Molecular Sciences, 2018. **19**(1):181.

[2] Leach, T.S., et al., *Tissue organoid models and applications*, in *Principles of Tissue Engineering*. 2020. p. 1537-1549.

[3] McGonigle, P. and B. Ruggeri, *Animal models of human disease: Challenges in enabling translation.* Biochemical Pharmacology, 2014. **87**(1): p. 162-171.

[4] Zhou, J., et al., *Microfluidic device for primary tumor spheroid isolation.* Experimental Hematology & Oncology, 2017. **6**(1).

[5] Ben-David, U., et al., *Patient-derived xenografts undergo mouse-specific tumor evolution.* Nature Genetics, 2017. **49**(11): p. 1567-1575.

[6] Rossi, G., A. Manfrin, and M.P. Lutolf, *Progress and potential in organoid research.* Nature Reviews Genetics, 2018. **19**(11): p. 671-687.

[7] Clevers, H., *Modeling Development and Disease with Organoids.* Cell, 2016. **165**(7): p. 1586-1597.

[8] Fatehullah, A., S.H. Tan, and N. Barker, *Organoids as an in vitro model of human development and disease.* Nature Cell Biology, 2016. **18**(3): p. 246-254.

[9] Kelava, I. and M.A. Lancaster, *Dishing out mini-brains: Current progress and future prospects in brain organoid research.* Developmental Biology, 2016. **420**(2): p. 199-209.

[10] Shi, Y., et al., *Induced pluripotent stem cell technology: a decade of progress.* Nature Reviews Drug Discovery, 2016. **16**(2): p. 115-130.

[11] Vlachogiannis, G., et al., *Patient-derived organoids model treatment response of metastatic gastrointestinal cancers.* Science, 2018. **359**(6378): p. 920-926.

[12] Simian, M. and M.J. Bissell, *Organoids: A historical perspective of thinking in three dimensions.* Journal of Cell Biology, 2017. **216**(1): p. 31-40.

[13] Schutgens, F. and H. Clevers, *Human Organoids: Tools for Understanding Biology and Treating Diseases.* Annual Review of Pathology: Mechanisms of Disease, 2020. **15**(1): p. 211-234.

[14] Artegiani, B. and H. Clevers, *Use and application of 3D-organoid technology.* Human Molecular Genetics, 2018. **27**(R2): p. R99-R107.

[15] Xu, H., et al., *Organoid technology in disease modelling, drug development, personalized treatment and regeneration medicine.* Experimental Hematology & Oncology, 2018. **7**: 30.

[16] Takasato, M., et al., *Kidney organoids from human iPS cells contain multiple lineages and model human nephrogenesis.* Nature, 2015. **526**(7574): p. 564-568.

[17] Zacharias, W.J., et al., *Regeneration of the lung alveolus by an evolutionarily conserved epithelial progenitor.* Nature, 2018. **555**(7695): p. 251-255.

[18] Chen, Y.W., et al., *A three-dimensional model of human lung development and disease from pluripotent stem cells.* Nature Cell Biology, 2017. **19**(5): p. 542-549.

[19] Dye, B.R., et al., *In vitro generation of human pluripotent stem cell derived lung organoids.* eLife, 2015. **4**.

[20] Sachs, N., et al., *Long-term expanding human airway organoids for*

*disease modeling.* The EMBO Journal, 2019. **38**(4).

[21] Fujii, M., et al., *Human Intestinal Organoids Maintain Self-Renewal Capacity and Cellular Diversity in Niche-Inspired Culture Condition.* Cell Stem Cell, 2018. **23**(6): p. 787-793.e6.

[22] Lancaster, M.A., et al., *Cerebral organoids model human brain development and microcephaly.* Nature, 2013. **501**(7467): p. 373-379.

[23] Drost, J., et al., *Organoid culture systems for prostate epithelial and cancer tissue.* Nature Protocols, 2016. **11**(2): p. 347-358.

[24] Devarasetty, M., et al., *Optical Tracking and Digital Quantification of Beating Behavior in Bioengineered Human Cardiac Organoids.* Biosensors, 2017. **7**(3): 24.

[25] Nakano, T., et al., *Self-Formation of Optic Cups and Storable Stratified Neural Retina from Human ESCs.* Cell Stem Cell, 2012. **10**(6): p. 771-785.

[26] Kim, J., B.-K. Koo, and J.A. Knoblich, *Human organoids: model systems for human biology and medicine.* Nature Reviews Molecular Cell Biology, 2020. **21**(10): p. 571-584.

[27] Sridhar, A., et al., *A Perspective on Organoids for Virology Research.* Viruses, 2020. **12**(11).

[28] Ettayebi, K., et al., *Replication of human noroviruses in stem cell-derived human enteroids.* Science, 2016. **353**(6306): p. 1387-1393.

[29] Pyrc, K., et al., *Culturing the Unculturable: Human Coronavirus HKU1 Infects, Replicates, and Produces Progeny Virions in Human Ciliated Airway Epithelial Cell Cultures.* Journal of Virology, 2010. **84**(21): p. 11255-11263.

[30] Dijkman, R., et al., *Human Bocavirus Can Be Cultured in Differentiated Human Airway Epithelial Cells.* Journal of Virology, 2009. **83**(15): p. 7739-7748.

[31] Hao, W., et al., *Infection and Propagation of Human Rhinovirus C in Human Airway Epithelial Cells.* Journal of Virology, 2012. **86**(24): p. 13524-13532.

[32] Jazaeri Farsani, S.M., et al., *Culturing of respiratory viruses in well-differentiated pseudostratified human airway epithelium as a tool to detect unknown viruses.* Influenza and Other Respiratory Viruses, 2015. **9**(1): p. 51-57.

[33] Tapparel, C., et al., *Growth and characterization of different human rhinovirus C types in three-dimensional human airway epithelia reconstituted in vitro.* Virology, 2013. **446**(1-2): p. 1-8.

[34] Bochkov, Y.A., et al., *Mutations in VP1 and 3A proteins improve binding and replication of rhinovirus C15 in HeLa-E8 cells.* Virology, 2016. **499**: p. 350-360.

[35] Meerovitch, K., R. Nicholson, and N. Sonenberg, *In vitro mutational analysis of cis-acting RNA translational elements within the poliovirus type 2 5′ untranslated region.* Journal of Virology, 1991. **65**(11): p. 5895-5901.

[36] Lulla, V., et al., *An upstream protein-coding region in enteroviruses modulates virus infection in gut epithelial cells.* Nature Microbiology, 2018. **4**(2): p. 280-292.

[37] Drummond, C.G., et al., *Enteroviruses infect human enteroids and induce antiviral signaling in a cell lineage-specific manner.* Proceedings of the National Academy of Sciences, 2017. **114**(7): p. 1672-1677.

[38] Essaidi-Laziosi, M., et al., *Propagation of respiratory viruses in human airway epithelia reveals persistent virus-specific signatures.* Journal of

Allergy and Clinical Immunology, 2018. **141**(6): p. 2074-2084.

[39] Bai, J., et al., *Phenotypic Responses of Differentiated Asthmatic Human Airway Epithelial Cultures to Rhinovirus.* Plos One, 2015. **10**(2).

[40] Kessler, M., et al., *Chronic Chlamydia infection in human organoids increases stemness and promotes age-dependent CpG methylation.* Nature Communications, 2019. **10**(1).

[41] Clevers, H., *COVID-19: organoids go viral.* Nature Reviews Molecular Cell Biology, 2020. **21**(7): p. 355-356.

[42] Milewska, A., et al., *Replication of Severe Acute Respiratory Syndrome Coronavirus 2 in Human Respiratory Epithelium.* Journal of Virology, 2020. **94**(15).

[43] Pizzorno, A., et al., *Characterization and Treatment of SARS-CoV-2 in Nasal and Bronchial Human Airway Epithelia.* Cell Reports Medicine, 2020. **1**(4).

[44] Lamers, M.M., et al., *SARS-CoV-2 productively infects human gut enterocytes.* Science, 2020. **369**(6499): p. 50-54.

[45] Wu, Y., et al., *Prolonged presence of SARS-CoV-2 viral RNA in faecal samples.* The Lancet Gastroenterology & Hepatology, 2020. **5**(5): p. 434-435.

[46] DosSantos, M.F., et al., *Neuromechanisms of SARS-CoV-2: A Review.* Frontiers in Neuroanatomy, 2020. **14**.

[47] Zhang, B.-Z., et al., *SARS-CoV-2 infects human neural progenitor cells and brain organoids.* Cell Research, 2020. **30**(10): p. 928-931.

[48] Ramani, A., et al., *SARS-CoV-2 targets neurons of 3D human brain organoids.* The EMBO Journal, 2020. **39**(20).

[49] Pellegrini, L., et al., *Human CNS barrier-forming organoids with cerebrospinal fluid production.* Science, 2020. **369**(6500).

[50] Heukelbach, J., et al., *Zika virus outbreak in Brazil.* The Journal of Infection in Developing Countries, 2016. **10**(02): p. 116-120.

[51] Heymann, D.L., et al., *Zika virus and microcephaly: why is this situation a PHEIC?* The Lancet, 2016. **387**(10020): p. 719-721.

[52] Ming, G.-l., H. Tang, and H. Song, *Advances in Zika Virus Research: Stem Cell Models, Challenges, and Opportunities.* Cell Stem Cell, 2016. **19**(6): p. 690-702.

[53] Tang, H., et al., *Zika Virus Infects Human Cortical Neural Progenitors and Attenuates Their Growth.* Cell Stem Cell, 2016. **18**(5): p. 587-590.

[54] Garcez, P.P., et al., *Zika virus impairs growth in human neurospheres and brain organoids.* Science, 2016. **352**(6287): p. 816-818.

[55] Qian, X., et al., *Using brain organoids to understand Zika virus-induced microcephaly.* Development, 2017. **144**(6): p. 952-957.

[56] Kelava, I. and Madeline A. Lancaster, *Stem Cell Models of Human Brain Development.* Cell Stem Cell, 2016. **18**(6): p. 736-748.

[57] Stanifer, M.L., et al., *Asymmetric distribution of TLR3 leads to a polarized immune response in human intestinal epithelial cells.* Nature Microbiology, 2019. **5**(1): p. 181-191.

[58] Roodsant, T., et al., *A Human 2D Primary Organoid-Derived Epithelial Monolayer Model to Study Host-Pathogen Interaction in the Small Intestine.* Frontiers in Cellular and Infection Microbiology, 2020. **10**.

[59] Shih, S.R., et al., *Exosomes Facilitate Transmission of Enterovirus A71 From*

*Human Intestinal Epithelial Cells.* The Journal of Infectious Diseases, 2020. **222**(3): p. 456-469.

[60] Zhu, N., et al., *A Novel Coronavirus from Patients with Pneumonia in China, 2019.* N Engl J Med, 2020. **382**(8): p. 727-733.

[61] Zhou, P., et al., *A pneumonia outbreak associated with a new coronavirus of probable bat origin.* Nature, 2020. **579**(7798): p. 270-273.

[62] Huang, C., et al., *Clinical features of patients infected with 2019 novel coronavirus in Wuhan, China.* Lancet, 2020. **395**(10223): p. 497-506.

[63] Chan, J.F., et al., *Genomic characterization of the 2019 novel human-pathogenic coronavirus isolated from a patient with atypical pneumonia after visiting Wuhan.* Emerg Microbes Infect, 2020. **9**(1): p. 221-236.

[64] Lu, R., et al., *Genomic characterisation and epidemiology of 2019 novel coronavirus: implications for virus origins and receptor binding.* Lancet, 2020. **395**(10224): p. 565-574.

[65] Zhu, Z., et al., *From SARS and MERS to COVID-19: a brief summary and comparison of severe acute respiratory infections caused by three highly pathogenic human coronaviruses.* Respiratory Research, 2020. **21**(1).

[66] Zamorano Cuervo, N. and N. Grandvaux, *ACE2: Evidence of role as entry receptor for SARS-CoV-2 and implications in comorbidities.* eLife, 2020. **9**.

[67] Wilkinson, D.C., et al., *Development of a Three-Dimensional Bioengineering Technology to Generate Lung Tissue for Personalized Disease Modeling.* STEM CELLS Translational Medicine, 2017. **6**(2): p. 622-633.

[68] Zhou, J., et al., *Differentiated human airway organoids to assess infectivity of emerging influenza virus.* Proceedings of the National Academy of Sciences, 2018. **115**(26): p. 6822-6827.

[69] Elbadawi, M. and T. Efferth, *Organoids of human airways to study infectivity and cytopathy of SARS-CoV-2.* The Lancet Respiratory Medicine, 2020. **8**(7): p. e55-e56.

[70] Han, Y., et al., Identification of Candidate COVID-19 Therapeutics using hPSC-derived Lung Organoids, 2020.

[71] Mulay, A., et al., SARS-CoV-2 infection of primary human lung epithelium for COVID-19 modeling and drug discovery, Cell Rep, 2021. **35**(5): p. 109055

[72] Guan, W.J., et al., *Clinical Characteristics of Coronavirus Disease 2019 in China.* N Engl J Med, 2020. **382**(18): p. 1708-1720.

[73] Lechien, J.R., et al., *Olfactory and gustatory dysfunctions as a clinical presentation of mild-to-moderate forms of the coronavirus disease (COVID-19): a multicenter European study.* European Archives of Oto-Rhino-Laryngology, 2020. **277**(8): p. 2251-2261.

[74] Yuen, K.-Y., et al., *Olfactory Dysfunction in Coronavirus Disease 2019 Patients: Observational Cohort Study and Systematic Review.* Open Forum Infectious Diseases, 2020. **7**(6).

[75] Zhang, A.J., et al., *Severe Acute Respiratory Syndrome Coronavirus 2 Infects and Damages the Mature and Immature Olfactory Sensory Neurons of Hamsters.* Clinical Infectious Diseases, 2020. ciaa995

[76] Helms, J., et al., *Neurologic Features in Severe SARS-CoV-2 Infection.* New England Journal of Medicine, 2020. **382**(23): p. 2268-2270.

[77] Puelles, V.G., et al., *Multiorgan and Renal Tropism of SARS-CoV-2.* New England Journal of Medicine, 2020. **383**(6): p. 590-592.

[78] Pamies, D., *A human brain microphysiological system derived from induced pluripotent stem cells to study neurological diseases and toxicity.* Altex, 2017: p. 362-376.

[79] Chen, R., et al., 2020.

[80] Hoffmann, M., et al., *SARS-CoV-2 Cell Entry Depends on ACE2 and TMPRSS2 and Is Blocked by a Clinically Proven Protease Inhibitor.* Cell, 2020. **181**(2): p. 271-280.e8.

[81] Brann, D.H., et al., *Non-neuronal expression of SARS-CoV-2 entry genes in the olfactory system suggests mechanisms underlying COVID-19-associated anosmia.* Science Advances, 2020. **6**(31).

[82] Zhou, H., et al., *A Novel Bat Coronavirus Closely Related to SARS-CoV-2 Contains Natural Insertions at the S1/S2 Cleavage Site of the Spike Protein.* Current Biology, 2020. **30**(11): p. 2196-2203.e3.

[83] Kanberg, N., et al., *Neurochemical evidence of astrocytic and neuronal injury commonly found in COVID-19.* Neurology, 2020. **95**(12): p. e1754-e1759.

[84] Bullen, C.K., *Infectability of Human BrainSphere Neurons Suggests Neurotropism of SARS-CoV-2*.* Altex, 2020.

[85] Wei, X.-S., et al., *Diarrhea Is Associated With Prolonged Symptoms and Viral Carriage in Corona Virus Disease 2019.* Clinical Gastroenterology and Hepatology, 2020. **18**(8): p. 1753-1759.e2.

[86] Hikmet, F., et al., *The protein expression profile of ACE2 in human tissues.* Molecular Systems Biology, 2020. **16**(7).

[87] Xiao, F., et al., *Evidence for Gastrointestinal Infection of SARS-CoV-2.* Gastroenterology, 2020. **158**(6): p. 1831-1833.e3.

[88] Wang, W., et al., *Detection of SARS-CoV-2 in Different Types of Clinical Specimens.* Jama, 2020.

[89] Xiao, F., et al., *Evidence for Gastrointestinal Infection of SARS-CoV-2.* Gastroenterology, 2020. **158**(6): p. 1831-1833 e3.

[90] Xu, Y., et al., *Characteristics of pediatric SARS-CoV-2 infection and potential evidence for persistent fecal viral shedding.* Nat Med, 2020. **26**(4): p. 502-505.

[91] Zhou, J., et al., *Infection of bat and human intestinal organoids by SARS-CoV-2.* Nature Medicine, 2020. **26**(7): p. 1077-1083.

[92] Zang, R., et al., *TMPRSS2 and TMPRSS4 promote SARS-CoV-2 infection of human small intestinal enterocytes.* Sci Immunol, 2020. **5**(47).

[93] Sato, T., et al., *Single Lgr5 stem cells build crypt-villus structures in vitro without a mesenchymal niche.* Nature, 2009. **459**(7244): p. 262-5.

[94] Spence, J.R., et al., *Directed differentiation of human pluripotent stem cells into intestinal tissue in vitro.* Nature, 2010. **470**(7332): p. 105-109.

[95] Holloway, E.M., et al., *Differentiation of Human Intestinal Organoids with Endogenous Vascular Endothelial Cells.* Developmental Cell, 2020. **54**(4): p. 516-528.e7.

[96] Krüger, J., et al., *Drug Inhibition of SARS-CoV-2 Replication in Human Pluripotent Stem Cell–Derived Intestinal Organoids.* Cellular and Molecular Gastroenterology and Hepatology, 2021. **11**(4): p. 935-948.

[97] Zhang, H., et al., *Angiotensin-converting enzyme 2 (ACE2) as a SARS-CoV-2 receptor: molecular mechanisms and potential therapeutic target.* Intensive Care Medicine, 2020. **46**(4): p. 586-590.

[98] Monteil, V., et al., *Inhibition of SARS-CoV-2 Infections in Engineered Human Tissues Using Clinical-Grade Soluble Human ACE2.* Cell, 2020. **181**(4): p. 905-913.e7.

[99] Wimmer, R.A., et al., *Human blood vessel organoids as a model of diabetic vasculopathy.* Nature, 2019. **565**(7740): p. 505-510.

[100] Pei, G., et al., *Renal Involvement and Early Prognosis in Patients with COVID-19 Pneumonia.* J Am Soc Nephrol, 2020. **31**(6): p. 1157-1165.

[101] Garreta, E., et al., *Fine tuning the extracellular environment accelerates the derivation of kidney organoids from human pluripotent stem cells.* Nature Materials, 2019. **18**(4): p. 397-405.

[102] Lou, Y.-R. and A.W. Leung, *Next generation organoids for biomedical research and applications.* Biotechnology Advances, 2018. **36**(1): p. 132-149.

Section 3

# COVID-19 in Clinics

Chapter 6

# Chest Imaging in Coronavirus Disease-19 (COVID-19)

*Arshed Hussain Parry and Abdul Haseeb Wani*


## Abstract

Coronavirus disease-19 (COVID-19), a highly contagious viral disease caused by severe acute respiratory syndrome coronavirus 2 (SARS-CoV-2) affects many organ systems causing a vast range of clinical manifestations. However, involvement of lungs is the most common manifestation and is the main cause of mortality. Detection of viral nucleic acid in the respiratory secretions is the corner stone of the diagnosis of COVID-19 infection; however, imaging plays a critical role in clinching diagnosis of reverse transcriptase polymerase chain reaction (RT-PCR) negative cases and those with atypical presentation. More importantly imaging has a pivotal role in the detection of complications and their appropriate management. Chest radiography, computed tomography (CT) and magnetic resonance imaging (MRI) all have a role in the diagnosis of COVID-19 pneumonia and detection of various thoracic complications related to this disease. This chapter comprehensively discusses the thoracic manifestations of COVID-19 and the role of imaging in their diagnosis and effective management.


**Keywords:** COVID-19, chest manifestations, CXR, CT, MRI, CT perfusion, PET-CT

## 1. Introduction

Coronavirus disease 2019 (COVID-19) first emerged in Wuhan, China in late 2019 and spread rapidly across the world. COVID-19 has touched vast swathes of land affecting 220 countries across the world. The disease has infected an estimated 57.7 million people and claimed 1.37 million lives as on 23 November, 2020. The World Health Organization (WHO) declared COVID-19 a pandemic on 11 March, 2020 [1].

COVID-19 is a viral disease. The causative agent is a novel enveloped single-stranded RNA virus belonging to betacoronavirus group and is referred to as severe acute respiratory syndrome coronavirus 2 (SARS-CoV-2) [2]. SARS-CoV-2 is believed to have originated from bats which act as the natural reservoir. The disease spreads through human-to-human contact via respiratory route [3]. Coronaviruses (CoVs) are classified into three genera of alphacoronavirus, betacoronavirus, and gammacoronavirus [4]. CoVs infect animals and humans and cause respiratory, gastrointestinal and neurological diseases of various degrees of severity. CoVs exhibit the genetic characteristics of mutation and recombination which confers them the ability to adapt to new hosts and ecological niches [5].

Respiratory system is the primary target organ of SARS-CoV-2 [6]. However, the virus also affects other organ systems including gastrointestinal system, neurological system, cardiac and vascular systems [7–11]. Many infected patients do not develop any symptoms. 19–50% patients have been reported to have an asymptomatic infection [12]. Asymptomatic patients act as covert transmitters and constitute a potential contagious source of SARS-CoV-2 as they unknowingly transmit the virus to others [13–17]. However, many patients who are asymptomatic at the time of initial diagnosis become symptomatic later and are referred to as pre-symptomatic cases [16].

Detection of viral nucleic acid in the respiratory secretions by reverse transcriptase polymerase chain reaction (RT-PCR) is the mainstay of diagnosis [13, 15]. RT-PCR has a reported sensitivity of 60–71 percent with a very high specificity [17]. However, the performance of RT-PCR is limited by various factors including specimen collection, type of specimen, transportation of specimen and the processing time which results in many false negative results [18, 19].

Imaging plays a key role in the diagnosis of various manifestations of COVID-19 and detection of its associated complications. An effective utilization of imaging would require a comprehensive understanding and appropriate interpretation of the typical and atypical imaging features of the disease. In this chapter we first elaborate chest manifestations of COVID-19 and subsequently we discuss the role of various chest imaging modalities in their management.

## 2. Chest manifestations of COVID-19

SARS-CoV-2 which is acquired through the inhalation route primarily targets the respiratory system. The symptoms attributable to respiratory system include cough, breathlessness, expectoration, sore throat, chest discomfort or pain and hemoptysis. Non-specific symptoms include fever, fatigue, and myalgia [20].

SARS-CoV-2 expresses various spike proteins on its outer surface which avidly binds to angiotensin converting enzyme-2 (ACE-2). ACE-2 is expressed in alveolar pneumocytes and vascular endothelium in abundance. The virus binds to ACE-2 and enters into the cell where it replicates and causes cell death with consequent release of inflammatory cytokines in profusion which cause damage to the host [21, 22].

The primary manifestation of COVID-19 is pneumonia. The pneumonia is usually bilateral and peripheral with a predilection for lung bases. Mild to moderate disease constitutes the bulk of cases (80%) and is characterized by constitutional symptoms and development of mild pneumonia, whereas severe disease occurs in approximately 15% and is generally characterized by more than 50% lung involvement and presents with dyspnea and hypoxia [21]. Critically ill patients constitute a small portion (5%) of infections and present with respiratory failure, shock and multiorgan dysfunction. Apart from affliction of lungs the bronchial tree is also affected by this disease leading to inflammation of bronchial walls [23, 24].

Pulmonary vascular involvement is commonly reported in COVID-19. Frequent involvement of pulmonary vessels is a unique feature of COVID-19 which makes it different from other viral and bacterial causes of pneumonia [18]. Pulmonary embolism frequently occurs in severely ill COVID-19 cases. The underlying mechanisms include the triad of Virchow including hypercoagulability induced by infection and hypoxia, immobility and vascular endothelial injury [25, 26]. However, besides involvement of major pulmonary vessels affection of small pulmonary vessels has been described as a unique distinguishing feature of COVID-19 pneumonia [27].

In various autopsy studies of COVID-19 patients small vessel involvement has been reported to be the hallmark of COVID-19 pneumonia [28]. Small pulmonary vessel thrombosis is commonly found in COVID-19 pneumonia. The putative mechanism put forth to explain this includes immunothrombosis [29]. Vascular endothelial injury caused by SARS-CoV-2 upon binding with ACE-2, which is expressed abundantly on endothelial cells, leads to severe endothelialitis and thrombosis of these small vessels [28–30].

Cardiac manifestations in COVID-19 include arrhythmias, myocarditis, cardiomyopathy, carcinogenic shock and cardiac arrest and sudden death. Myocarditis and cardiomyopathy has been reported in 7% and 7–33% of severely ill COVID-19 cases, respectively [31, 32]. Myocardial dysfunction evidenced by elevated serum troponin levels is associated with poor clinical outcome. Various mechanisms have been put forth to explain cardiac injury in COVID-19. COVID-19 can cause direct injury to myocardium leading to myocarditis which is a dreaded complication with high mortality [32]. Severe infection can induce plaque rupture and coronary artery thrombosis leading to myocardial ischemia. Infection associated hypoxia and vasoconstriction can affect coronary vessels leading to critical myocardial ischemia and cardiac dysfunction [33]. Alternately, disseminated intravascular coagulation (DIC) induced by severe SARS-CoV-2 infection can precipitate coronary artery thrombosis and cause myocardial infarction [33]. Lastly, stress induced cardiomyopathy can also explain myocardial dysfunction in COVID-19 [34].

### 2.1 Chest X-ray radiography (CXR)

Chest X-ray radiography (CXR) is the preliminary imaging modality employed in the initial workup of suspected COVID-19 pneumonia cases [35]. CXR has a multitude of unique advantages and limitations. CXR is widely available in almost all health facilities including emergency rooms (ER), intensive care units (ICU) and wards. Due to the small size of equipment it has the advantage of portability which circumvents the transfer of patients away from ICU or wards for performance of imaging thereby minimizing the requirements of staff and chances of spread of infection [35, 36]. CXR equipment is easy to disinfect. CXR entails a small radiation dose to the patient which makes it preferable for children and pregnant patients. Owing to these advantages major medical societies across the world have advocated the use of CXR in the workup of individuals suspected of having COVID-19. American College of Radiology supported the use of CXR for the evaluation of suspected individuals to facilitate triage and monitoring the course of illness [36, 37].

However, CXR has some major limitations. It has a low sensitivity and specificity in the detection of COVID-19 pneumonia. The sensitivity of CXR has been reported in the range of 33–69% [38–40]. CXR is insensitive especially in mild cases and during the early stages of disease [40]. To address the issue of low sensitivity and specificity attempts have been made to take advantage of artificial intelligence by developing deep learning algorithms [41, 42]. Deep learning algorithms have been found to improve the accuracy of CXR in the detection of COVID-19 pneumonia. Most of the patients have a normal CXR during the initial stages of infection, however, with the passage of time the positivity rate of CXR increases. It has been reported that approximately 80% patients will have a positive CXR at some point during the course of hospitalization [43, 44].

A postero-anterior or an antero-posterior CXR is obtained. A slight modification of conventional technique has been made by interposing a glass door between the patient and film to reduce exposure of radiographer to infection [44]. This technique has been found to produce optimal image quality and at the same time minimizing the exposure of radiographer to infection.

The typical findings at CXR include consolidations and ground glass opacification (GGO) with a peripheral and basal predilection (**Figure 1**). Peripheral distribution of pulmonary opacities is one of the specific features of COVID-19 pneumonia [45]. Diffuse lung opacification may be seen in patients with severe disease or acute

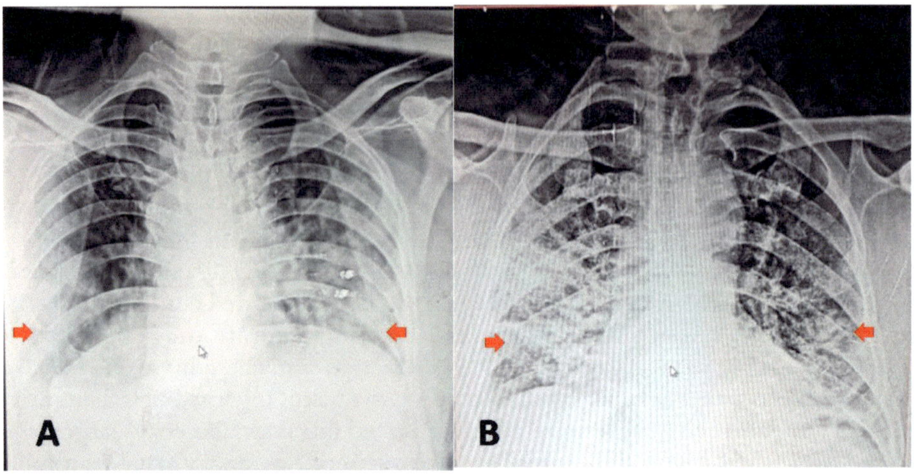

**Figure 1.**
*CXR in two different RT-PCR confirmed COVID-19 cases showing bilateral ground glass opacification (red arrows in A) and multifocal consolidations (red arrows in B) with lower zone predominance.*

respiratory distress syndrome (ARDS) [46, 47]. Initially the CXR may be normal; however, lung opacities may evolve rapidly reaching a peak at around 6–12 days [48, 49]. Pleural effusion, pericardial effusion and mediastinal lymphadenopathy is seen infrequently in severe cases [44]. The degree of pulmonary opacification on CXR has been reported to predict the need for hospitalization or intubation with patients having GGO in two lung zones more likely to require hospitalization and those with opacification of three or more zones likely to undergo intubation [46]. Bilateral lung involvement is seen commonly (73%) whereas, a unilateral lung involvement is seen less frequently (<25%) [43, 44]. It is a good clinical practice to look beyond lungs when assessing a CXR. Position of tubes (endotracheal tube and nasogastric tube) and lines (central venous line) must be assessed on CXR [46].

The two most common radio-opacities of GGO and consolidation are not specific to COVID-19 and are seen in many other infectious and non-infectious pulmonary pathologies [47, 48]. Non-COVID-19 viral pneumonias like influenza, Middle East Respiratory Syndrome (MERS) and other viral pneumonias must be included in the differential diagnosis in cases of bilateral pulmonary affection [49]. Bacterial pneumonia must be considered in the differential diagnosis particularly in cases of unilateral lung involvement [50]. Non-infectious causes of pulmonary opacities like pulmonary edema, aspiration, pulmonary hemorrhage, inflammation (like pulmonary eosinophilia) and pulmonary vasculitides should be considered in the differential diagnosis in appropriate clinical setting [43, 48].

The British Society of Thoracic Imaging (BSTI) guidelines recommend performance of CXR in all patients with a oxygen saturation of less than 94% and those who do not meet this criterion, CXR should be performed in them when "clinically required" [45]. COVID-19 survivors who recover from acute illness require clinico-radiological follow-up. BSTI guidelines recommend that patients who required ICU or high dependency unit (HDU) admission or were managed as in-ward patients with severe pneumonia should be assessed virtually at 4-6 weeks post-discharge and then face-to-face if needed and subsequently a face-to-face clinical assessment along with a CXR must be undertaken at 12 weeks. Patients who did not require ICU or HDU admission and were managed as mild–moderate pneumonia should undergo a follow-up CXR at 12 weeks [45]. Follow-up CXR are essential to pick any residual lung abnormalities sufficiently early to ensure their management to avert any long-term fibrotic pulmonary sequelae.

### 2.2 Lung ultrasound (LUS)

Due to its rapidity, easy availability, portability, repeatability and lack of ionizing radiation there has been a resurgent use of LUS in COVID-19 pandemic. It has been used mostly as a complementary and sometimes as an alternative modality in the detection of pulmonary involvement in COVID-19 cases. LUS usage has been particularly rewarding in critically ill patients who need a bedside modality which could circumvent their transfer out of the intensive care unit (ICU) room [46, 47].

The most common imaging features of LUS in pulmonary involvement in COVID-19 include B-lines, thick irregular pleura and subpleural consolidations [46]. B-lines are an imaging surrogate of subpleural interlobular septal thickening which occurs due to accumulation of fluid in pulmonary interstitium and alveolar spaces [48]. B-lines are hyperechoic linear lines, oriented vertically from pleural surface into the depths of lung. These lines spread like rays down the ultrasound screen and maintain their brightness throughout without fading. B-lines may be separate or coalescent. When multiple lines coalesce together they produce what is referred to as shining white lung. B-lines should move or slide with respiratory excursions [49]. Lack of this sliding movement should alert one to consider the possibility of underlying pneumothorax [49].

LUS can be used in emergency room (ER) for prompt detection of pulmonary involvement in symptomatic patients suspected of COVID-19 as soon as they arrive in the ER. LUS features typical of pulmonary involvement will ensure rapid detection, prompt isolation and timely treatment of these patients before RT-PCR results are available [50].

LUS can prove handy in monitoring the course of illness in inward patients by demonstrating the degree of lung involvement. The presence of a few widely separated B-lines in limited areas of chest suggests a mild disease whereas multiple clumped lines spread in multiple chest areas is indicative of a more severe form of disease [50, 51]. Similarly, in ICU setting LUS can help in monitoring the progression of disease and additionally help in detection of complications like pleural or pericardial effusion [51]. LUS can also be used in detection of complications of mechanical ventilation like pneumothorax. Ultrasound can also be used in the diagnosis of arterial and venous thrombosis, a complication which is frequently seen in severe COVID-19 cases [52].

Echocardiography, a specialized form of ultrasound, can aid in detection of cardiac complications of COVID-19 like myocarditis, cardiomyopathy, cardiac failure, intracardiac thrombosis and major pulmonary artery embolism [53]. Echocardiography can be used in this specific disease for the detection of major pulmonary embolism and its prognostication [54]. Detection of thrombus in right heart, right ventricular outflow tract or main pulmonary artery, akinesis of free wall of right ventricle (McConnell's sign), hypercontractility of right ventricular apical wall, dilatation of right ventricle (ventricular diameter of >42 mm at base and > 35 mm at mid-cavitary level) and paradoxical motion of interventricular septum are specific echocardiographic signs of pulmonary embolism [55, 56]. Echocardiography can also detect cardiac dysfunction in myocarditis, myocardial ischemia and cardiac failure [56].

### 2.3 Computed tomography (CT)

CT is a cross-sectional imaging modality which uses x-rays projected through multiple angles at the patient to generate an image [22]. The use of CT for the diagnosis and screening of COVID-19 has been universally discouraged by various radiological societies across the world citing reasons such as lack of specificity of CT for precise diagnosis with overlap seen between COVID-19 pneumonia and other viral infections on CT [16, 19]. Secondly, CT entails transfer of patients from wards or ICU to CT suite. Finally there is a possibility that CT suites may act as a vector of cross infection. The consensus guidelines of American College of Radiology (ACR) and European Society of Radiology (ESR) and the European Society of Thoracic Imaging (ESTI) do not recommend performance of CT for the diagnosis or screening of COVID-19 [16, 22, 31]. CT has thus been reserved for a small subset of patients with severe disease, those showing respiratory worsening during illness or to monitor the course of disease. However, in some selected circumstances CT may also be helpful in patients with milder symptoms who have pre-existing co-morbidities, such as diabetes mellitus, chronic respiratory disease, obesity, chronic kidney disease etc. [57]. Performance of repeat CTs is not routinely indicated during recovery. However, a repeat CT may be warranted in cases with suspicion of complications likely superadded infection and pulmonary embolism [57].

Notwithstanding the recommendations, CT has been widely performed in COVID-19 cases and has been used to support the diagnosis, assess severity, detect complications, choose appropriate treatment and monitor response to therapy [41]. CT has greatly helped in understanding the natural course of the disease. While CXR is considered the first line tool in the initial screening or assessment of COVID-19 cases, CT is still employed widely owing to its high sensitivity in the detection of pneumonia [43]. In many cases subtle imaging findings which are difficult to detect on CXR are readily identifiable on CT.

Typical CT findings include multifocal and bilateral GGOs and or consolidations with peripheral and lower lobe predominance (**Figures 2** and **3**) [34, 36, 38]. Unilateral lung involvement is less common [43]. On CT, GGO is defined as increased lung attenuation with preservation of underlying vascular and bronchial structures [58]. Consolidation is defined as increased lung attenuation with obscuration of underlying bronchial and vascular structures [58]. Other additional features seen on CT include crazy paving pattern which is a GGO with superimposed interlobular septal thickening producing a pavement like appearance [59, 60]. The relative frequency of type and distribution of lung lesions varies across different studies. A systematic analysis of 34 published studies including 4121 patients revealed bilateral lung involvement in 73% [61]. Multilobar lung involvement was seen in 67% patients. GGOs were seen in 68%, consolidation in 32% and crazy-paving pattern in 35% patients [61]. Additional findings reported were air bronchogram sign (44%), pleural thickening (27%), pleural effusion (5%) and lymphadenopathy (5%) [61]. Some

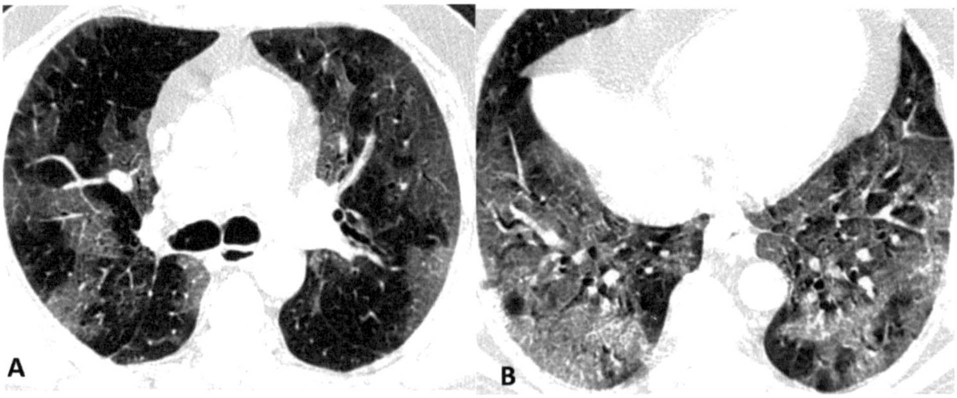


**Figure 2.**
*Axial chest CT images at slightly different levels (A, B) in lung window settings of a 56-year-old COVID-19 patient showing diffuse ground glass opacification in both lungs with a peripheral distribution.*

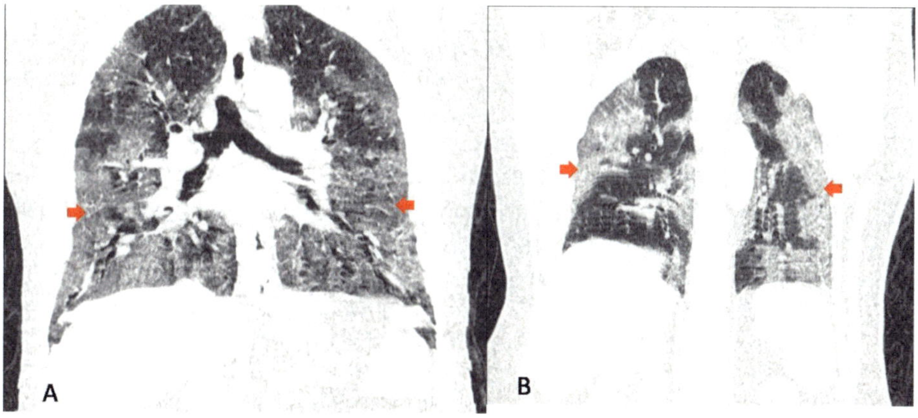

**Figure 3.**
*Coronal chest CT images at slightly different levels (A, B) in lung window settings of a 61-year-old COVID-19 patient showing diffuse ground glass opacification in both lungs with both upper and lower lobe involvement.*

symptomatic patients may have a normal CT, especially during the early stages of disease. Similarly, asymptomatic patients may have an abnormal chest CT [62–64].

CT findings evolve rapidly after symptom onset and reach a peak at around 6–13 days of illness [63]. There is increase in the extent of lung involvement and change in the appearance of pulmonary opacities. GGOs may progress into crazy paving pattern or consolidations [64]. Thereafter the findings may remain stable for some time and then gradually resorb [65]. However, in some cases there may be rapid progression into ARDS [66]. The pulmonary opacities during resolution phase start organizing and lead to secondary organizing pneumonia which manifests as reverse halo or atoll sign and perilobular opacities [61]. In one study nearly half of the patients had residual lung abnormalities consisting of fibrosis 3 months after discharge [66]. Other findings observed on CT include segmental or subsegmental vascular enlargement (defined as greater than 3 mm diameter) within the lung opacities. It has been observed in up to 89% COVID-19 pneumonia [28]. This sign of segmental or subsegmental vascular enlargement is a relatively specific sign of COVID-19 pneumonia with a diagnostic significance [41]. Presence of vascular enlargement sign may help confidently diagnose COVID-19 pneumonia. The underlying pathophysiological mechanism for vascular enlargement sign may be related to severe vascular inflammation, vasodilatory effect of proinflammatory cytokines or small vessel thrombosis [65–67].

Other less common findings observed on CT include reverse halo sign or atoll sign, bronchial wall thickening, nodules and halo sign [34]. Reverse halo sign is defined as a relatively lucent GGO surrounded by a dense ring of consolidation [51]. This finding is typically seen in resorptive stage of the disease. Pleural effusion, pericardial effusion and mediastinal lymphadenopathy is seen infrequently particularly in severe disease [18]. Presence of cavitation or tree in bud nodules are not observed in COVID-19 and should arouse suspicion of an alternate diagnosis. CT has been reported to have a high sensitivity of around 94% in detecting COVID-19 [54]. However, the specificity of CT is limited (39%) [68]. The dominant findings of GGO and consolidation observed in COVID-19 are seen in many other infectious and non-infectious diseases of lung [69, 70]. A comprehensive and detailed clinical information and exposure history is essential during interpretation of CT to increase the diagnostic confidence.

To determine the severity of lung inflammation in COVID-19 and help in identifying the patients in need of special care, severity scoring systems have been devised [71]. Anatomically there are five lobes in two lungs. Each lobe is assessed individually to determine the degree of pulmonary opacification. Each lobe is scored visually from 0 to 5. A score of 0 is assigned if there is no involvement, score of 1 for <5% involvement, score 2 for 5–25% involvement, score 3 for 26–50% involvement, score 4 for 51–75% involvement and score 5 for >75% involvement. The individual scores of all 5 lobes are added to provide a final CT severity score. CT severity scores of 1–5 are categorized as mild disease, 6–14 as moderate disease and 15–25 as severe disease [71, 72]. The disease severity as determined on CT correlates with short-term clinical outcome with higher CT severity scores associated with worse outcomes [73].

CT imaging features of COVID-19 overlap with many other pulmonary infections, predominantly viral infections, but it also exhibits some characteristic imaging features which are seen infrequently in other infections [65]. The Radiological Society of North America (RSNA) Expert Consensus Statement on Reporting proposed a standardized nomenclature and included four categories to determine the chances of a pulmonary opacity being COVID-19 [74]. The four categories are typical appearance, indeterminate appearance, atypical appearance and negative for pneumonia (**Table 1**) [74]. In March, 2020, the Dutch Radiological Society developed a standardized CT based reporting format known as COVID-19 reporting and data system (CO-RADS) to ensure uniformity in reporting and to improve communication between radiologists and physicians [75]. CO-RADS provides a level of suspicion for lung involvement in COVID-19. The degree of suspicion increases from CO-RADS category 1 (very low suspicion) to CO-RADS-5 (very high suspicion). The two peripheral categories of 0 and 6 are invoked when a CT is technically inferior and insufficient for diagnosis or to label a scan in a patient with positive RT-PCR result for SARS-CoV-2, respectively (**Table 2**) [74–76].

## 2.4 CT pulmonary angiography (CTPA)

CTPA has demonstrated pulmonary embolism in up to 30% of COVID-19 patients [61]. The location of these emboli has been reported in main pulmonary artery (22%), lobar pulmonary artery (34%), segmental pulmonary artery (28%) and subsegmental arteries (16%) [77, 78]. In cases with a severe disease with sudden respiratory worsening or hemodynamic instability, CTPA is indicated to detect pulmonary embolism [77]. Pulmonary embolism is a life-threatening complication of COVID-19. However, if diagnosed early and treated appropriately improved outcomes are observed. CTPA entails administration of a bolus of non-ionic iodinated contrast and performance of CT during passage of contrast through the pulmonary vascular tree. To ensure optimal timing of scanning a bolus tracking technique is used. Pulmonary embolism manifests as a filling defect within a contrast filled pulmonary artery [79]. Besides the direct visualization of embolus some indirect signs in lungs and heart can be seen. Pulmonary infarction can be seen as a wedge shaped peripheral consolidation [80]. Similarly, bowing of interventricular septum, dilatation of right ventricle and reflux of contrast into inferior vena cava or hepatic veins may be seen and indicates increased pulmonary artery pressure [80, 81].

## 2.5 CT perfusion angiography

Besides pulmonary macroembolism, involvement of pulmonary microvasculature is a unique feature of COVID-19. Micro vascular dysfunction of pulmonary and non-pulmonary organ systems has been widely reported in COVID-19 [66]. It is believed that binding of viral spike proteins to ACE-2 on endothelial cells incites severe endothelialitis and precipitates microthrombosis of these small vessels. This microthrombotic phenomenon also referred to as immunothrombosis has been

| Category | CT findings |
|---|---|
| Typical appearance | 1. GGOs+/−consolidations or visible intralobular lines (crazy-paving pattern) with a bilateral and peripheral distribution.<br>2. Multifocal GGOs of rounded morphology +/− consolidation or visible intralobular lines (crazy paving pattern)<br>3. Reverse halo or atoll sign or other findings of organizing pneumonia (like perilobular opacities) |
| Indeterminate appearance | Absence of typical CT findings and the presence of either of the following:<br>1. Multifocal, perihilar, diffuse or unilateral GGOs +/− consolidation which lack a specific distribution and are non-rounded or non-peripheral<br>2. Few very small GGOs with a non-rounded and non-peripheral distribution |
| Atypical appearance | Absence of typical or indeterminate findings and the presence of<br>1. Lobar or segmental consolidation without GGO<br>2. Discrete small lung nodules (e.g. centrilobular, tree-in-bud appearance)<br>3. Lung cavitation<br>4. Smoother interlobular septal thickening with pleural effusion |
| Negative for pneumonia | No CT features of pneumonia (like absence of GGO and consolidation) |

**Table 1.**
*RSNA expert consensus guidelines for reporting CT in patients suspected of COVID-19.*

| CO-RADS category | Level of suspicion | CT findings |
|---|---|---|
| 0 | Not interpretable | Low quality, technically insufficient scan for assigning a score |
| 1 | Very low | Normal or non-infectious pathology (like mass) |
| 2 | Low | Typical for other infection but not COVID-19 |
| 3 | Equivocal/unsure | CT features are ambiguous; compatible with both COVID-19 and non-COVID-19 causes of pneumonia |
| 4 | High | Suspicious for COVID-19 |
| 5 | Very high | Typical for COVID-19 |
| 6 | RT-PCR proven | CT findings of pneumonia with RT-PCR positive for SARS-CoV-2 |

**Table 2.**
*COVID-19 reporting and data system (CO-RADS).*

confirmed by various autopsy studies [15, 23]. This microthrombotic angiopathy causes obliteration of vascular bed and results in hypoxemia [29]. Non-contrast CT or CTPA cannot detect this condition. The direct visualization of occlusion of micro vascular bed is not possible on CTPA as it is beyond the resolution thresholds of currently available technology [80]. CT perfusion angiography is an advanced CT technology which demonstrates micro vascular thrombosis by detecting pulmonary perfusion defects [81]. However, this technology is limited by its availability. It has been suggested that CT perfusion angiography may also have a role in COVID-19 survivors who demonstrate residual respiratory dysfunction by detecting residual clot burden [82, 83].

## 2.6 Magnetic resonance imaging (MRI)

MRI is not recommended for the detection of pulmonary involvement in COVID-19. However, in many cases MRI performed for other indications may accidentally pick up pulmonary changes consistent with COVID-19 [84]. On MRI, pulmonary parenchymal changes of increased signal intensity on both T1-weighted and T2-weighted sequences correspond to GGO and consolidation seen on CXR and CT [84, 85]. MRI has found use in the evaluation of cardiac complications of COVID-19. MRI has the capability to demonstrate changes of myocarditis or ischemia precipitated by COVID-19 infection and also to provide a quantitative measure of various cardiac functional indices [85]. In myocarditis, a diffuse increase in myocardial signal intensity on T2-weighted sequence, increase in T1-relaxation values on T1-mapping can be seen [84]. Post-contrast studies may reveal late gadolinium enhancement in a mid-myocardial or transmural pattern. Cine steady state free precession (SSFE) sequences will reveal regional or global wall motion abnormalities with reduced ejection fraction [86].

### 2.7 Positron emission tomography/computed tomography (PET-CT)

Although PET-CT is not currently indicated in the management of COVID-19 cases, however, reports of pulmonary findings consistent with COVID-19 have emerged when PET-CT was used for other conditions particularly oncology imaging [87]. The lung opacities of GGO and consolidation demonstrate increased 18-fluorodeoxyglucose (FDG) uptake [88]. Standard uptake values (SUV) of 4.6 to 12.2 have been reported [88]. Increased FDG uptake has also been demonstrated in normal sized mediastinal and hilar nodes in COVID-19. In future, FDG-PET may find use in the monitoring of response to treatment and prediction of recovery as FDG uptake may help determine the degree of residual inflammation [89, 90].

## 3. Conclusion

Pulmonary and extra-pulmonary thoracic organ involvement lies at the heart of COVID-19 disease manifestation. Chest imaging, although not a substitute for microbiological diagnosis of COVID-19, has helped tremendously in understanding the natural course of disease and its management. Imaging supports the diagnosis, helps in triage, detects complications, guides treatment and is useful in monitoring the response to therapy. A varying combination of CXR, CT, LUS, CTPA and MRI performed individually or in different combinations depending on the clinical presentation has played a pivotal role in the management of COVID-19 disease.

## Author details

Arshed Hussain Parry[1]* and Abdul Haseeb Wani[2]

1 Department of Radiodiagnosis, Sher-i-Kashmir Institute of Medical Sciences, Srinagar, Jammu and Kashmir, India

2 Department of Radiodiagnosis, Government Medical College, Srinagar, Jammu and Kashmir, India

*Address all correspondence to: arshedparry@gmail.com

## References

[1] World Health Organization. WHO coronavirus disease (COVID-19) dashboard. https://covid19.who.int/ Accessed 24 November 2020.

[2] Chen Y, Li L. SARS-CoV-2: virus dynamics and host response. The Lancet Infectious Diseases. 2020 Mar 23.

[3] Kong WH, Li Y, Peng MW, Kong DG, Yang XB, Wang L, Liu MQ. SARS-CoV-2 detection in patients with influenza-like illness. Nature Microbiology. 2020 Apr 7:1-4.

[4] Yang Y, Yang M, Shen C, et al. Evaluating the accuracy of different respiratory specimens in the laboratory diagnosis and monitoring the viral shedding of 2019-nCoV infections. 2020. doi:10.1101/2020.02.11.20021493.

[5] Wu A, Peng Y, Huang B, Ding X, Wang X, Niu P, Meng J, Zhu Z, Zhang Z, Wang J, Sheng J. Genome composition and divergence of the novel coronavirus (2019-nCoV) originating in China. Cell host & microbe. 2020 Feb 7.

[6] Guan WJ, Ni ZY, Hu Y, Liang WH, Ou CQ, He JX, Liu L, Shan H, Lei CL, Hui DS, Du B. Clinical characteristics of coronavirus disease 2019 in China. New England journal of medicine. 2020 Apr 30;382(18):1708-1720.

[7] Jin X, Lian JS, Hu JH, Gao J, Zheng L, Zhang YM, Hao SR, Jia HY, Cai H, Zhang XL, Yu GD. Epidemiological, clinical and virological characteristics of 74 cases of coronavirus-infected disease 2019 (COVID-19) with gastrointestinal symptoms. Gut. 2020 Jun 1;69(6):1002-1009.

[8] Mao L, Jin H, Wang M, Hu Y, Chen S, He Q, Chang J, Hong C, Zhou Y, Wang D, Miao X. Neurologic manifestations of hospitalized patients with coronavirus disease 2019 in Wuhan, China. JAMA neurology. 2020 Apr 10.

[9] Parry AH, Wani AH, Yaseen M. Acute mesenteric ischemia in severe coronavirus-19 (COVID-19): possible mechanisms and diagnostic pathway. Academic radiology. 2020 Aug 1;27(8):1190.

[10] Parry AH, Wani AH, Yaseen M. Neurological dysfunction in coronavirus disease-19 (COVID-19). Academic Radiology. 2020 Jun 10.

[11] Shafi AM, Shaikh SA, Shirke MM, Iddawela S, Harky A. Cardiac manifestations in COVID-19 patients—A systematic review. Journal of cardiac surgery. 2020 Aug;35(8):1988-2008.

[12] Parry AH, Wani AH, Yaseen M, Shah NN, Dar KA. Clinicoradiological course in coronavirus disease-19 (COVID-19) patients who are asymptomatic at admission. BJR|Open. 2020 Jul;2:20200033.

[13] Arons MM, Hatfield KM, Reddy SC, Kimball A, James A, Jacobs JR, Taylor J, Spicer K, Bardossy AC, Oakley LP, Tanwar S. Presymptomatic SARS-CoV-2 infections and transmission in a skilled nursing facility. New England Journal of Medicine. 2020 Apr 24.

[14] Bai Y, Yao L, Wei T, Tian F, Jin DY, Chen L, Wang M. Presumed asymptomatic carrier transmission of COVID-19. Jama. 2020 Apr 14;323(14):1406-1407.

[15] Meng H, Xiong R, He R, Lin W, Hao B, Zhang L, Lu Z, Shen X, Fan T, Jiang W, Yang W. CT imaging and clinical course of asymptomatic cases with COVID-19 pneumonia at admission in Wuhan, China. Journal of Infection. 2020 Apr 12.

[16] Qiu J. Covert coronavirus infections could be seeding new outbreaks. Nature. 2020 Mar 20.

[17] Gandhi M, Yokoe DS, Havlir DV. Asymptomatic transmission, the Achilles' heel of current strategies to control COVID-19.

[18] Yang Y, Yang M, Shen C, et al. Evaluating the accuracy of different respiratory specimens in the laboratory diagnosis and monitoring the viral shedding of 2019-nCoV infections. 2020. doi:10.1101/2020.02.11.20021493.

[19] Fang Y, Zhang H, Xie J, Lin M, Ying L, Pang P, Ji W. Sensitivity of chest CT for COVID-19: comparison to RT-PCR. Radiology. 2020 Feb 19:200432.

[20] Allotey J, Stallings E, Bonet M, Yap M, Chatterjee S, Kew T, Debenham L, Llavall AC, Dixit A, Zhou D, Balaji R. Clinical manifestations, risk factors, and maternal and perinatal outcomes of coronavirus disease 2019 in pregnancy: living systematic review and meta-analysis. bmj. 2020 Sep 1;370.

[21] Ozma MA, Maroufi P, Khodadadi E, Köse Ş, Esposito I, Ganbarov K, Dao S, Esposito S, Dal T, Zeinalzadeh E, Kafil HS. Clinical manifestation, diagnosis, prevention and control of SARS-CoV-2 (COVID-19) during the outbreak period. Infez Med. 2020 Jan 1;28(2):153-165.

[22] Luo W, Yu H, Gou J, Li X, Sun Y, Li J, Liu L. Clinical pathology of critical patient with novel coronavirus pneumonia (COVID-19). Preprints. 2020 Mar;2020:2020020407.

[23] Polak SB, Van Gool IC, Cohen D, Jan H, van Paassen J. A systematic review of pathological findings in COVID-19: a pathophysiological timeline and possible mechanisms of disease progression. Modern Pathology. 2020 Nov;33(11):2128-2138.

[24] Bohn MK, Hall A, Sepiashvili L, Jung B, Steele S, Adeli K. Pathophysiology of COVID-19: mechanisms underlying disease severity and progression. Physiology. 2020 Sep 1;35(5):288-301.

[25] Gąsecka A, Borovac JA, Guerreiro RA, Giustozzi M, Parker W, Caldeira D, Chiva-Blanch G. Thrombotic Complications in Patients with COVID-19: Pathophysiological Mechanisms, Diagnosis, and Treatment. Cardiovascular drugs and therapy. 2020 Oct 19:1-5.

[26] Leonard-Lorant I, Delabranche X, Severac F, Helms J, Pauzet C, Collange O, Schneider F, Labani A, Bilbault P, Moliere S, Leyendecker P. Acute pulmonary embolism in COVID-19 patients on CT angiography and relationship to D-dimer levels. Radiology. 2020 Apr 23.

[27] Parry AH, Wani AH. Segmental Pulmonary Vascular Changes in COVID-19 Pneumonia. American Journal of Roentgenology. 2020 May 8:W1-.

[28] Parry AH, Wani AH, Yaseen M, Dar MI. Demystifying pulmonary vascular complications in severe coronavirus disease-19 pneumonia (COVID-19) in the light of clinico-radiologic-pathologic correlation. Thrombosis Research. 2020 Jun 27.

[29] Wichmann D, Sperhake JP, Lütgehetmann M, Steurer S, Edler C, Heinemann A, Heinrich F, Mushumba H, Kniep I, Schröder AS, Burdelski C. Autopsy findings and venous thromboembolism in patients with COVID-19: a prospective cohort study. Annals of internal medicine. 2020 May 6.

[30] Ackermann M, Verleden SE, Kuehnel M, Haverich A, Welte T, Laenger F, Vanstapel A, Werlein C, Stark H, Tzankov A, Li WW. Pulmonary vascular endothelialitis, thrombosis, and angiogenesis in Covid-19. New England Journal of Medicine. 2020 May 21.

[31] Zeng JH, Wu WB, Qu JX, Wang Y, Dong CF, Luo YF, Zhou D, Feng WX, Feng C. Cardiac manifestations of COVID-19 in Shenzhen, China. Infection. 2020 Dec;48(6): 861-870.

[32] Kochi AN, Tagliari AP, Forleo GB, Fassini GM, Tondo C. Cardiac and arrhythmic complications in patients with COVID-19. Journal of Cardiovascular Electrophysiology. 2020 May;31(5):1003-1008.

[33] Bandyopadhyay D, Akhtar T, Hajra A, Gupta M, Das A, Chakraborty S, Pal I, Patel N, Amgai B, Ghosh RK, Fonarow GC. COVID-19 pandemic: cardiovascular complications and future implications. American Journal of Cardiovascular Drugs. 2020 Jun 23:1-4.

[34] Gavriatopoulou M, Korompoki E, Fotiou D, Ntanasis-Stathopoulos I, Psaltopoulou T, Kastritis E, Terpos E, Dimopoulos MA. Organ-specific manifestations of COVID-19 infection. Clinical and experimental medicine. 2020 Jul 27:1-4.

[35] Toussie D, Voutsinas N, Finkelstein M, Cedillo MA, Manna S, Maron SZ, Jacobi A, Chung M, Bernheim A, Eber C, Concepcion J. Clinical and chest radiography features determine patient outcomes in young and middle age adults with COVID-19. Radiology. 2020 May 14:201754.

[36] Cleverley J, Piper J, Jones MM. The role of chest radiography in confirming covid-19 pneumonia. bmj. 2020 Jul 16;370.

[37] Hui TC, Khoo HW, Young BE, Mohideen SM, Lee YS, Lim CJ, Leo YS, Kaw GJ, Lye DC, Tan CH. Clinical utility of chest radiography for severe COVID-19. Quantitative imaging in medicine and surgery. 2020 Jul;10(7):1540.

[38] Jacobi A, Chung M, Bernheim A, Eber C. Portable chest X-ray in coronavirus disease-19 (COVID-19): A pictorial review. Clinical Imaging. 2020 Apr 8.

[39] Hui TC, Khoo HW, Young BE, Mohideen SM, Lee YS, Lim CJ, Leo YS, Kaw GJ, Lye DC, Tan CH. Clinical utility of chest radiography for severe COVID-19. Quantitative imaging in medicine and surgery. 2020 Jul;10(7):1540.

[40] Wong HY, Lam HY, Fong AH, Leung ST, Chin TW, Lo CS, Lui MM, Lee JC, Chiu KW, Chung T, Lee EY. Frequency and distribution of chest radiographic findings in COVID-19 positive patients. Radiology. 2020 Mar 27:201160.

[41] Zhang R, Tie X, Qi Z, Bevins NB, Zhang C, Griner D, Song TK, Nadig JD, Schiebler ML, Garrett JW, Li K. Diagnosis of covid-19 pneumonia using chest radiography: Value of artificial intelligence. Radiology. 2020 Sep 24:202944.

[42] Wang L, Lin ZQ, Wong A. Covid-net: A tailored deep convolutional neural network design for detection of covid-19 cases from chest x-ray images. Scientific Reports. 2020 Nov 11;10(1):1-2.

[43] Zhang R, Tie X, Qi Z, Bevins NB, Zhang C, Griner D, Song TK, Nadig JD, Schiebler ML, Garrett JW, Li K. Diagnosis of covid-19 pneumonia using chest radiography: Value of artificial intelligence. Radiology. 2020 Sep 24:202944.

[44] Narin A, Kaya C, Pamuk Z. Automatic detection of coronavirus

disease (covid-19) using x-ray images and deep convolutional neural networks. arXiv preprint arXiv:2003.10849. 2020 Mar 24.

[45] Cleverley J, Piper J, Jones MM. The role of chest radiography in confirming covid-19 pneumonia. bmj. 2020 Jul 16;370.

[46] Denina M, Scolfaro C, Silvestro E, Pruccoli G, Mignone F, Zoppo M, Ramenghi U, Garazzino S. Lung ultrasound in children with COVID-19. Pediatrics. 2020 Jul 1;146(1).

[47] Soldati G, Smargiassi A, Inchingolo R, Buonsenso D, Perrone T, Briganti DF, Perlini S, Torri E, Mariani A, Mossolani EE, Tursi F. Is there a role for lung ultrasound during the COVID-19 pandemic?. Journal of Ultrasound in Medicine. 2020 Mar 20.

[48] Soldati G, Smargiassi A, Inchingolo R, Buonsenso D, Perrone T, Briganti DF, Perlini S, Torri E, Mariani A, Mossolani EE, Tursi F. Proposal for international standardization of the use of lung ultrasound for COVID-19 patients; a simple, quantitative, reproducible method. J ultrasound Med. 2020 Mar 30;10.

[49] Nouvenne A, Zani MD, Milanese G, Parise A, Baciarello M, Bignami EG, Odone A, Sverzellati N, Meschi T, Ticinesi A. Lung ultrasound in COVID-19 pneumonia: Correlations with chest CT on hospital admission. Respiration. 2020;99(7):617-624.

[50] Smith MJ, Hayward SA, Innes SM, Miller AS. Point-of-care lung ultrasound in patients with COVID-19–a narrative review. Anaesthesia. 2020 Apr 10.

[51] Buonsenso D, Pata D, Chiaretti A. COVID-19 outbreak: less stethoscope, more ultrasound. The Lancet Respiratory Medicine. 2020 May 1;8(5):e27.

[52] Parry AH, Wani AH. Pulmonary embolism in coronavirus disease-19 (COVID-19) and use of compression ultrasonography in its optimal management. Thrombosis Research. 2020 May 16.

[53] Vrettou AR, Parissis J, Ikonomidis I. The Dual Role of Echocardiography in the Diagnosis of Acute Cardiac Complications and Treatment Monitoring for Coronavirus Disease 2019 (COVID-19). Frontiers in cardiovascular medicine. 2020;7.

[54] Zhang L, Wang B, Zhou J, Kirkpatrick J, Xie M, Johri AM. Bedside Focused Cardiac Ultrasound in COVID-19 from the Wuhan Epicenter: The Role of Cardiac Point-of-Care Ultrasound, Limited Transthoracic Echocardiography, and Critical Care Echocardiography. Journal of the American Society of Echocardiography. 2020 Jun 1;33(6):676-682.

[55] Dandel M. Cardiac manifestations of COVID-19 infection: the role of echocardiography in patient management. Infection. 2020 Aug 24:1-3.

[56] Zoghbi WA, DiCarli MF, Blankstein R, Choi AD, Dilsizian V, Flachskampf FA, Geske JB, Grayburn PA, Jaffer FA, Kwong RY, Leipsic JA. Multimodality cardiovascular imaging in the midst of the COVID-19 pandemic: ramping up safely to a new normal. JACC: Cardiovascular Imaging. 2020 Jul 1;13(7):1615-1626.

[57] Revel MP, Parkar AP, Prosch H, Silva M, Sverzellati N, Gleeson F, Brady A, European Society of Radiology (ESR). COVID-19 patients and the Radiology department–advice from the European Society of Radiology (ESR) and the European Society of Thoracic Imaging (ESTI). European Radiology. 2020 Apr 20:1.

[58] Yu M, Xu D, Lan L, Tu M, Liao R, Cai S, Cao Y, Xu L, Liao M, Zhang X, Xiao SY. Thin-section Chest CT Imaging of Coronavirus Disease 2019 Pneumonia: Comparison Between Patients with Mild and Severe Disease. Radiology: Cardiothoracic Imaging. 2020 Apr 23;2(2):e200126.

[59] Yang R, Gui X, Xiong Y. Comparison of clinical characteristics of patients with asymptomatic vs symptomatic coronavirus disease 2019 in Wuhan, China. JAMA Network Open. 2020 May 1;3(5):e2010182-.

[60] Salehi S, Abedi A, Balakrishnan S, Gholamrezanezhad A. Coronavirus disease 2019 (COVID-19): a systematic review of imaging findings in 919 patients. American Journal of Roentgenology. 2020 Mar 14:1-7.

[61] Parry AH, Wani AH, Yaseen M, Dar KA, Choh NA, Khan NA, Shah NN, Jehangir M. Spectrum of chest computed tomographic (CT) findings in coronavirus disease-19 (COVID-19) patients in India. European Journal of Radiology. 2020 Aug 1;129:109147.

[62] Zhu J, Zhong Z, Li H, Ji P, Pang J, Li B, Zhang J. CT imaging features of 4121 patients with COVID-19: A meta-analysis. Journal of Medical Virology. 2020 Jul;92(7):891-902.

[63] Wang Y, Dong C, Hu Y, Li C, Ren Q, Zhang X, Shi H, Zhou M. Temporal changes of CT findings in 90 patients with COVID-19 pneumonia: a longitudinal study. Radiology. 2020 Mar 19:200843.

[64] Parry AH, Wani AH, Shah NN, Yaseen M, Jehangir M. Chest CT features of coronavirus disease-19 (COVID-19) pneumonia: which findings on initial CT can predict an adverse short-term outcome?. BJR|Open. 2020 Jun;2:20200016.

[65] Middleton EA, He XY, Denorme F, Campbell RA, Ng D, Salvatore SP, Mostyka M, Baxter-Stoltzfus A, Borczuk AC, Loda M, Cody MJ. Neutrophil extracellular traps contribute to immunothrombosis in COVID-19 acute respiratory distress syndrome. Blood, The Journal of the American Society of Hematology. 2020 Sep 3;136(10):1169-1179.

[66] Nicolai L, Leunig A, Brambs S, Kaiser R, Weinberger T, Weigand M, Muenchhoff M, Hellmuth JC, Ledderose S, Schulz H, Scherer C. Immunothrombotic dysregulation in COVID-19 pneumonia is associated with respiratory failure and coagulopathy. Circulation. 2020 Sep 22;142(12):1176-1189.

[67] Nakazawa D, Ishizu A. Immunothrombosis in severe COVID-19. EBioMedicine. 2020 Sep 1;59.

[68] Fang Y, Zhang H, Xie J, Lin M, Ying L, Pang P, Ji W. Sensitivity of chest CT for COVID-19: comparison to RT-PCR. Radiology. 2020 Feb 19:200432.

[69] Long C, Xu H, Shen Q, Zhang X, Fan B, Wang C, Zeng B, Li Z, Li X, Li H. Diagnosis of the Coronavirus disease (COVID-19): rRT-PCR or CT?. European journal of radiology. 2020 Mar 25:108961.

[70] Raptis CA, Hammer MM, Short RG, Shah A, Bhalla S, Bierhals AJ, Filev PD, Hope MD, Jeudy J, Kligerman SJ, Henry TS. Chest CT and coronavirus disease (COVID-19): a critical review of the literature to date. American Journal of Roentgenology. 2020 Mar 26:1-4.

[71] Yang R, Li X, Liu H, Zhen Y, Zhang X, Xiong Q, Luo Y, Gao C, Zeng W. Chest CT severity score: an imaging tool for assessing severe COVID-19. Radiology: Cardiothoracic Imaging. 2020 Mar 30;2(2):e200047.

[72] Lessmann N, Sánchez CI, Beenen L, Boulogne LH, Brink M, Calli E, Charbonnier JP, Dofferhoff T, van Everdingen WM, Gerke PK, Geurts B. Automated assessment of CO-RADS and chest CT severity scores in patients with suspected COVID-19 using artificial intelligence. Radiology. 2020 Jul 30:202439.

[73] Inui S, Fujikawa A, Jitsu M, Kunishima N, Watanabe S, Suzuki Y, Umeda S, Uwabe Y. Chest CT findings in cases from the cruise ship "Diamond Princess" with coronavirus disease 2019 (COVID-19). Radiology. Cardiothoracic Imaging. 2020 Mar 17;2(2).

[74] Li K, Wu J, Wu F, Guo D, Chen L, Fang Z, Li C. The clinical and chest CT features associated with severe and critical COVID-19 pneumonia. Investigative radiology. 2020.

[75] Prokop M, van Everdingen W, van Rees Vellinga T, Quarles van Ufford J, Stöger L, Beenen L, Geurts B, Gietema H, Krdzalic J, Schaefer-Prokop C, van Ginneken B. CO-RADS–A categorical CT assessment scheme for patients with suspected COVID-19: definition and evaluation. Radiology. 2020 Apr 27:201473.

[76] Fujioka T, Takahashi M, Mori M, Tsuchiya J, Yamaga E, Horii T, Yamada H, Kimura M, Kimura K, Kitazume Y, Kishino M. Evaluation of the usefulness of CO-RADS for chest CT in patients suspected of having COVID-19. Diagnostics. 2020 Sep;10(9):608.

[77] Xie Y, Wang X, Yang P, Zhang S. COVID-19 complicated by acute pulmonary embolism. Radiology: Cardiothoracic Imaging. 2020 Mar 16;2(2):e200067.

[78] Rotzinger DC, Beigelman-Aubry C, Von Garnier C, Qanadli S. Pulmonary embolism in patients with COVID-19: time to change the paradigm of computed tomography. Thrombosis research. 2020 Jun 1;190:58-59.

[79] Leonard-Lorant I, Delabranche X, Severac F, Helms J, Pauzet C, Collange O, Schneider F, Labani A, Bilbault P, Moliere S, Leyendecker P. Acute pulmonary embolism in COVID-19 patients on CT angiography and relationship to D-dimer levels. Radiology. 2020 Apr 23.

[80] Jalaber C, Revel MP, Chassagnon G, Bajeux E, Lapotre T, Croisille P, Lederlin M. Role of upfront CT pulmonary angiography at admission in COVID-19 patients. Thrombosis Research. 2020 Dec 1;196:138-140.

[81] Parry AH, Wani AH, Yaseen M. Pulmonary embolism in coronavirus disease-19 (COVID-19): rational and stepwise use of clinical data and imaging in its diagnosis. Clinical and Translational Imaging. 2020 Oct;8(5):299-301.

[82] Oudkerk M, Kuijpers D, Oudkerk SF, van Beek EJ. The vascular nature of COVID-19. The British journal of radiology. 2020 Sep 1;93(1113): 20200718.

[83] Patel BV, Arachchillage DJ, Ridge CA, Bianchi P, Doyle JF, Garfield B, Ledot S, Morgan C, Passariello M, Price S, Singh S. Pulmonary angiopathy in severe COVID-19: physiologic, imaging, and hematologic observations. American Journal of Respiratory and Critical Care Medicine. 2020 Sep 1;202(5):690-699.

[84] Inciardi RM, Lupi L, Zaccone G, Italia L, Raffo M, Tomasoni D, Cani DS, Cerini M, Farina D, Gavazzi E, Maroldi R. Cardiac involvement in a patient with coronavirus disease 2019 (COVID-19). JAMA cardiology. 2020 Mar 27.

[85] Hameed S, Elbaaly H, Reid CE, Santos RM, Shivamurthy V, Wong J,

Jogeesvaran KH. Spectrum of imaging findings on chest radiographs, US, CT, and MRI images in multisystem inflammatory syndrome in children (MIS-C) associated with COVID-19. Radiology. 2020 Jun 25:202543.

[86] Rudski L, Januzzi JL, Rigolin VH, Bohula EA, Blankstein R, Patel AR, Bucciarelli-Ducci C, Vorovich E, Mukherjee M, Rao SV, Beanlands R. Multimodality Imaging in Evaluation of Cardiovascular complications in Patients with COVID-19. Journal of the American College of Cardiology. 2020 Jul 22.

[87] Zou S, Zhu X. FDG PET/CT of COVID-19. Radiology. 2020 Mar 6:200770.

[88] Deng Y, Lei L, Chen Y, Zhang W. The potential added value of FDG PET/CT for COVID-19 pneumonia. European Journal of Nuclear Medicine and Molecular Imaging. 2020 Mar 21:1-2.

[89] Joob B, Wiwanitkit V. 18F-FDG PET/CT and COVID-19. European Journal of Nuclear Medicine and Molecular Imaging. 2020 Mar 12:1-.

[90] Parry AH, Wani HA, Choh NA, Shah NN, Jehangir M. Spectrum of chest CT manifestations of coronavirus disease (COVID-19): a pictorial essay. The Indian Journal of Radiology & Imaging. 2021 Jan;31(Suppl 1):S170.

Chapter 7

# COVID-19 and Cardiovascular Disease: Mechanisms and Implications

*Irena Mitevska*


## Abstract

We are living and fighting serious COVID-19 pandemic, which is caused by the severe acute respiratory syndrome coronavirus-2 (SARS-CoV-2) virus. Cardiovascular diseases are highly prevalent in the infected individuals, which modifies their treatment and prognosis. The injury of the myocardium is reported in over 15% of hospitalized severely ill patients, mostly presented in the form of acute heart failure, acute coronary syndrome, cardiac arrythmias, myocarditis and thromboembolic complications. All these complications may appear at early in the course of the disease, during the disease progress or in the later stage of the COVID-19 disease. Thromboembolic complications accompany more severe cases, caused by excessive inflammation, platelet activation, endothelial dysfunction, and stasis. This new virus pandemic is a global challenge for health care system where we still have much to learn.


**Keywords:** COVID-19, pandemic, myocardial injury, cardiovascular disease

## 1. Introduction

The COVID-19 pandemic has opened up many serious challenges to the world. The pandemic has put enormous pressure on healthcare systems worldwide. There are many unknown puzzles the virus imposes to us as medical professionals. Most data we have come from China, Italy, France and USA and management is guided by the expert opinion. While COVID-19 primarily affects the lungs, causing interstitial pneumonitis and severe acute respiratory distress syndrome (ARDS), it can also affect multiple organs, particularly cardiovascular system. Mortality and complications risk is increased by the presence of several comorbidities: cardiovascular disease, hypertension, diabetes, obesity, chronic pulmonary disease, and cancer [1]. Cardiovascular system in COVID-19 infection is affected in up to 15% of severely ill patients on multiple levels, which leads to increased morbidity but also it might induce myocardial injury leading to myocardial dysfunction [2]. The most common complications include arrhythmia (atrial fibrillation, ventricular tachyarrhythmia, and ventricular fibrillation), cardiac injury (elevated highly sensitive troponin I (hs-TnI) and creatine kinase (CK) levels, NT pro-BNP levels), fulminant myocarditis, heart failure, pulmonary embolism, and disseminated intravascular coagulation (DIC) [3].

Patients with established heart disease constitute a particularly challenging group, with conditions that may be life-threatening if proper treatment or intervention is inadequately delayed, which is the base for increased complications risk and worsened disease prognosis. COVID-19 case fatality rate is significantly different around the world. Patients with several comorbidities have significantly increased case fatality rate (CFR): 10.5% for cardiovascular disease (CVD); 7.3% for diabetes mellitus; 6.3% for chronic obstructive pulmonary disease (COPD); around 6% for hypertension patients with cancer [4]. The mortality rates are different in different world regions and are influenced by several technical and quality measures of the healthcare systems, number of tests performed, demographic characteristics of the tested population and their health status. These aspects underline the importance of the need for multidisciplinary assessment and treatment, including cardiovascular evaluation and therapy aimed to reduce the COVID-19 mortality.

## 2. COVID-19 and cardiovascular system

Published data about disease manifestation and progression showed that patients with established cardiovascular disease are among the highest risk individuals for severe manifestation of COVID 19 and death. In a series of 44 672 confirmed patients with COVID-19 from China, 14.2% were reported to have cardiovascular disease, but also 22,7% of all deaths were in patients with underlying cardiovascular disease [5, 6]. The presence of common risk factors, such as hypertension, diabetes, coronary artery disease (CAD) increase the risk for COVID-19 induced complications as shown in **Figure 1**. It is of greater concern and importance the fact that COVID-19 can lead to cardiac injury even in individual not reporting previous cardiovascular disease. There is a need for proper understanding of the pathophysiological mechanisms of the cardiovascular damage caused by COVID-19 disease. This will enable on time effective patient's management and mortality reduction. The affection of the cardiovascular system by the infection is followed by release of inflammatory markers such as highly sensitive troponin and natriuretic peptides, which modifies prognosis, particularly in patients with continuous rise of those markers [7]. Cytokines such as IL-6 causes inflammation of the vascular system that result in generalized endotheliopathy and immune induced thrombosis. Inflammation in the myocardium can lead to myocarditis, heart failure, cardiac arrhythmias, and sudden death [7, 8]. Down-regulation of ACE2 with viral infection may predispose to relatively unopposed angiotensin II effects, which and cause new or worsened hypertension. After infection with common RNA viruses, most infected patients may experience only a transient viral syndrome with no significant cardiac dysfunction. However, depending on the immune response it can manifest as acute myocarditis with heart failure or cardiogenic shock, accompanied by cytokine storm and inflammatory cell infiltration of the heart. With proper treatment some patients can recover, but others can develop inflammatory cardiomyopathy [9].

A place of the initial *SARS-CoV-2* virus entrance to our organism is virus attachment to the angiotensin converting-enzyme 2 (ACE-2) membrane-linked aminopeptidase receptor on the epithelial cells of the lungs. However, these receptors are expressed in many human organs including myocardium making them vulnerable to the virus [10]. The studies showed higher expression of ACE-2 receptors in diabetic and hypertensive patients, which might be one of the causes of more severe forms of the disease in those individuals. While ACE2 is essential for viral invasion, there is no evidence that ACE inhibitors or angiotensin receptor blockers (ARBs) worsen prognosis. Hence, patients should not discontinue their use, based on recommendations for COVID-19 and cardiovascular disease treatment from several cardiology associations. Moreover, renin–angiotensin–aldosterone system (RAAS) inhibitors might be beneficial in COVID-19 [10]. Initial immune and inflammatory

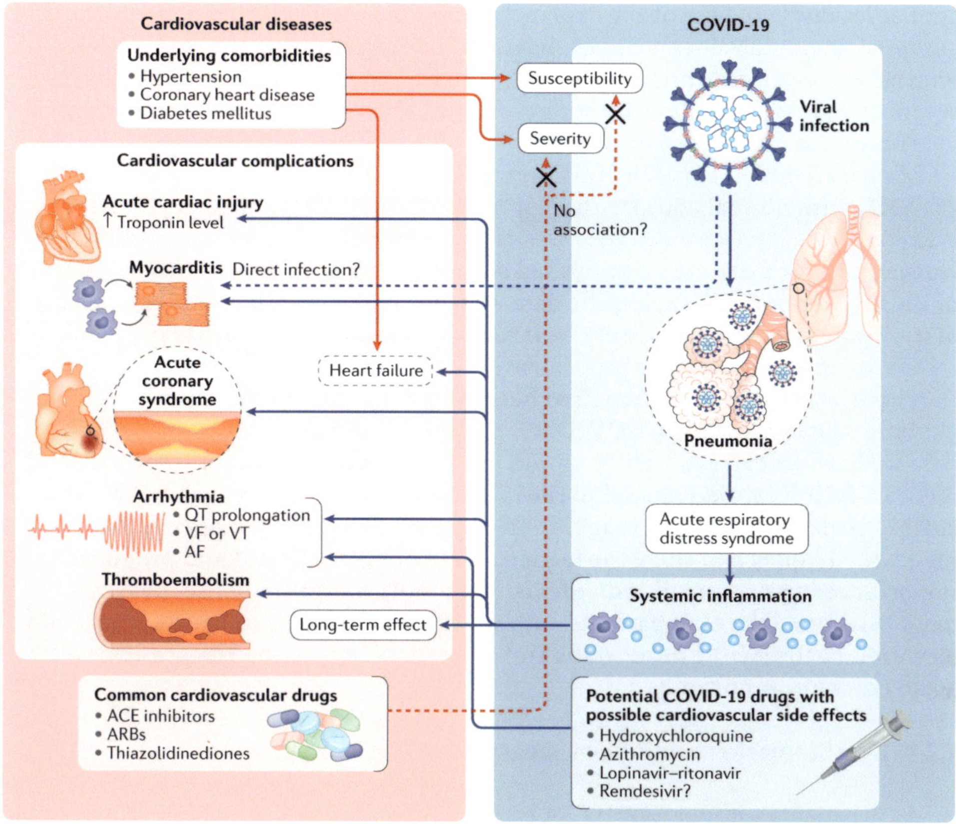


**Figure 1.**
*In COVID-19 disease patients' cardiovascular comorbidities are the cause of the increased mortality. Angiotensin-converting enzyme (ACE) inhibitors and angiotensin II receptor blockers (ARBs) which are established drugs for reduction of the cardiovascular risk have many positive effects that might modify the course of the COVID-19 disease. Nature Reviews Cardiology volume 17, pages 543–558(2020), ref. [7].*

responses induce a severe cytokine storm during the rapid progression phase of COVID-19. Early evaluation and continued monitoring of cardiac damage using the values of high sensitive cardiac troponin I (hs-cTn I), N-terminal *pro* b-type natriuretic peptide (NT-proBNP) and coagulation (D-dimer) after hospitalizationmay identify patients with cardiac injury and predict COVID-19 complications [11]. Severe inflammation is assumed as a cause of underlying generalized endothelial disfunction (endotheliopathy), which serves as a basis for development of microvascular thrombosis.

## 2.1 Cardiac injury caused by COVID-19 infection

The data from published studies showed that patients with myocardial injury (elevated cardiac troponin), have up to three times higher hospital mortality [12]. Increased hospital values of the high-sensitivity cardiac troponin I are found in over 50% of fatal COVID-19 disease cases. Elevation of the troponin values parallel the elevation of N-terminal pro-B-type natriuretic peptide and C-reactive protein and markers of cardiac injury and inflammation. Data showing the rise of the troponin in the same time with other inflammatory biomarkers (D-dimer, ferritin, interleukin-6 (IL-6), lactate dehydrogenase), lead to conclusion that isolated myocardial injury mediated through ACE-2 is not the only mechanism of COVID-19 induced cardiac lesions [13]. One of the explanations is the presence of cytokine storm. The curves of troponin values changes show slow elevation during the first 2 weeks, with steep elevation during the third week in severely and critical ill patients with severe disease forms. Follow up studies showed that hs- Troponin I value in survivors have no significant changes [14].

Many patients' cases with of ST segment elevation myocardial infarctions (STEMI) with normal coronary angiography findings are published [15] which is explained as injury caused by stress cardiomyopathy or acute myocarditis. However, so far there are no published data of the signs of direct virus infiltration of the myocardium. The scientific data we have indicates inflammation as a cause of multi-organ damage, not only myocardial damage. Use of cardiac magnetic resonance imaging may give more answers to these questions.

There are evidences of impaired heart function due to myocardial injury in patients who recover from COVID-19, mostly due to myocarditis. Based on all data we have we can evaluate troponin levels as markers on disease severity and myocardial injury, also related to the underlying mechanisms such as cytokine storm, tissue hypoxia, and coagulation disturbances [16]. Management of the myocardial injury and their consequences are of great clinical and prognostic importance in critically ill individuals. We should not initially use invasive diagnostic procedures in patients with COVID-19 disease and isolated troponin elevation in absence of other signs and symptoms suggesting the presence of acute coronary syndrome.

### 2.2 Which biomarkers should we measure?

As in patients without COVID-19, cardiac troponin T and troponin I values should be measured based on clinical presentations when T1 type myocardial infarction (MI) is suspected [17]. Normal high -sensitive cardiac troponin values depend on gender and essay analyses used. Diagnostic algorithms for rapid rule out and/or rule-in of MI in patients with acute chest discomfort such as the high-sensitivity cardiac troponin (hs-cTn) T or I 0/1 hour algorithm is expected to provide comparable performance and add to diagnosis in other challenging subgroups with higher baseline concentrations such patients with renal dysfunction: very high safety for rule-out and high accuracy for rule-in, but reduced efficacy with a higher percentage of patients remaining in the observe zone [17, 18]. Clinical assessment including chest pain characteristics, hs-cTn T or I measurement at 3 hours, and cardiac imaging using echocardiography are the key elements for the identification of STEMI in the setting of COVID-19 infection. Hs-cTn I should be measured in patients with confirmed pulmonary embolism, as a marker for risk stratification and prognosis [19].

Similarly, B-type natriuretic peptide (BNP) and NT-proBNP should be measured whenever clinically heart failure is suspected [19]. Rule-in cut-offs for heart failure (HF) maintain high positive predictive value even in patients with pneumonia, who are not critically ill. Having in mind that most of the critical ill patients have significantly higher BNP/NT-proBNP values, it is therefore not recommended to use current cut-off values applied for heart failure patients. Increased BNP/NT-proBNP levels in severely ill patients with COVID-19 disease are explained by the presence of hemodynamic stress and myocardial injury leading to heart failure [20]. Cardiac injury, as assessed by several serum analysis parameters (lactate dehydrogenase, cardiac troponin I, creatine kinase (-MB) and myoglobin), were associated with poor prognosis in COVID-19 infection, assessed in. the retrospective multicenter study from Xie and coworkers, as shown in **Figure 2** [21].

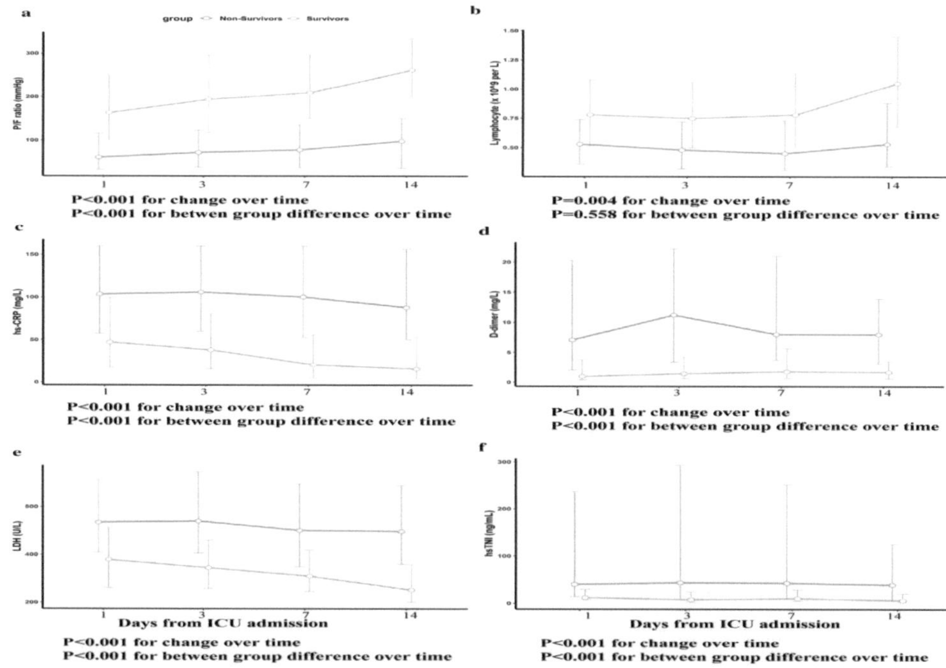


**Figure 2.**
*Dynamic changes in laboratory markers of severely ill patients with COVID-19 disease hospitalized in the intensive care units (ICU). The figure describes changes in the arterial pO2 ("P") from the ABG divided by the FIO2 ("F") (P/F ratio) which includes the values of lymphocytes, high sensitive C reactive protein (hs-CRP), D-dimer, lactate dehydrogenase (LDH) and high sensitive troponin I (hs-troponin I) (a-f). At all-time points shown, there were significant differences between survivors and non-survivors. Intensive care medicine volume 46, pages1863–187, 2020 (ref [21].*

## 2.3 COVID-19 and Heart failure

COVID-19 infection might present as new or worsened previously established heart failure. It is a challenge for every physician to make differential diagnoses between decompensated heart failure (HF), often complicated with pulmonary infection and COVID-19 infection, prior to laboratory-confirmation. There are significant similarities between chest computer tomography (CT) findings of the patients with heart failure and those with COVID-19 disease. Higher ratios of central ground glass opacity are found in patients with heart failure, comparing to the more peripheral gradient distribution in patients with COVID-19 infection [22].

Scientific data reports up to 25% of case fatality rate in patients with extreme elevation of NTproBNP levels caused by heart failure and cardiac arrest [23]. In a large cohort from China, heart failure was reported in 23% of infected patients and the prevalence was significantly higher among non-survivors (52% vs. 12%, $p < 0.0001$) [23].

From the evidences we have so far, patients with previous heart failure will have more complicated pulmonary disease and COVID-19 infection course. Acute heart failure and myocarditis might be one of the clinical presentations of COVID-19 disease. Some of the explanations of the underlying mechanisms of the heart dysfunction are initial structural changes in the early stage of the disease with preserved left ejection fraction in parallel with pulmonary complications and the development of acute heart failure with reduction of systolic function in the later stage of the disease as a response to cytokine storm.

Heart failure has been reported as an outcome in 23% of COVID subjects in a recent report from in-hospital Chinese subjects. Approximately 52% of non-survivors had heart failure as compared with 12% of survivors [24, 25] Mechanisms underlying myocardial injury remain unknown and it is unclear whether they reflect systemic, local, ischemic or inflammatory process. It is still not known whether acute injury is a primary infective phenomenon or secondary to lung disease.

Elderly patients with heart failure may have left ventricular hypertrophy, diastolic dysfunction or systolic dysfunction and are prone to higher pulmonary vascular pressure in case of overload with fluid infusions and administration of parenteral therapy. Myocardial injury is observed in more than 20% of hospitalized patients with COVID-19 [26]. Increased levels of brain natriuretic peptide or N-terminal pro brain natriuretic peptide may be found in COVID-19 patients and may suggest concomitant impairment of cardiac function and poorer clinical course. Patients with elevated troponin levels have higher rates of major complications, including cardiac arrhythmias, acute kidney injury, ARDS, need for mechanical ventilation, and death [26].

Most patients with heart failure have elevated C-reactive protein, erythrocyte sedimentation rate and other indexes of inflammation and thrombogenicity, such as ferritin, interleukin-6, lactate dehydrogenase, fibrinogen, and D-dimer. An increase in these markersis associated with high mortality [27]. All these markers are higher with continuing increase during the hospitalization in high risk patients who do not survive the disease. Contrary in lower risk stable patients who survive all these parameters remains stable and relatively low. Procalcitonin must be measured when bacterial superinfection is suspected. Echocardiography must be considered in all patients with HF and suspected or confirmed COVID-19 infection to assess cardiac function and to detect concomitant causes of HF, either pre-existing or COVID-19-related (e.g. right ventricular dysfunction secondary to pulmonary embolism). Treatment of heart failure patients should be based on the latest guidelines from several cardiology societies [17, 28].

## 2.4 COVID-19 and Coronary artery disease

Patients with coronary artery disease, stabile or unstable, are prone to complications during COVID-19 infection, due to coronary plaque rupture or stent-thrombosis secondary to pro-coagulant effects of systemic inflammation [28]. Around 6% of patients with severe COVID-19 disease report the history of previous coronary artery disease (CAD), comparing with 1.8% prevalence of CAD in patients with non-severe disease forms [18].

It is important to underline that many individuals with COVID-19 disease initially presents with chest pain, palpitation and dyspnea instead of cough, fever and other related respiratory symptoms. Normal coronary angiography in patients presenting with chest pain and suspected acute coronary syndrome, should raise the first suspicion of infection with COVID-19. However, elevated troponin during COVID-19 infection, if followed by typical symptoms and signs of myocardial infarction should lead to guideline-directed interventions, fibrinolysis, or coronary angioplasty in designated hospitals [18, 28]. There are evidences of high expression of angiotensin II receptors in the heart muscle [29]. These findings explain the SARS-CoV-2 infection repercussion on the myocardium in the form of locally induced microvascular inflammation and dysfunction leading to myocardial infarction without the obstruction of the coronary arteries (MINOCA). All these pathophysiological mechanisms could explain the scientific data we have obtained concerning the clinical course of patients presenting with myocardial infarction signs during the COVID-19 disease [30]. Additionally, cytokine storm significantly contributes for the development of the endotheliopathy through well described mechanisms. The global finding during the COVID-19 pandemic is significant reduction of number of acute myocardial infarction by 30–50%, mostly due to fear for on time search of medical help [31]. The late patient's presentation leads to significant increase of acute myocardial infarction complications, especially heart failure.

Several pathways associated with viral diseases may contribute to destabilize plaques in COVID-19 patients [32]. Viral illness can potentially destabilize atherosclerotic plaques through systemic inflammatory responses, cytokine storm, as well as specific changes of immune cell polarization towards more unstable phenotypes. In patients with viral infections, type 2 myocardial infarction is the most common subtype, were the usefulness of invasive treatment with coronary revascularization is limited.

In patients with acute coronary syndrome (ACS) and COVID-19 disease the final treatment decision weather invasive or medical management is applied should be carefully considered. Primary percutaneous coronary intervention (PCI) is the standard treatment for patients presenting to PCI centers within 90 minutes of first medical contact [28, 33]. It is important to underline that all patients presenting with a suspected STEMI should be considered COVID-19 possible. Testing for SARS-CoV-2 should be performed as soon as possible following first medical contact, irrespective of treatment strategy, in order to allow to implement adequate protective measures and management pathways [28]. Some of these patients may have a "STEMI-mimicker" such as focal myocarditis or stress cardiomyopathy known to be associated with COVID-19 illness.

Treatment of patients with non-ST segment elevation myocardial infarction non-STEMI should be guided by risk stratification. Patients with Troponin rise and no acute clinical signs of instability (ECG changes, recurrence of pain) might be managed with a primarily conservative approach. For patients at high risk, medical strategy aims at stabilization whilst planning an early (< 24 hours) invasive strategy.

The use of timely reperfusion in STEMI patients should not be compromised by the COVID-19 pandemic. Based on the recommendations from the latest guidelines of the European Society of Cardiology (ESC), reperfusion therapy is indicated in STEMI patients with ischemia symptoms in duration <12 hours and persistent ST segment elevation in at least 2 ECG leads, and these recommendations remain the same for COVID -19 disease patients with STEMI. The maximum delay from STEMI diagnosis to reperfusion of 120 minutes should remain the goal for reperfusion therapy with primary PCI when feasible within this time frame and performed in facilities approved for the treatment of COVID-19 patients [28]. If primary PCI performing hospital is no not available or target time cannot be met and fibrinolysis is not contraindicated, fibrinolysis should then become first line therapy [28, 34].

### 2.5 COVID-19 and myocarditis

Injury of the myocardium and acute myocardial inflammation are well documented complications of acute viral infections. One of the underlying mechanisms of the injury, obtained from the cardiac muscle autopsy specimens are myocytes necrosis with mononuclear cell infiltrates [35]. These findings together with the cases of fulminant myocarditis, lead as to conclude that myocarditis is an important cause of acute myocardial injury in patients with COVID-19 disease. However, the true prevalence, the exact mechanisms and clinical significance of acute myocarditis in COVID-19 patients still remains unclear. We do not have solid evidence of direct myocardial cytotoxic effects of the virus. The real prevalence of this complication still remains unclear. Myocarditis appears in COVID-19 patients after a prolonged period up to two weeks after the symptom's onset.

Clinically, COVID-19 myocarditis may manifest only as mild chest discomfort, palpitation and fatigue, which may be impossible to distinguish from other causes in most patients. In some patients, myocarditis results in fulminant disease, which may be the cause of arrhythmias, conduction block, myocardial dysfunction or even death. In many cases myocarditis is suspected when cardiac injury is present in the absence of ACS [36]. Acute myocarditis diagnosis can be confirmed by the presence of typical acute myocardial injury signals detected by cardiac magnetic resonance imaging (MRI). However Cardiac MRI and EMBs as diagnostic tools are likely to be inappropriate during the current COVID-19 pandemic but should be considered in the later phase to confirm diagnosis.

This cardiac injury in COVID 19 infected patients leads to activation of the innate immune response with release of proinflammatory cytokines. Proteins released through cell lysis might display epitopes similar to the viral antigens and be presented via the major histocompatibility complex [37]. An acquired immune response is the predominant mechanism evidenced by activation of antibodies and T lymphocytes. In the final stage, there is either recovery or low levels of chronic inflammation with concomitant development of left ventricular dysfunction. The most important question for potential therapeutic targets is the extent to which myocardial injury results from viral replication, is immune mediated, or is due to other mechanisms. Patients that develop heart failure have poor prognosis and should be treated based on heart failure guidelines [28]. Clinical follow up, with biomarkers and echocardiography are important for patient's treatment and prognosis [38].

### 2.6 Arrhythmias and sudden cardiac death

In-hospital and out-of-hospital sudden cardiac arrests have also been reported in patients with COVID-19 [39]. The contribution of COVID-19 disease for induction of cardiac arrhythmias remains uncertain, having in mind that atrial and ventricular arrhythmias can also be triggered by myocardial injury, other infections, fever, sepsis, hypoxia and electrolyte abnormalities. Arrhythmias can be induced by concomitant antiviral and antibiotic therapy used in patients with COVID-19 disease. Increase heart rate is reported as one of the main symptom in COVID-19 disease patients without other symptoms such as fever or caught. The presence of cardiac arrhythmias was reported in 17% of patient from the cohort of 138 COVID-19 cases in the study from Wuhan, China, and 44% of them were hospitalized in the ICU units [39]. Another study from Wuhan which includes 187 hospitalized COVDI-19 patients, showed that patients with elevated troponin T values were more likely to develop serious arrhythmias, including ventricular tachycardia and fibrillation, comparing to those with normal troponin T levels (12% vs. 5%) [40]. Treatment of all systemic causes and underlying heart injury having in mind drug interactions should remain the arrhythmias management goals in COVID 19 patients [28]. Hospital data from China revealed that hospitalized COVID-19 patients with elevated troponin levels had more frequent malignant arrhythmias (11.5% vs. 5.2%) and higher overall mortality (59.6% vs. 8.9%) [41].

### 2.7 COVID-19 and coagulation abnormalities

Thromboembolic complications are highly prevalent in patients with COVID-19 infection. Disseminated intravascular coagulation (DIC) and pulmonary embolism, characterized by increased D-dimer levels and fibrin degradation products, are the most characteristic clinical presentations. DIC has been observed in 71.4% of non-survivors [42]. Pulmonary embolism (PE) has been reported in up to 30% of hospitalized patients [41, 43]. Those percentages might not be surprising given the critical condition of these subjects. The clinical and scientific data we have from several world centers indicates that D-dimer values are highly predictive of adverse events in patients with COVID-19 disease. Results from retrospective cohort study showed that elevated D-dimer values (>1 g/L) are strongly associated with intrahospital mortality, which was confirmed as a relationship in the multivariate analysis (OR 18.4, 95% CI 2.6–128.6; p = 0.003) [44]. Additionally, Chinese and Italian experience emphasizes that in the earlier stage of the disease more discrete D-dimer changes are observed, which precede the rapid rise of D-dimer as disease progresses. Recommended diagnostic algorithms combing pre-test probability assessment and D dimer tests can be used in case of suspected acute PE.

Hypercoagulability caused by inflammation and cytokine release are the underlying cause for pulmonary embolism in COVID-19 infected patients [45]. Advanced age, bedridden, stasis, endothelial injury and hemostatic abnormalities are factors associated with increased risk for venous thromboembolism. Inflammatory activation in COVID-19 leads to frequent abnormalities in the coagulation system [45]. It is assumed that COVID -19 infection lead to generalized endotheliopathy as a one of the underlying mechanisms for impaired vascular function and hypercoagulability. For risk stratification purposes and prognosis as well as identification of the patients with increased thrombotic risk, markers of inflammation and thrombotic risk should be measured at baseline and repeated every 2–3 days if abnormal and whenever clinical deterioration is suspected.

The index of suspicion for VTE should be high in the case of typical deep vein thrombosis (DVT) symptoms, hypoxemia disproportionate to known respiratory pathologies, acute unexplained right ventricular dysfunction, new or unexplained tachycardia and new onset of ECG changes suggestive of PE, fall in blood pressure not attributable to tachyarrhythmia, hypovolemia or sepsis [46].

A diagnostic challenge arises among patients with COVID-19, as imaging studies used to diagnose DVT or PE may not be performed given risk of transmitting infection to other patients or health care workers and potentially due to patient instability. Prophylactic anticoagulation is recommended in all patients admitted with COVID-19 infection. When acute PE is confirmed, treatment should be guided by risk stratification in accordance with the current European Society of Cardiology (ESC) guidelines [28]. The novel oral non-vitamin K antagonists (NOACs) may show some interactions with the some of the drugs used in COVID-19 disease patients, mainly with lopinavir/ritonavir and in those cases NOACs should be avoided. There are no major interactions reported between investigational drugs for COVID-19 and the use of heparin as anticoagulant therapy [47].

## 3. Treatment in the light of cardiovascular disease

Regarding the treatment of the COVID-19 infection there are many trials from the beginning of April 2020. Based on the evidence we have so far, the treatment depends on clinical presentation, laboratory and imaging findings as indicated. Supportive care, starting from symptomatic measures, up to complete intensive care support is recommended [48].

There is a need of more research concerning the relationship between rennin-angiotensin-aldosterone blockade and COVID-19 disease in patients with cardiovascular conditions. From the recommendations and guidelines of the major cardiology societies we have so far, therapy with ACE inhibitors or angiotensin receptor blockators for other indications should not be discontinued [28, 49]. The evidences we have do not indicate increased risk of infection or worse clinical course in patient treated with these medications. From other side we have strong warnings that discontinuation of the therapy with these drugs, which modifies prognosis in patients with cardiovascular disease, may increase cardiovascular mortality rates [50]. In heart failure patients the use of drugs that may alter salt and water balance and cause excessive fluid accumulation, such as non-steroid anti-inflammatory drugs (NSAID) should be avoided. Advanced heart failure should be treated and monitored by cardiologists, based on the latest guidelines for the management of heart failure [28].

In patients with COVID-19 disease and established CAD the use of drugs that stabilize plaques and modifies prognosis (statins, aspirin, beta blockers, ACE inhibitors) should be used as indicated in the current guidelines [51, 52]. We should minimize or avoid the use of diagnostic tests that are unnecessary and will not change the diagnostic and treatment decisions. Unnecessary diagnostic tests should be minimized, or in some cases avoided. These tests should be used in circumstances in which they could add to the management of patients with COVID-19. Prophylactic anticoagulation should be applied in all hospitalized patients with COVID-19 infection. Patients with acute confirmed PE should be treated based on risk stratification as recommended in the latest European Society of Cardiology (ESC) guidelines and National PERT Consortium [28, 46, 47].

### 3.1 Knowledge gaps and future directions

COVID-19 has emerged as a new disease almost one year ago and it is still impossible to discuss long-term outcome in patients recovering from infection. Impaired heart function due to myocardial damage in acute phase leads to poor prognosis in these patients. Follow up studies and more data are needed to make conclusions.

There are still many challenges, undiscovered mechanisms, pathobiology, clinical characteristics and prognostic markers of the COVID -19 disease which are continuously studied. Early signs and markers of myocardial injury and presence of new or worsened heart failure are bad prognostic parameters. Long term COVID-19 syndrome and post COVID cardiovascular repercussions are another field of ongoing and future research. Special attention should be taken on timely diagnosis, management and follow up of the cardiovascular complications of COVID-19 disease.

The current evidence of association between renin-angiotensin-aldosterone medications and ACE-2 levels with clinical outcome in COVID-19 infection is insufficient. More information needs to be generated.

## 4. Conclusion

Preexisting cardiovascular disease are common in patients with COVID-19 and those patients are at higher risk of morbidity and mortality. Myocardial injury is present in more than a 15% of severely ill patients. The interaction between the virus S protein and ACE 2 is believed to have important role in disease pathogenesis, especially in cardiovascular manifestations, that could be potential target for the prevention and treatment of COVID-19 infection. The continuation of clinically indicated ACEi or ARB therapy is recommended by many heart associations, based on the currently available evidence. Reduced physical activity due to lockdown measures also contribute to worsened control of cardiovascular risk factors. Having in mind the prevalence of cardiovascular complications our main strategy to fight the pandemic remains social distancing, personal protection, vaccination and regular therapy for all cardiovascular disease patients.

*DOI: http://dx.doi.org/10.5772/intechopen.99332*

## Author details

Irena Mitevska
University Cardiology Clinic, Skopje, North Macedonia

*Address all correspondence to: peovskai@yahoo.com

## References

[1] Wu Z, McGoogan JM. Characteristics of and important lessons from the coronavirus disease 2019 (COVID-19) outbreak in China: summary of a report of 72314 cases from the Chinese Center for Disease Control and Prevention. JAMA 2020;doi: 10.1001/jama.2020.2648

[2] Zheng Y-Y, Ma Y-T, Zhang J-Y and Xie X. COVID-19 and the cardiovascular system. Nat Rev Cardiol. March 5, 2020. doi: 10.1038/s41569-020-0360-5

[3] Zhou P, Yang XL, Wang XG et.al. A pneumonia outbreak associated with a new coronavirus of probable bat origin. Nature 2020; 579:270-273

[4] Zhou F., Yu T., Du R. Clinical course and risk factors for mortality of adult inpatients with COVID-19 in Wuhan, China: a retrospective cohort study. Lancet. 2020

[5] Huayan X, Keke H, Rong X et al. Clinical Characteristics and Risk Factors of Cardiac Involvement in COVID-19. J Am Heart Assoc 2020 Sep 15;9(18)

[6] Zhonghua L, Xing B, Xue Z. Novel Coronavirus Pneumonia Emergency Response Epidemiology Team. The epidemiological characteristics of an outbreak of 2019

[7] Masataka N, Dao WW, Yaling H, David Bl, Joseph CW. COVID-19 and cardiovascular disease: from basic mechanisms to clinical perspectives. Nat Rev Cardiol 2020 Sep;17(9):543-558

[8] Shi S, Qin M, Shen B, et al. Association of cardiac Injury with mortality in hospitalized patients with COVID-19 in Wuhan, China. JAMA Cardiol 2020

[9] Xiong T.Y., Redwood S., Prendergast B., Chen M. Coronaviruses and the cardiovascular system: acute and long-term implications. Eur Heart J. 2020

[10] Kuba K, Imai Y, Rao S, et al. A crucial role of angiotensin converting enzyme 2 (ACE2) in SARS coronavirus-induced lung injury. Nat Med 2005; 11:875-79

[11] Juan-Juan Q , Xu C , Feng Z et al. Redefining Cardiac Biomarkers in Predicting Mortality of Inpatients With COVID-19. Hypertension 2020 Oct;76(4):1104-1112

[12] Michael B, Norbert F, Evangelos G, Karen S,and Andreas M. Zeiher Coronavirus Disease 2019 (COVID-19) and its implications for cardiovascular care: expert document from the German Cardiac Society and the World Heart Federation. Clin Res Cardiol. 2020 May 27: 1-14

[13] Tomasz JG, Saidi AM, Anthony D et al. COVID-19 and the cardiovascular system: implications for risk assessment, diagnosis, and treatment options. Cardiovasc Res. 2020 Aug 1; 116(10): 1666-1687

[14] Shi S, Qin M, Shen B, et al. Association of cardiac injury with mortality in hospitalized patients with COVID-19 in Wuhan, China. JAMA Cardiol 2020; doi: 10.1001/jamacardio.2020.0950

[15] Guo T, Fan Y, Chen M, Wu X, Zhang L, He T, Wang H, Wan J, Wang X, Lu Z. Cardiovascular implications of fatal outcomes of patients with Coronavirus Disease 2019 (COVID-19) JAMA Cardiol. 2020 doi: 10.1001/jamacardio.2020.1017

[16] Shi S, Qin M, Shen B, Cai Y, Liu T, Yang F, Gong W, Liu X, Liang J, Zhao Q, Huang H, Yang B, Huang C. Association of cardiac injury with mortality in hospitalized patients with COVID-19 in Wuhan, China. JAMA Cardiol. 2020 doi: 10.1001/jamacardio.2020.0950

[17] Sarju G, Sourbha SD, Sachin S. Management of Cardiovascular Disease During Coronavirus Disease (COVID-19) Pandemic. Trends Cardiovasc Med. 2020 Aug; 30(6): 315-325

[18] Zhou F, Yu T, Du R, Fan G, Liu Y, Liu Z. Clinical course and risk factors for mortality of adult inpatients with COVID-19 in Wuhan. China: a retrospective cohort study. Lancet. 2020 28 March-3 April; 395(10229): 1054-1062

[19] Peter AK, Ola H, Andrew W, Stephen WS, Fred SA. Cardiac Troponin Testing in Patients with COVID-19: A Strategy for Testing and Reporting Results. *Clinical Chemistry*, hvaa225, https://doi.org/10.1093/clinchem/hvaa225

[20] He XW, Lai JS, Cheng J, et al. Impact of complicated myocardial injury on the clinical outcome of severe or critically ill COVID-19 patients]. Zhonghua Xin Xue Guan Bing Za Zhi 2020;48(0):E011

[21] Jianfeng Xe, Wenjuan W, Shusheng L, et al. Clinical characteristics and outcomes of critically ill patients with novel coronavirus infectious disease (COVID-19) in China: a retrospective multicenter study. Intensive Care Med (2020) 46:1863-1872

[22] Kai-Cai L, Ping X Wei-Fu L, et al. CT manifestations of coronavirus disease-2019: A retrospective analysis of 73 cases by disease severity. European Journal of Radiology 126 (2020) 108941

[23] Mehra MR, Ruschitzka F, COVID-19 Illness and Heart Failure: A Missing Link? JACC: Heart Failure (2020), doi: https://doi.org/10.1016/j.jchf.2020.03.004

[24] Guan WJ, Ni ZY, Hu Y, et al. Clinical characteristics of coronavirus disease 2019 in China. N Engl J Med 2020

[25] Fei Zhou , Ting Yu , Ronghui Du. Clinical course and risk factors for mortality of adult in patients with COVID-19 in Wuhan, China: a retrospective cohort study. Lancet, 2020 Mar 28;395(10229):1054-1062

[26] Kensuke M, Benjamin M, Laurence J, Patrick O, and Olivier M. Impact of COVID-19 on the Cardiovascular System: A Review. J Clin Med. 2020 May; (5): 1407

[27] Muhammed K, Raveena KK, Kiran PZ and Amer H· The role of biomarkers in diagnosis of COVID-19 – A systematic review. Life Sci. 2020 Aug 1; 254: 117788

[28] ESC Guidance for the Diagnosis and Management of CV Disease during the COVID-19 Pandemic. https://www.escardio.org/Education/COVID-19-and-Cardiology/ESC-COVID-19-Guidance

[29] Liang C, Xiangjie L, Mingquan CYi F, and Chenglong X. The ACE2 expression in human heart indicates new potential mechanism of heart injury among patients infected with SARS-CoV-2. Cardiovasc Res. 2020 Mar 30: cvaa078. doi: 10.1093/cvr/cvaa078

[30] Francesca G, Kyriazoula Ch, Annamaria M et al. Acute Myocardial Infarction in the Time of COVID-19: A Review of Biological, Environmental, and Psychosocial Contributors. Int J Environ Res Public Health, 2020 Oct 9;17(20):7371.

[31] Jules M, Yves C, Pierre C, et al. Hospital admissions for acute myocardial infarction before and after lockdown according to regional prevalence of COVID-19 and patient profile in France: a registry study. Lancet Public Health. 2020 Oct;5(10):e536-e542.

[32] Oren O, Kopecky SL, Gluckman TJ et al. Coronavirus Disease 2019 (COVID-19): Epidemiology, Clinical Spectrum and Implications for the Cardiovascular Clinician. Available at:-https://www.acc.org/latest-in-cardiology/

articles/2020/04/06/11/08/covid-19-epidemiology-clinical-spectrum-and-implications-for-the-cv-clinician[Accessed 10 April 2020]

[33] Panayotis KV, Anastasios T, Ioannis K.˙ Concerns for management of STEMI patients in the COVID-19 era: a paradox phenomenon. J Thromb Thrombolysis. 2020 Jul 30: 1-5

[34] Sukhjinder SN, Ricardo P, Sayan S. Optimal management of acute coronary syndromes in the era of COVID-19. Heart. 2020 Oct; 106(20): 1609-1616

[35] Xin-xin W, Chen Sh, Xiao-jie Huang, Lin S, Ling-jia Meng, Hui Liu, Shi-jie Zhang, Hong-jun Li, Fu-dong Lv. Histopathological features of multiorgan percutaneous tissue core biopsy in patients with COVID-19. J Clin Pathol 2020 Aug 26; jclinpath-2020-206623

[36] Doyen D, Moceri P, Ducreux D, Dellamonica J. Myocarditis in a patient with COVID-19: a cause of raised troponin and ECG changes. Lancet. 2020;395(10235):1516

[37] Imazio M, Klingel K, Kindermann I, Brucato A, De Rosa FG, Adler Y, et al. COVID-19 pandemic and troponin: indirect myocardial injury, myocardial inflammation or myocarditis? Heart. 2020;heartjnl-2020-317186. doi: 10.1136/heartjnl-2020-317186

[38] Bhurint S, Saman N, Daniele M et al. Recognizing COVID-19–related myocarditis: The possible pathophysiology and proposed guideline for diagnosis and management. Heart Rhythm. 2020 Sep; 17(9): 1463-1471

[39] Rakesh Y. COVID-19 and sudden cardiac death: A new potential risk. Indian Heart J. 2020 Sep-Oct; 72(5): 333-336

[40] Mohit KT, Daniel M, Martin EG al. Malignant Arrhythmias in Patients With COVID-19. Incidence, Mechanisms, and Outcomes. Circulation: Arrhythmia and Electrophysiology. 2020 Nov; 13(11): e008920

[41] Guo T., Fan Y., Chen M. Cardiovascular implications of fatal outcomes of patients with Coronavirus disease 2019 (COVID-19) JAMA Cardiol. 2020;5(7):811-818

[42] David L. Disseminated intravascular coagulation in patients with 2019-nCoV pneumonia. J Thromb Haemost. 2020 Apr; 18(4): 786-787

[43] Yasser S, Manuela G, Marc L et al. Pulmonary embolism in patients with coronavirus disease-2019 (COVID-19) pneumonia: a narrative review. Ann Intensive Care. 2020; 10: 124

[44] Yumeng Yao, Jiatian Cao, Qingqing Wang, et al. D-dimer as a biomarker for disease severity and mortality in COVID-19 patients: a case control study. J Intensive Care. 2020; 8: 49

[45] Mouhamed Yazan Abou-Ismail, Akiva Diamond, Sargam Kapoor. The hypercoagulable state in COVID-19: Incidence, pathophysiology, and management. Thromb Res. 2020 Oct; 194: 101-115

[46] Rachel P. Rosovsky, Charles Grodzin, Richard Channick. Diagnosis and Treatment of Pulmonary Embolism During the Coronavirus Disease 2019 Pandemic A Position Paper From the National PERT Consortium: Chest. 2020 Aug 27, doi: 10.1016/j.chest.2020.08.2064

[47] Stavros V K, Guy M, Cecilia B et al. 2019 ESC Guidelines for the diagnosis and management of acute pulmonary embolism developed in collaboration with the European Respiratory Society (ERS): The Task Force for the diagnosis and management of acute pulmonary embolism of the European Society of Cardiology (ESC). *European Heart Journal*, Volume 41, Issue 4, 21 January 2020, Pages 543-603

[48] Maria N, Niamh O, Catrin Sohrabi, Mehdi Khan, Maliha Agha, and Riaz Agha. Evidence based management guideline for the COVID-19 pandemic - Review article. Int J Surg. 2020 May; 77: 206-216

[49] Lopes RD, Macedo AVS, de Barros e Silva PGM, Moll-Bernardes RJ et al. BRACE CORONA Investigators. Continuing versus suspending angiotensin-converting enzyme inhibitors and angiotensin receptor blockers: impact on adverse outcomes in hospitalized patients with severe acute respiratory syndrome coronavirus 2 (SARS-CoV-2)–The BRACE CORONA Trial. Am Heart J 2020;226:49-59

[50] Devan K, Katherine M, and Kathryn V. Update Alert: Risks and Impact of Angiotensin-Converting Enzyme Inhibitors or Angiotensin-Receptor Blockers on SARS-CoV-2 Infection in Adults. Ann Intern Med. 2020 Jun 25: L20-0887

[51] Sarju G, Sourbha SD, Sachin S et al. Management of Cardiovascular Disease During Coronavirus Disease (COVID-19) Pandemic. Trends Cardiovasc Med. 2020 Aug; 30(6): 315-325

[52] Charan Y, Brian CC, Brian J. Forrestal et al. Treatment of ST-Segment Elevation Myocardial Infarction During COVID-19 Pandemic. Cardiovasc Revasc Med. 2020 Aug; 21(8): 1024-1029

Chapter 8

# Management of Covid-19 Disease in Pediatric Oncology Patients

*Hatice Mine Cakmak*


## Abstract

Pediatric cancer patients are immunocompromised, and the risks are higher in this population. Confirmed cases are defined as PCR (polymerase chain reaction) positive patients. The severity of infection is divided into four groups: asymptomatic/mild, moderate, severe, and critical, based on the clinical, laboratory, and radiological features. In the pediatric population, the COVID-19 disease has a mild course. Chemotherapy courses can be interrupted according to the symptoms and severity of the disease. Azithromycin, antivirals are used as a single agent or in combination. In critical patients, convalescent plasma, mesenchymal stem cells, tocilizumab, and granulocyte transfusions are administered. In recent studies, having hematological malignancy, stem cell transplantation, a mixed infection, and abnormal computerized tomography findings increase the severity of the disease and the need for an intensive care unit. Therefore, the patients and their families should be aware of a higher risk of severe forms than immunocompetent children.


**Keywords:** chemotherapy, COVID-19, immunocompromised, immunotherapy, pediatric oncology

## 1. Introduction

Coronaviruses are zoonotic RNA viruses. SARS-CoV-2 (severe acute respiratory syndrome coronavirus 2), the novel coronavirus, belongs to the Betacoranovirus subgroup [1]. SARS-CoV-2's incidence in children varies (China: 2-12.3%, Italy: 1.2%, USA: 5%). The infection in pediatric cases is asymptomatic or mild. The median incubation period is 5-7 days. The primary source of transmission is respiratory droplets and direct contact. The primary tool for diagnosis is a real-time polymerase chain reaction test (RT-PCR) on samples. Eighty percent of children had household contact; ten percent were asymptomatic, fifty percent had a fever. Other symptoms are cough, respiratory distress, fatigue, myalgias, vomiting, diarrhea, anosmia, ageusia, sore throat. Children generally recover in 1-2 weeks. The case fatality rate in children is zero percent [2]. This benign course of the disease is related to the immune preparedness of children to a new pathogen. Immunologic mechanisms are also different in children compared with adults [3, 4]. Multisystem Inflammatory Syndrome in Children (MIS-C) is a rare postinfectious complication of SARS-CoV-2 infections; it is RT-PCR negative for SARS-CoV-2 virus but antibody positive [5].

Cancer treatment includes various immunosuppressive drugs [6]. It is well known that immunocompromised children have higher mortality and morbidity rates than the healthy population due to viral respiratory infections [7]. In the pediatric oncology setting, the mortality rate in COVID-19 is reported up to 4% [8]. In COVID-19 relevant areas, the virus transmission rate is low in children with cancer. Cancer diagnosis, treatment, palliative care, hospital visits are interrupted because of the pandemic. Another concern is delayed cancer diagnosis, chemotherapy shortages, decreased availability of surgery, radiotherapy, supportive treatment, inadequate personal productive equipment, and drugs, especially in low-middle income countries [9, 10]. The most common cancer in the pediatric population is acute leukemia. In industrialized countries, the incidence of acute leukemia is a 40-60 age-standardized rate per million, one-third of all childhood cancers. Brain and spinal tumors are the second; lymphomas are the third most common tumors in industrialized countries [11]. Therefore, urgent treatment is critical and life-saving, especially in leukemia and lymphoma induction therapy [12]. Here we present an explanatory review of different approaches and experiences in this unique population.

## 2. SARS-CoV-2 infection in pediatric oncology

The incidence of COVID-19 among cancer patients varies %1 to 7% [13–15]. In SARS-CoV-2 Infection, cancer patients' hospitalization rate is four times more than the healthy population [16]. Madhusoodhan et al. reported that mortality and morbidity rates in COVID-19 positive children with cancer were higher than the average population. The most common underlying malignancy was acute lymphoblastic leukemia (ALL) (53%). Severe infection and critical support need rates are also higher. Among hospitalized patients with cancer, oxygen support and intensive care unit (ICU) admission rates were significantly higher than the non-cancer group. Sixty-seven percent of positive cases' chemotherapy courses were interrupted between 2 and 78 days. Forty-six percent delays in surgery, thirty percent delays in transplant were noted. The mortality rate was 4.1%, not solely associated with the COVID-19 disease [17].

### 2.1 Risk of SARS-CoV2 infection in children with cancer

Cancer patients are immunocompromised due to tumor growth and treatment. Chemotherapy reduces immunoglobulin levels and causes qualitative and quantitative T cell dysfunction. Immunocompromised patients have a higher risk of developing severe disease. Therefore, the leading practices are basic hygiene rules, avoiding crowded places, and possible infection and handwashing situations [18]. Patients with cancer have a higher risk of symptomatic or severe COVID-19 disease. Chemotherapy, surgery in the last month, and immunotherapy administration increase COVID-19 disease severity and associated deaths. However, radiotherapy was not associated with adverse outcomes. Developing symptoms are rapidly, and hospitalization rates and duration were higher in cancer patients. Cancer survivors' signs are more extreme than the average because immune recovery is not completed [19]. In one study, male sex, older age; obesity rates were slightly higher in severe COVID-19 cases with cancer [17]. The United States Centers for Disease Control and Prevention published the risk factors for the severity of COVID-19. Medical complexity, genetic, chronic health conditions, and immunosuppression are presented as possible severity risk factors [18].

### 2.2 Variants of COVID-19

The mutations in the SARS-CoV2 genome may change its phenotype (transmissibility, virulence). Alfa (B.1.1.7 lineage) variant (20I/501Y.V1) has increased transmission compared with previous strains. Some studies suggest this variant is also associated with severity. Delta (B.1.617.2 lineage), first identified in India, is more transmissible and has more hospitalization rates than the alfa variant. Vaccine effectiveness is also altered in this variant but is high in preventing hospitalization and severe disease. Beta (B.1.351 variant) was identified first in South Africa; vaccine effectiveness may be reduced with this mutation. Gama (P.1 lineage) variant may increase transmissibility. Epsilon variants (B.1.427 and B..1.429) are associated with higher viral mRNA levels on nasal swabs [20].

### 2.3 Clinical presentation

Clinical features are mild in neonates and children worldwide. However, fever, respiratory symptoms, gastrointestinal symptoms, and neurologic manifestations are observed among COVID-19 cases. The severity of the disease is divided into five groups (asymptomatic, mild, moderate, severe, critical) [21]. Covid toes are described as reddish nodules in distal digits in children and adolescents. The other dermatologic manifestations are morbilliform rah, livedo reticularis-like vascular lesions, and urticarial [22]. Multisystem Inflammatory Syndrome In Children (MIS-C) is a past-infection complication of COVID-19 infection. MIS-C features are persistent fever >38°C, history of SARS-CoV2 disease, at least two of the following symptoms (rash, gastrointestinal, edema of the hands and feet, oral mucosa changes, conjunctivitis, lymphadenopathy, and neurologic symptoms). Arrhythmias and ventricular dysfunction are other presentations of MIS-C [23].

### 2.4 Diagnosis

Whole-genome sequencing led to finding newer genes for RT-PCR. RT-PCR test on upper and lower respiratory secretions is routinely used for diagnosis. This test should be repeated in clinically suspected cases. Gaita samples can also be positive by RT-PCR. Serology is essential for the previous infection for SARS-CoV2 and common coronaviruses. Laboratory findings may be lymphopenia, thrombocytopenia, neutropenia. In severe cases, lactate dehydrogenase, coagulation parameters, and D-dimers are elevated. C.T. (computerized tomography) findings include multiple patchy, nodular, ground-glass, or reticular opacities and infiltrations [24].

#### *2.4.1 Testing of patients with cancer*

Symptoms of COVID-19 (fever, cough, dyspnea, diarrhea, etc.) and suspected exposure are essential for testing cancer patients. According to IDSA (Infectious Diseases Society of America) guidelines, the first higher priority includes unexplained viral pneumonia or respiratory failure in critically ill patients in ICU. Also, fever or lower respiratory tract illness in immunosuppressed, older, or have underlying chronic health conditions is an indication. The other symptoms in the first higher priority are fever or lower respiratory tract illness in patients with COVID-19 contact within 14 days or in health care workers, public health care workers, and other essential leaders. Non-ICU hospitalized patients with unexplained fever, and lower tract illness are in the second level of priority. The third priority consists of outpatients with criteria of influenza testing (chronic diseases and immunocompromising conditions), pregnant women, and children with similar risk factors. Public health and infectious diseases authorities' decisions are the fourth priority [25]. Before cytotoxic chemotherapy, solid organ and stem cell transplantation, cellular immunotherapy, or high-dose corticosteroids, SARS-CoV2 RNA testing is recommended in several guidelines [26].

## 2.5 Treatment and outcome of SARS-CoV2 infection in children with cancer

### *2.5.1 Guideline recommendations for children*

Treatment recommendations of COVID-19 for childhood cancer are the same with children without cancer. Supportive treatment (hydration, nutrition, oxygen supplementation) is essential in COVID-19 treatment. In the COVID-19 treatment guidelines panel, remdesivir is recommended for hospitalized children ≥12 years with risk factors of severe disease and increasing demand for oxygen. In addition, this panel recommends dexamethasone for children with high flow oxygen, mechanical ventilation, or extracorporeal membrane oxygenation in COVID-19 disease. If dexamethasone is not available, other glucocorticoids can also be given. The dose of dexamethasone is 0.15 mg/kg/dose (maximum 6 mg) for up to ten days. Convalescent plasma is used for mechanical ventilated COVID-19 positive children. Anti-SARS-CoV2 monoclonal antibodies (bamlanivumab plus etesevimab or casarivimab plus imdevimab) studies are insufficient in the pediatric population. However, ≥ 16 aged and hospitalized patients having at least one high risk of severe disease can be consulted for pediatric infectious disease. The safety of baricitinib has not been evaluated in pediatric patients; the data of baricitinib and remdesivir combination is insufficient for hospitalized children who have a contraindication for corticosteroids. The use of tocilizumab for severe pediatric cases has been described; there is inadequate data for recommending tocilizumab in MIS-C or hospitalized children with COVID-19. All of these therapies can be discussed for selected patients [23]. Increased D-dimer and high risk of thrombosis are indications for anticoagulation in childhood cancer with COVID-19 disease [27].

In MIS-C, IVIG (intravenous immunoglobin) and corticosteroids are in the first-line treatment. High-dose IVIG (typically 2 g/kg, based on ideal body weight) is used. In severe cases, low-moderate dose glucocorticosteroids (1-2 mg/kg/day) should be given with IVIG. Interleukin-1 antagonists are given in refractory instances in patients with MIS-C. Features of macrophage activation syndrome or contraindications for glucocorticosteroids are indications of it. Therefore, high-dose steroids are used for refractory patients. Antiplatelet therapy is used at least for weeks after diagnosis. In case of indefinite treatment and documented thrombosis, anticoagulation is recommended [23, 28].

### *2.5.2 The COVID-19 treatment guideline panel recommendations for adult patients with cancer*

Vaccination for COVID-19 is recommended for adults with active cancer and those receiving treatment for cancer. The vaccination should be done at least two weeks before starting chemotherapy. In adults with hematologic malignancies, vaccination should be done after neutrophil recovery for those receiving intensive chemotherapy. Vaccination should be done at least after three months of hematopoietic stem cell transplantation and chimeric T-cell therapy.

For signs and symptoms of COVID-19 and before chemotherapy, radiotherapy, and all invasive procedures, testing with PCR should be performed. Treatment delays for curable cancers like pediatric lymphoblastic leukemia should be avoided. If regimens with similar results are preferable, orally administered drugs or regimens with fewer days should be chosen. Regimens should not be altered even in COVID-19 patients with cancer. In radiotherapy guidelines, the daily dose by a fraction is increased to lower the days of treatment. For patients with febrile neutropenia, a PCR test for COVID-19 should be performed. National Comprehensive Cancer

Network guidelines should be followed. Treatment of COVID-19 in cancer patients is the same with the general population. Drug interactions are essential [23].

### *2.5.3 COVID-19 experience in pediatric oncology*

Early data from China revealed that children positive for COVID-19 had a low (2.8%) rate of severe disease [29]. However, in COVID-19 positive children, ICU admission rates were 33.2% in the COVID-NET group study and 35% in another study [30, 31]. Furthermore, in a systemic review (June 2020), the survival rate was %100 among children with cancer and COVID-19 [32].

In a multicenter, retrospective study of 578 children with cancer, 98 were positive for COVID-19. Asymptomatic (n = 25), mild (n = 45), moderate (n = 11), severe (n = 17) disease were observed. Twenty-eight were hospitalized, seven needed mechanical ventilation. Hydroxychloroquine (n = 15), azithromycin (n = 15), tocilizumab (n = 5), remdesivir (n = 4) were given [17]. In a systematic review of 204 children with cancer, 96 were hospitalized because of COVID-19 infection. Thirty-two percent had oxygen requirements. Pneumothorax, pleural effusion, pulmonary arterial hypertension, bronchiolitis obliterans, diffuse alveolar hemorrhage, septic shock, and acute respiratory distress syndrome are other complications. Forty-one patients received hydroxychloroquine; nine took steroids, five took lopinavir/ritonavir combination. Azithromycin (n = 4), remdesivir (n = 4), and tocilizumab (n = 3) were used. Twenty-one required intensive care unit admission. Out of 15 deaths, four of them were not related to COVID-19. Thus, the mortality rate was 4.9% [33]. Millen et al. reported 54 positive children of COVID-19 with cancer. The majority (53.7%) of the patients had ALL (acute lymphoblastic leukemia). Four of them had acute myeloid leukemia, five had central nervous system tumors, six had neuroblastoma. None of them died of COVID-19 disease. Twenty-one percent were taking very myelosuppressive chemotherapy; twenty-one were receiving a less intense regimen. Twenty-six had targeted therapies. None received high-dose chemotherapy and stem-cell transplantation within 28 days of this infection [34]. In a resource-limited country, Peru, the epidemiologic data was similar. Among 69 children with cancer, 36 had ALL, 5 had NHL (non-Hodgkin lymphoma), 5 had brain tumors, and COVID 19. Ivermectin, azithromycin, corticosteroids were used for COVID-19 treatment. Unfortunately, seven of them died and, COVID-19 lethality is 10% in this study [35]. Graetz et al. reported that out of 79 countries and 213 centers, 88% had SARS-CoV2 testing opportunities, 43% of centers declined in new cancer diagnosis. Reduction in surgery (72%), chemotherapy changes (57%), disruption in radiotherapy (28%) has been a great deal. In low-middle income countries, unavailability of chemotherapy agents, lag in treatment, and radiotherapy was more common [36].

In another cross-sectional study, 51 children with cancer were examined, and they had COVID-19. Sixty point eight percent had hematologic malignancies; six underwent stem cell transplantation, 17 had moderate or severe disease, nine had a critical illness. Delay in treatment (chemotherapy, radiotherapy, surgery) and reduction in chemotherapy doses were reported in 40-58% of the cases [37]. Kebudi et al. said the mortality rate was 1.9% in COVID-19 infection of pediatric oncology patients. Hematologic malignancies, HSCT, a mixed condition, increased the severity of COVID-19 disease [38]. COVID-19 recommendations are rapidly changing, guidelines of the Ministry of health were used in this study. Recent proposals for immunocompromised children in this guideline are; mild cases with possible worsening respiratory failure should be treated. Here, drug interactions should be carefully examined. These patients older than twelve receive favipiravir with a loading dose of 1600 mgr twice a day, and a maintenance dose of 600 mg, once a day. Hydroxychloroquine ± azithromycin is deleted currently but previously given in this guideline [39].

### 2.6 Managing hematologic malignancies in COVID-19 pandemic

European Society for Blood and Marrow Transplantation (EBMT) reported their recommendations (June 2020). Steroids that may cause viral rebounds and adverse events are the main component of acute lymphoblastic leukemia treatment. Dose reduction is not recommended in prophase, induction, and consolidation. Asparaginase has thrombotic complications that are also observed in COVID infections. Treatment delay is not recommended for drugs, blinatumomab or inotuzumab. Tyrosine kinase inhibitors are the mainstay treatment in Philadelphia-positive ALL; this treatment should not be delayed. As well as acute promyelocyte leukemia should be treated immediately. Acute myeloid leukemia with adverse cytogenetic risks and a suitable donor for allogeneic stem cell transplantation needs intensive therapy. Patients with favorable or intermediate-risk factors should also be treated, but some modifications in doses can be preferred after induction. This procedure cannot be postponed for patients with a risk of progression or relapse without allogeneic stem cell transplantation. Controversial indications should be reconsidered [40]. Passamonti et al. reported that outcomes were worse in hematological malignancies with COVID-19. The leading diagnoses with worse survival were acute myeloid leukemia, indolent NHL, aggressive NHL, or plasma cell neoplasms. In addition, the mortality rate of hematological malignancies was four times higher than the general population with COVID-19. This rate was also 41 times higher than the hematologic malignancies without COVID-19. Thus, disease type and status are essential for outcome [41]. Retrospective studies support a mortality rate up to %62 in hematological malignancies with COVID-19. Prolonged persistence of the RNA up to 32.7 days is reported.

Acute leukemias, especially acute myeloid leukemia (AML), myeloproliferative neoplasms, myelodysplastic syndromes, lymphomas, have the worst complications and outcomes. Chemotherapy was not generally associated with worse results. PCR ± C.T. of the chest is recommended before treatment. Induction treatment should not be delayed. In case of a positive test, a multidisciplinary team containing a pediatric hematology-oncologist and pediatric infectious diseases specialists should decide the time of others courses. With a positive test, the period of chemotherapy can be postponed for two weeks. In high-risk AML, allogeneic stem cell transplantation should not be delayed. Recommendations of EBMT should be followed [42]. Tyrosine kinase inhibitors (TKIs) are the mainstay treatment in chronic myeloid leukemia (CML). The cessation of these drugs needs a deep and stable response to treatment and close follow-up. In the COVID-19 pandemic, termination of therapy is not a helpful approach. The interaction of remdesivir with imatinib, dasatinib, and nilotinib is essential. In CML blastic phase, TKIs plus intensive chemotherapy is an urgent treatment [42].

Newly diagnosed aggressive NHL like Burkitt lymphoma and Diffuse large B cell Lymphoma need acute treatment, and delay is inappropriate. DA-EPOCH-R (dose-adjusted etoposide, cyclophosphamide, vincristine, doxorubicin, prednisone) is the standard treatment for PMBCL (primary mediastinal B-cell lymphoma). Because of the severe immunosuppressive effect of this regimen, alternatives are recommended, like R-CHOP with radiotherapy consolidation. RICE (rituximab, ifosfamide, carboplatin, etoposide) can be given as a salvage regimen in a relapsed refractory setting. However, less myelotoxic regimens can be preferred. In Hodgkin lymphoma treatment, bleomycin and checkpoint inhibitors have adverse pulmonary toxicity events. In adults, the omission of bleomycin can be an option for complete remission after the second course. Guidelines for radiotherapy should be followed [39]. Bendamustine as an option in relapsed refractory patients is associated with mortality in COVID-19 positive lymphomas [43].

### 2.7 Treatment of brain tumors in COVID-19 pandemic

The mainstay treatment in children is surgery; the delay in treatment leads to neurologic sequela, decreases survival, increases morbidity. Late diagnoses are other challenges. Early intervention is essential [44].

### 2.8 Treatment of SARS-CoV2 infection for children receiving bone marrow transplantation and current recommendations

Of 318 HSCT receipts with COVID-19 infection, 184 with allogeneic HSCT, 134 with autologous HSCT were included in one study. In the allogeneic HSCT group, fifteen cases were ≤ ten years old; eleven were between 11 and 20 years old. Three patients were ≤ ten years old; none were 11-20 years old in the other group. Therefore, AML, ALL, MDS are the leading diagnoses for allogeneic HSCT. Fifty-five patients had a severe presentation of COVID-19 infection requiring mechanical ventilation. In the allogeneic HSCT group, 42% had a myeloablative regimen, 56% took a reduced-intensity conditioning regimen (RIC), 45% received TBI (total body irradiation) based conditioning regimen. In moderate–severe cases, COVID-19 convalescent plasma remdesivir, tocilizumab, Hydroxychloroquine, azithromycin were commonly used. In addition, Lopinavir, ritonavir, methylprednisolone, oseltamivir, ribavirin, acyclovir, famciclovir, antibacterial agents were also used. After 30 days of transplantation, overall survival was 68% for the allogeneic HSCT group, 67% for autologous HSCT receipts. Male sex, age older than 50, and COVID-19 within 12 months of transplantation was strongly associated with mortality [45].

The COVID-19 Treatment Guidelines include the following recommendations for HSCT and cellular therapy receipts and donors;

- For adults, vaccination for SARS-COV2 is recommended.
- In the presence of signs and symptoms of COVID-19, PCR testing is recommended. If COVID-19 infection is suspected, time donation or transplantation should be re-checked.
- In transplant and cellular therapy patients, COVID-19 treatment should be consulted by a transplantation specialist. In addition, drug interactions of immunosuppressants with other medications should be investigated [23].

## 3. Covid-19 vaccines in children

BNT162b2 (Pfizer; BioNTech) is the first vaccine approved in children (12-15 years) with 100% efficacy. A trial of this vaccine for six months to eleven years of age is ongoing. Moderna's mRNA-1273 vaccine also has 100% efficacy in adolescents (12-17 years aged). Sinovac's mRNA vaccine is approved in China for children more than three years of age. Protection may be lower against some variants. However, BNT162b2 and AZD122 vaccines have excellent results in reducing hospitalization and severe disease. Phase III trials for beta variants include BNT162b2s01 (Pfizer; BioNTech), Moderna's mRNA-1273.351, and mRNA-1273.211 vaccines [46]. More recent studies revealed that the third dose of vaccine is warranted for active use of chemotherapy for cancer, hematologic malignancies, hematopoietic stem cell transplantation. Administration of some drugs (rituximab etc.) should be postponed until two-four weeks after vaccination completion if possible [47, 48]. FDA has recently approved BNT162b2 (Pfizer; BioNTech) for individuals aged 16 years and older. It is still under emergency use for children between 12-15 years of age [49].

## 4. Conclusions

COVID-19 infection is mild in children. However, the outcomes of COVID-19 in children with cancer are worse than the healthy children. Therefore, cancer treatment initiation should not be postponed for curable cancers. Treatment of COVID-19 in children with cancer is the same with healthy children with COVID-19. Therefore, Hydroxychloroquine plus azithromycin is no longer used; in the panel, remdesivir is recommended. In Turkey, favipiravir is used. MIS-C is a critical and late complication of COVID-19. Vaccination is recommended. However, the vaccine studies of COVID 19 in children are not completed [50]. Following the recent guidelines, multidisciplinary teamwork is essential for deciding the management of children with cancer.

## Conflict of interest

The authors declare no conflict of interest.

## Author details

Hatice Mine Cakmak
Department of Pediatric Hematology-Oncology, Eskisehir City Hospital, Eskisehir, Turkey

*Address all correspondence to: h.m.tokuc@hotmail.com

## References

[1] Zimmerman, P. & Curtis, N. Coronavirus infections in children including COVID-19: an overview of the epidemiology, clinical features, diagnosis, treatment, and prevention options in children. Pediatr. Infect. Dis. J. 39, 355-368 (2020). DOI: 10.1097/INF.0000000000002660.

[2] Di Nardo M, van Leeuwen G, Loreti A, Barbieri MA, Guner Y, Locatelli F, Ranieri VM. A literature review of 2019 novel coronavirus (SARS-CoV2) infection in neonates and children. Pediatr Res. 2021;89(5):1101-1108. DOI: 10.1038/s41390-020-1065-5.

[3] Cristiani L, Mancino E, Matera L, Nenna R, Pierangeli A, Scagnolari C, Midulla F. Will children reveal their secret? The coronavirus dilemma. Eur Respir J. 2020; 55(4): 2000749. DOI: 10.1183/13993003.00749-2020.

[4] Carsetti R, Quintarelli C, Quinti I, Piano Mortari E, Zumla A, Ippolito G, Locatelli F. The immune system of children: the key to understanding SARS-CoV-2 susceptibility? Lancet Child Adolesc Health. 2020;4(6):414-416. DOI: 10.1016/S2352-4642(20)30135-8.

[5] Radia T, Williams N, Agrawal P, Harman K, Weale J, Cook J, Gupta A.Multi-system inflammatory syndrome in children & adolescents (MIS-C): A systematic review of clinical features and presentation. Paediatr Respir Rev. 2021;38:51-57. DOI: 10.1016/j.prrv.2020.08.001.

[6] Amicucci M, Mastronuzzi A, Ciaralli I, Piccioni F, Schiopu AC, Tiozzo E, Gawronski O, Biagioli V, Dall'Oglio I. The Management of Children with Cancer during the COVID-19 Pandemic: A Rapid Review. J Clin Med. 2020 Nov 21;9(11):3756. DOI: 10.3390/jcm9113756.

[7] Ogimi C, Englund JA, Bradford MC, Qin X, Boeckh M, Waghmare A. Characteristics and Outcomes of Coronavirus Infection in Children: The Role of Viral Factors and an Immunocompromised State. J Pediatric Infect Dis Soc. 2019; 28:21-28. DOI: 10.1093/jpids/pix093.

[8] The Global COVID-19 Observatory and Resource Center for Childhood Cancer. Global Registry of COVID-19 in pediatric cancer. 2020. From: https://global.stjude.org/en-us/global-covid-19-observatory-and-resource-center-for-childhood-cancer/registry.html [Accessed: 31-October- 2020).

[9] Kaspers GJL. COVID-19: how will this impact children with cancer, now and in the future? Expert Rev Anticancer Ther. 2020;20:527-529. DOI: 10.1080/14737140.2020.1781621.

[10] Slone JS, Ozuah N, Wasswa P. Caring for Children with Cancer in Africa during the COVID-19 Crisis: Implications and Opportunities. Pediatr Hematol Oncol. 2020 Oct;37(7):549-553. DOI: 10.1080/08880018.2020.

[11] Stiller CA, Gatta G. The epidemiology of cancer in children and adolescents. In: Caron HN, Biondi A, Boterberg T, Doz F editors. Oxford Textbook of Cancer in Children. 7th ed. United Kingdom: Oxford University Press:2020. P.1-11. ISBN: 0192517694, 9780192517692

[12] Hus I, Salomon-Perzyński A, Tomasiewicz K, Robak T. The management of hematologic malignancies during the COVID-19 pandemic. Expert Opin Pharmacother. 2021;22(5):565-582. DOI: 10.1080/14656566.2020.1849143.

[13] Liang W, Guan W, Chen R, Wang W, Li J, Xu K, et al. Cancer patients in SARS-CoV-2 infection: a nationwide

analysis in China. Lancet Oncol. 2020;21:335. DOI:10.1016/S1470-2045(20)30096-6.

[14] Amicucci M, Mastronuzzi A, Ciaralli I, Piccioni F, Schiopu A.C, Tiozzo E, Gawronski O, Biagioli V, Dall'Oglio I. The Management of Children with Cancer during the COVID-19 Pandemic: A Rapid Review. J. Clin. Med. 2020, *9*, 3756. https://doi.org/10.3390/jcm9113756.

[15] Rogado J, Obispo B, Pangau C, Serrano-Montero G, Martin Marino A, Peres-Perez M, et al. Covid-19 transmission, outcome and associated risk factors in cancer patients at the first month of the pandemic in a Spanish Hospital in Madrid. Clin Transl Oncol. 2020;22:2364. DOI:10.1007/s12094—020-02381-z.

[16] Fillmore NR, La J, Szalat RE, Tuck DP, Nguyen V, Yildirim C, Do NV, Brophy MT, Munshi NC. Prevalence and Outcome of Covıd-19 Infection in Cancer Patients: A National Veterans Affairs Study. J Natl Cancer Inst. 2021;113:691-698. DOI:10.1093/jnci/djjaa159.

[17] Madhusoodhan, PP, Pierro, J, Musante, J, et al. Characterization of COVID-19 disease in pediatric oncology patients: The New York-New Jersey regional experience. Pediatr Blood Cancer. 2021; 68:e28843. https://doi.org/10.1002/pbc.28843

[18] Centers for Disease Control and Prevention, Underlying medical conditions associated with high risk for severe COVID-19: Information for healthcare providers. Avaliable at: https://www..cdc.gov/coronavirus/2019-ncov/hcp/clinical-care/underlyingconditions.html (Accessed on April 5, 2021)

[19] Ruggiero A, Romano A, Attinà G. Covid-19 and children with cancer: are they at increased risk of infection? Pediatr Res. 2021 Feb;89(3):398. DOI: 10.1038/s41390-020-0919-1.

[20] Cantón R, De Lucas Ramos P, García-Botella A, García-Lledó A, Gómez-Pavón J, González Del Castillo J et.al. New variants of SARS-CoV-2. Rev Esp Quimioter. 2021 Jun 2:canton02jun2021. doi: 10.37201/req/071.2021. Epub ahead of print. PMID: 34076402.

[21] Dong Y, Mo X, Hu Y, Qi X, Jiang F, Jiang Z, Tong S. Epidemiology of COVID-19 Among Children in China. Pediatrics. 2020 Jun;145(6):e20200702. DOI: 10.1542/peds.2020-0702.

[22] Suchonwanit P, Leerunyakul K, Kositkuljorn C. Cutaneous manifestations in COVID-19: Lessons learned from current evidence. J Am Acad Dermatol. 2020 Jul;83(1):e57-e60. DOI: 10.1016/j.jaad.2020.04.094.

[23] COVID-19 Treatment Guidelines Panel Coronaviruses Disease 2019 (COVID-19) Treatment Guidelines. National Institutes of Health. Avaliable at: https://www.covid19treatmentguidelines.nih.gov/. Accessed [insert date]

[24] Zare-Zardini H, Soltaninejad H, Ferdosian F, Hamidieh AA, Memarpoor-Yazdi M. Coronavirus Disease 2019 (COVID-19) in Children: Prevalence, Diagnosis, Clinical Symptoms, and Treatment. Int J Gen Med. 2020 July 28;13:477-482. DOI: 10.2147/IJGM.S262098.

[25] Infectious Diseases Society of America. COVID-19. Prioritization of Diagnostic Testing. Available at: http://www.idsociety.org/globallassetsss/idsa/public-health/covid-19-prioritization-of-dx-testing..pdf (Accessed on March 26, 2020)

[26] Infectious Diseases Society of America Guidelines on the diagnosis of COVID-19. Avaliable at: http://www.

idsociety.org/practice-guideline-diagnostics/ (Accessed on May 08, 2020)

[27] Shen KL, Yang YH, Jiang RM, Wang TY, Zhao DC, Jiang Y, Lu XX, Jin RM, Zheng YJ, Xu BP, Xie ZD, Liu ZS, Li XW, Lin LK, Shang YX, Shu SN, Bai Y, Lu M, Lu G, Deng JK, Luo WJ, Xiong LJ, Liu M, Cui YX, Ye LP, Li JF, Shao JB, Gao LW, Wang YY, Wang XF; China National Clinical Research Center for Respiratory Diseases; National Center for Children's Health, Beijing, China; Group of Respirology, Chinese Pediatric Society, Chinese Medical Association; Chinese Medical Doctor Association Committee on Respirology Pediatrics; China Medicine Education Association Committee on Pediatrics; Chinese Research Hospital Association Committee on Pediatrics; China Non-government Medical Institutions Association Committee on Pediatrics; China Association of Traditional Chinese Medicine, Committee on Children's Health and Medicine Research; China News of Drug Information Association, Committee on Children's Safety Medication; Global Pediatric Pulmonology Alliance. Updated diagnosis, treatment and prevention of COVID-19 in children: experts' consensus statement (condensed version of the second edition). World J Pediatr. 2020 Jun;16(3):232-239. DOI: 10.1007/s12519-020-00362-4.

[28] Henderson L, Canna S, Friedman K, Gorelik M, Lapidus S, Bassiri H, et al. (2020). American College of Rheumatology Clinical Guidance for Multisystem Inflammatory Syndrome in Children Associated With SARS-CoV-2 and Hyperinflammation in Pediatric COVID-19: Version 1. *Arthritis & rheumatology (Hoboken, N.J.)*, 72(11), 1791-1805. Avaliable at: http://dx.doi.org/10.1002/art.41454. (Accessed on July,23, 2020)

[29] Dong Y, Mo X, Hu Y, et al. Epidemiology of COVID-19 among children in China. Pediatrics. 2020;145(6):e20200702. DOI: https://doi.org/10.1542/peds.2020-0702

[30] Kim L, Whitaker M, O'Halloran A, et al. Hospitalization rates and characteristics of children aged <18 years hospitalized with laboratoryconfirmedCOVID-19 - COVID-NET, 14 States, March 1-July 25, 2020.MMWRMorbMortalWkly Rep. 2020;69(32):1081-1088. DOI: 10.15585/mmwr.mm6932e3.

[31] Kainth MK, Goenka PK, Williamson KA, et al. Early experience of COVID-19 in a U.S. children's hospital. *Pediatrics*. 2020;146(4):e2020003186. DOI: https://doi.org/10.1542/peds.2020-003186

[32] Dorantes-Acosta E, Ávila-Montiel D, Klünder-Klünder M, et al. survival in pediatric patients with cancer during the COVID-19 pandemic: scoping systematic review. Bol Med Hosp Infant Mex. 2020;77(5):234-241. DOI: 10.24875/BMHIM.20000174

[33] Meena JP, Kumar Gupta A, Tanwar P, Ram Jat K, Mohan Pandey R, Seth R. Clinical presentations and outcomes of children with cancer and COVID-19: A systematic review. Pediatr Blood Cancer. 2021 Jun;68(6):e29005. DOI: 10.1002/pbc.29005.

[34] Millen GC, Arnold R, Cazier JB, Curley H, Feltbower RG, Gamble A, Glaser AW, Grundy RG, Lee LYW, McCabe MG, Phillips RS, Stiller CA, Várnai C, Kearns PR. Severity of COVID-19 in children with cancer: Report from the United Kingdom Paediatric Coronavirus Cancer Monitoring Project. Br J Cancer. 2021 Feb;124(4):754-759. DOI: 10.1038/s41416-020-01181-0.

[35] Montoya J, Ugaz C, Alarcon S, Maradiegue E, García J, Díaz R, Zapata A, Chávez S, Morales R, Ordoñez K, Hernandez E, Reaño R,

Gutierrez C, Vargas MP, Sanchez K, Valdiviezo C, Maza I, Rojas N, Moore C, León E, Vásquez L. COVID-19 in pediatric cancer patients in a resource-limited setting: National data from Peru. Pediatr Blood Cancer. 2021 Feb;68(2):e28610. DOI: 10.1002/pbc.28610. Epub 2020 Jul 22.

[36] Graetz D, Agulnik A, Ranadive R, et al. Global effect of the COVID-19 pandemic on paediatric cancer care: a cross-sectional study. Lancet Child Adolesc Health. 2021;5(5):332-340. DOI:10.1016/S2352-4642(21)00031-6.

[37] Kebudi R, Kurucu N, Tuğcu D. Delays in Treatment Because of COVID-19 Infection in Children With Cancer and Stem-Cell Transplant Recipients in Turkey. JCO Oncol Pract. 2021 Jun;17(6):363-364. DOI: 10.1200/OP.21.00047.

[38] Kebudi R, Kurucu N, Tuğcu D, Hacısalihoğlu Ş, Fışgın T, Ocak S, Tokuç G, Nihal Özdemir G, Bozkurt C, İnce D, Aras S, Ayçiçek A, Aksoy BA, Karadaş N, Öztürk G, Orhan MF, Ataseven E, Akbayram S, Yılmaz E, Tüfekçi Ö, Vural S, Akyay A, Ayhan AC, Kılıç S, Uzel VH, Düzenli Y, Kazancı EG, Acıpayam C, Elli M, Tanyeli A, Karakas Z, Somer A, Kara A. COVID-19 infection in children with cancer and stem cell transplant recipients in Turkey: A nationwide study. Pediatr Blood Cancer. 2021 Jun;68(6):e28915. DOI: 10.1002/pbc.28915.

[39] Ministry of Health of Turkey, COVID 19 guidelines. 20.05.2021 Pediatric COVID 19 disease and it's management. https://covid19.saglik.gov.tr/TR-66301/covid-19-rehberi.html

[40] Brissot E, Labopin M, Baron F, Bazarbachi A, Bug G, Ciceri F, Esteve J, Giebel S, Gilleece MH, Gorin NC, Lanza F, Peric Z, Ruggeri A, Sanz J, Savani BN, Schmid C, Shouval R, Spyridonidis A, Versluis J, Nagler A, Mohty M. Management of patients with acute leukemia during the COVID-19 outbreak: practical guidelines from acute leukemia working party of the European Society for Blood and Marrow Transplantation. Bone Marrow Transplant. 2021 Mar;56(3):532-535. DOI: 10.1038/s41409-020-0970-x.

[41] Passamonti F, Cattaneo C, Arcaini L, Bruna R, Cavo M, Merli F et al.,; ITA-HEMA-COV Investigators. Clinical characteristics and risk factors associated with COVID-19 severity in patients with hematological malignancies in Italy: a retrospective, multicentre, cohort study. Lancet Haematol. 2020 Oct;7(10):e737-e745. DOI: 10.1016/S2352-3026(20)30251-9.

[42] Hus I, Salomon-Perzyński A, Tomasiewicz K, Robak T. The management of hematologic malignancies during the COVID-19 pandemic. Expert Opin Pharmacother. 2021 Apr;22(5):565-582. doi: 10.1080/14656566.2020.

[43] Lamure S, Duléry R, Di Blasi R, Chauchet A, Laureana C, Deau-Fischer B, Drenou B, Soussain C, Rossi C, Noël N, Choquet S, Bologna S, Joly B, Kohn M, Malak S, Fouquet G, Daguindau E, Bernard S, Thiéblemont C, Cartron G, Lacombe K, Besson C. Determinants of outcome in Covid-19 hospitalized patients with lymphoma: A retrospective multicentric cohort study. EClinicalMedicine. 2020 Oct;27:100549. DOI: 10.1016/j.eclinm.2020.100549.

[44] Capozza MA, Triarico S, Attinà G, Romano A, Mastrangelo S, Maurizi P, Frassanito P, Bianchi F, Verdolotti T, Gessi M, Balducci M, Massimi L, Tamburrini G, Ruggiero A; Gemelli Pediatric Neuro-Oncology Tumor Board. Managing children with brain tumors during the COVID-19 era: Don't stop the care! Comput Struct Biotechnol J. 2021 Jan 12;19:705-709. DOI: 10.1016/j.csbj.2021.01.005.

[45] Sharma A, Bhatt NS, St Martin A, Abid MB, Bloomquist J, Chemaly RF, Dandoy C, Gauthier J, Gowda L, Perales MA, Seropian S, Shaw BE, Tuschl EE, Zeidan AM, Riches ML, Shah GL. Clinical characteristics and outcomes of COVID-19 in hematopoietic stem-cell transplantation recipients: an observational cohort study. Lancet Haematol. 2021 Mar;8(3):e185-e193. DOI: 10.1016/S2352-3026(20)30429-4.

[46] Sharma K, Koirala A, Nicolopoulos K, Chiu C, Wood N, Britton PN. Vaccines for COVID-19: Where do we stand in 2021? Paediatr Respir Rev. 2021 Jul 12:S1526-0542(21)00065-8. DOI: 10.1016/j.prrv.2021.07.001. Epub ahead of print. PMID: 34362666; PMCID: PMC8274273.

[47] Emergency Use Authorization of the Pfizer-BioNTech COVID-19 Vaccine to Prevent Coronavirus. Fact sheet for health care providers administering vaccine. https://www.fda.gov/media/144413/download (Accessed on February 25, 2021)

[48] Emergency Use Authorization of the Moderna COVID-19 Vaccine to Prevent Coronavirus. Fact sheet for health care providers administering vaccine. https://www.fda.gov/media/144637/download?utm_medium=emailutm_source=govdelivery (Accessed on December 18, 2020).

[49] Tanne JH. Covid-19: FDA approves Pfizer-BioNTech vaccine in record time. BMJ. 2021 Aug 24;374:n2096. doi: 10.1136/bmj.n2096. PMID: 34429279.

[50] Kamidani S, Rostad CA, Anderson EJ. COVID-19 vaccine development: a pediatric perspective. Curr Opin Pediatr. 2021 Feb 1;33(1):144-151. DOI: 10.1097/MOP.0000000000000978.

Section 4

# Impact of COVID-19 in Health Care System

Chapter 9

# Economic, Health-Care and Teaching-Learning Impact of COVID-19 (SARS-CoV-2) on Dentistry

*Alba Pérez González, Cintia Chamorro Petronacci, Karem L. Ortega, Eva M. Otero Rey and Mario Pérez-Sayáns*

## Abstract

The aim of this chapter is to look more closely at the impact that the crisis generated by the SARS-CoV-2 is having on health, the economy and education in the field of dentistry. The considerations that must be taken into account in dental practice will be presented, as well as the usefulness that the use of teledentistry (TD) could have in times of pandemic, reflecting on the different specialties of dentistry that can benefit from this modality, as well as the advantages and disadvantages that its use can present. Likewise, teaching has been condemned to a lack of presence, having to resort to distance learning, both synchronous and non-synchronous, which can cause needs and deficiencies in undergraduate and postgraduate students. We will analyse the health risks in the dental field and the changes and needs for safe dentistry in times of pandemic. We will also break down the effect of the crisis on the medical-dental sector and the economy, from the point of view of patients and professionals, especially in times of increased restriction and confinement worldwide.

**Keywords:** oral health, protection, COVID-19, crisis, education, teledentistry, SARS-Cov-2, pandemics

## 1. Introduction

Severe acute respiratory syndrome coronavirus 2 (SARS-CoV-2), the causal agent of coronavirus disease (COVID-19), is a 60–140 nm single-stranded RNA virus that belongs to the genus β-Coronavirus, has a corona appearance because of the presence of glycoproteins in the envelope, and it is substantially different genetically from MERS-Cov but similar to SARS-CoV [1]. It can be transmitted between humans and its intermediate host is still under investigation [2]. The Covid-19 pandemic has caused huge changes in all fields, including dentistry.

It is known that several viruses, such as herpes simplex virus, cytomegalovirus and Zika are transmitted through saliva and are able to infect and replicate in the oral mucosa, causing painful ulcers. Currently some authors have reported oral manifestations of COVID-19 disease [3]. These can have a variety of clinical presentations, presumably supporting the hypothesis of thrombus formation and vasculitis [4]. These include necrotic ulcers and aphthous ulcerations that develop early in the course of the disease, as well as dysgeusia. Awareness of these oral manifestations is important because lesions may precede typical respiratory symptoms by several days, and worsening oral lesions may precede a more severe clinical scenario [3].

Saliva from asymptomatic persons with COVID-19 has also been observed to have potential for viral transmission and a positive correlation between salivary viral load and loss of taste [5]. SARS-CoV-2 utilises host entry factors, such as members of the ACE2 (angiotensin-converting enzyme, the major host cell receptor of SARS-CoV-2) and TMPRSS (TMPRSS2 and TMPRSS4) family that have been expressed in salivary glands and oral mucosal epithelia [5, 6]. These data demonstrate that the oral cavity is an important site for SARS-CoV-2 infection and implicate saliva as a possible route of SARS-CoV-2 transmission.

In addition, it is considered that some oral diseases could be exacerbated by COVID-19, especially those of autoimmune aetiology, as these are related to a compromised immune system or long-term pharmacotherapy, [7], which indicates that we should pay special attention to the dental care of these patients. Patients with oral psychosomatic illnesses are more susceptible to stress and this could be exacerbated in the current pandemic situation, so they may need emergency consultations and psychological counselling. The dentist must provide comprehensive care to patients and to this end, teleconsultation may be useful. [8].

Healthcare workers have a higher rate of exposure to the virus (face-to-face interaction, exposure to body fluids such as blood and saliva) which increases the risk of infection, as we try to illustrate in **Figure 1**. Dental practice presents a potential risk of cross-contamination and staff are at risk of transmission of infections. [9] In this situation, it may be advisable to use teleconsultations. The advantages of teledentistry (TD) during the COVID-19 crisis have been observed through a pilot study, where it was determined that TD allowed a monitoring of all patients, reducing costs and contact, therefore decreasing the risk of COVID-19 spreading [10]. The Australian Dental Association has published the guidelines for TD and it considers that teleconsultation is most suited to patients who require follow up, and, likewise it is very convenient for patients presenting with an acute dental problem that needs to be deal with outside of normal practising hours, for those who are unable to attend the clinic due to illness or quarantine, and for vulnerable patients

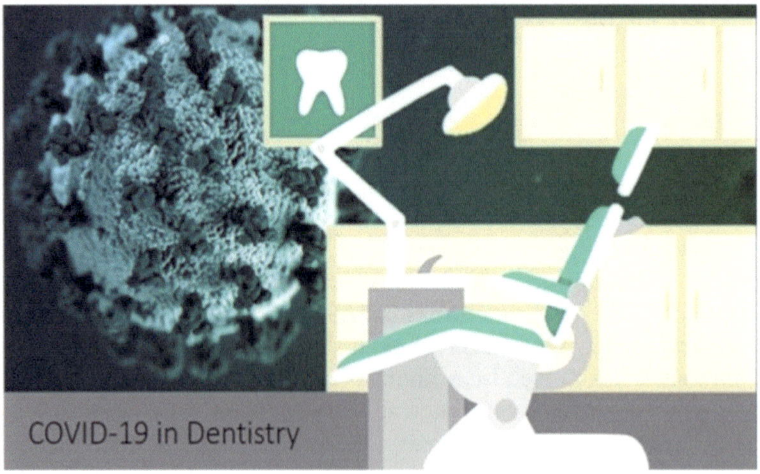


**Figure 1.**
*SARS-CoV-2 in dentistry.*

during the pandemic, including those who meet the triage protocol criteria for suspected Covid-19 infection [11].

## 2. Clinical considerations

Dental professionals must examine and detect potential high-risk patients to prevent the dissemination of infectious disease. No routine treatment should be carried out on patients in the early stages of infection [1].

### 2.1 Telephone triage

We will ask the following dichotomous questions over the phone and repeat them when the patient arrives at the clinic.

- Do you have fever or have you had one in the last 14 days (temperature > 37.5°C)?
- Have you had a cough or any other respiratory sign in the last 14 days?
- Have you had or do you have diarrhoea or other digestive problems in the last 14 days?
- Do you have or have you had a feeling of great tiredness or discomfort in the last 14 days?
- Have you noticed a loss of sense of taste or smell in the last 14 days?
- Have you been in contact or living with someone suspected or diagnosed to have coronavirus?
- Has COVID-19 disease passed?
- If so, are you still in quarantine?

In order to make a decision, we must act as follows:

- In the case of the 8 negative responses:
    - Patient with more than 37.5° (99.5°F) do not treat unless it is urgent, postpone 14 days to see evolution.
    - Patients with less than 37.5° will be treated with the indicated protocols
- At least one affirmative answer
    - Patient with more than 37.5° do not treat except as a matter of urgency
    - Patients with less than 37.5°, it is advisable to postpone the treatments for 14 days.
- If it is an emergency (cellulitis, abscess, haemorrhage, severe trauma...) the patient will be attended under maximum safety conditions.

When the patient is summoned by telephone, he/she must be informed of the recommendations for coming to the clinic:

- o The patient should go alone (unless he/she is a minor or a person in need of help).
- o Bracelets, rings, earrings, watches, etc. should be removed. The patient should arrive at the agreed time and avoid bringing bags and unnecessary personal objects.
- o As soon as the patient arrives, his your temperature will be taken by means of an infrared thermometer, he will be asked to rub his hands with hydroalcoholic gel for 20 seconds and to answer the questionnaire. The patient should maintain a distance of 2 metres if he or she crosses someone and should not wander.

The patient must be made aware of the importance of preventive measures. At the same time, we must convey to him/her the feeling that he/she is in a place where all preventive and safety measures are being followed.

### 2.2 Hand hygiene and personal protective equipment (PPE)

The WHO in 2012 recommends that hand hygiene should be performed before touching a patient, before any cleaning or aseptic procedure, after body fluid exposure risk, after touching a patient and after touching a patient's surroundings [12].

In the dental practice, the spread of micro-organisms is mainly radiated to the dentist's face, specifically to the eyes and around the nose [13] therefore personal protective equipment (PPE) should be used. PPE forms an effective barrier against most of the aerosols generated [14].

- Respirators.

Filtering facepiece respirators, also known as disposable respirators, are subject to different rules worldwide. Their use is recommended by dentists as they are continuously exposed to aerosols [15]. Before selecting one, users should consult their local regulations and requirements for respiratory protection.

The standardisation methods used in the different countries are as follows [16].

1. N95 (United States NIOSH-42CFR84).
2. Filtering facepiece particles 2 (FFP2) (Europe EN 149–2001).
3. KN95 (China GB2626–2006).
4. P2 (Australia/New Zealand AS/NZA 1716:2012).
5. Korea 1st class (Korea KMOEL-2017-2064).
6. DS (Japan JMHLW-Notification 214, 2018).

Under no circumstances should they include an exhalation valve, as in this case the air is exhaled directly into the environment without any retention, favouring the diffusion of the virus We must bear in mind that these should not be sterilised and at most can be disinfected through different methods depending on the type, which will not increase the number of times or time we can use it [17, 18].

- Gloves.

  They should always be used as usual in daily clinical activity. It is recommended to use gloves that protect against viruses (EN ISO 374-5) made of nitrile. For cleaning and disinfection tasks, it is recommended to use thicker, more break-resistant gloves.

- Eye and face protection.

  The eye protectors certified according to the UNE-EN 166:2002 standard for protection against liquids can be integral glasses or face shields. They should always be used as COVID-19 can be transmitted through eye contact, as infectious droplets could contaminate the conjunctival epithelium [19].

- Protective clothing,

  We should avoid using street clothes or shoes in the clinic, avoiding wearing earrings, rings, bracelets, watches and other elements, as they behave as reservoirs of COVID-19.

In **Table 1** we can see in what order we should put on and take off the PPE. With the PPE on we must keep our hands away from our face and avoid touching surfaces. When we remove the personal protective equipment, we must disinfect it. PPE must be kept in a proper place and different from the place where we leave our street clothes.

### 2.3 The patient in the cabinet

The patient must pass with the mask on and it will be removed at the time indicated by the professional.

#### *2.3.1 Rinses*

During dental practice, it is often difficult to avoid the generation of aerosols, which is why it is important to reduce their viral load. To this end, the preoperative use of antiseptic mouthwashes can be useful. SARS-CoV-2 is vulnerable to oxidation, so a pre-procedure mouthwash with oxidising agents such as 1% hydrogen peroxide or 0.2% povidone was initially suggested [1, 9], however, it was recently noted that there is no evidence to support the indication of hydrogen peroxide rinse to reduce viral load of SARS-CoV-2 [20]. A recently published systematic review

| Putting on PPE | Removing PPE |
|---|---|
| 1. Hand hygiene | 1. Protective gown |
| 2. Protective gown | 2. Gloves |
| 3. Mask or respirator | 3. Hand hygiene |
| 4. Check fit | 4. Eye protection |
| 5. Eye protection | 5. Hat: from the back |
| 6. Hat | 6.Respirator: from the back |
| 7. Gloves | 7. Hand hygiene |

**Table 1.**
*In what order should the PPE be put on and taken off.*

has highlighted the lack of scientific evidence to support the virucidal activity of hydrogen peroxide rinse, associated with its lack of substantivity and and its indication in dental care protocols should be reviewed [21] . As for povidone-iodine, it can be an effective measure, having demonstrated 99.99% activity when used against enveloped and non-enveloped viruses such as influenza, Ebola, MERS and SARS coronavirus [22], and has strong bactericidal and virucidal properties against pathogens, which cause oral and respiratory tract infections.

Regarding chlorhexidine, a rinse often used in dental practice, several studies have suggested that it had little or no effect against the virus compared to other rinses [1, 23], but other authors have noted that its use could be beneficial [24].

With regard to Cetylpyridinium chloride (CPC), it could be effective against enveloped viruses such as Sars-Cov 2 [25].

### *2.3.2 Aerosols*

We must bear in mind that any procedure that produces aerosols is potentially risky so high flow suction should be used, as it reduces the dispersion of aerosols, as well as suctioning as close as possible to the treated area. In addition, the cabinet door should remain closed and the cabinet should be aerated between patients.

High-speed rotating instruments must be equipped with an anti-retraction system, which prevents the release of debris and fluids that can accidentally be inhaled during clinical procedures [26]. During the current pandemic, the use of these instruments without an anti-retraction system should be avoided.

The risk of aerosol generation depends very much on the clinical activity performed. The ADA (American Dental Association) classifies the risk into 4 categories:

1. No risk of aerosols (no patient contact)

    - Extraoral radiological diagnosis

2. Low risk of aerosols (contact with patients but no aerosols

    - Diagnosis: clinical examination, intraoral x-rays
    - Prevention: fluoride, atraumatic restorations
    - Surgery: simple exodontia
    - Orthodontics: adjustments

3. Moderate/high risk of aerosols (contact with aerosols, controlled)

    - Prevention: manual tartrectomy, absolute isolation sealant, controlled polishing
    - Restorative: seals with absolute insulation
    - Periodontics: manual treatments
    - Removable prosthodontics: procedures without intraoral adjustments, adjustments after disinfection, prosthodontics on implants
    - Fixed prosthodontics: preparation with absolute isolation, cemented

- Orthodontics: minimum use of rotary

4. Very high risk of aerosols (contact with aerosols, very difficult to control)

   - Prevention: ultrasound tartrectomy
   - Restorative: seals with high speed or without absolute insulation
   - Endodontics: no absolute isolation
   - Periodontics: ultrasonic treatments
   - Removable prosthodontics: intraoral adjustments
   - Fixed prosthodontics: no absolute isolation
   - Surgery: surgical extraction
   - Orthodontics: with generation of aerosols

#### *2.3.3 Rubber dam*

One of the easiest and most useful ways to reduce contamination is isolation with rubber dams, especially in those procedures performed with high-speed instruments. This isolation provides a 70% reduction in drops around the surgical field [27]. When its use is not feasible, manual instruments should be used to keep aerosol generation to a minimum [28].

#### *2.3.4 X-rays*

X-rays are one of the most commonly used complementary tests. Intraoral x-rays are the most common, however they can stimulate saliva secretion and coughing [26]. Therefore, extraoral x-rays, such as panoramic x-ray and cone beam CT, are suitable alternatives [29].

#### *2.3.5 Disinfection of impressions and prostheses*

Before disinfecting it, it must be washed with water. After disinfecting it, rinse it again. The prints made with alginate must be sprayed with 1% sodium hypochlorite for 10 minutes, those made with elastomers (silicones and polyethers) with the same material for 15–20 minutes. Metal-ceramic prostheses and skeletal prostheses should be immersed in alcohol for 5 minutes, acrylics should be immersed in 1% sodium hypochlorite for 10 minutes.

It should be remembered that solutions prepared with sodium hypochlorite have a 24-hour efficacy and should therefore be prepared daily.

#### *2.3.6 Surface disinfection*

Human coronaviruses, such as SARS and MERS, can persist on inanimate surfaces for up to 9 days and yet can be efficiently inactivated by surface disinfectants within one minute. Surfaces should be disinfected after each patient visit, especially surfaces near work areas.

Ethanol between 62% and 71%, and sodium hypochlorite between 0.1% and 0.5% are considered to be the most effective [23, 26].

Initially Kampf et al. have suggested that 0.5% hydrogen peroxide applied for one minute could be effective against the virus [23] however a study by our group has observed that this is not the case [20] There is no study in the literature demonstrating its effect at this concentration during that time and the authors portrayed themselves shortly afterwards, indicating that their results can only be attributed to 0.5% hydrogen peroxide in an accelerated form [30].

### *2.3.7 Environmental disinfection*

The greatest number of SARS-CoV 2 infections occur in closed spaces, such as the dental cabinet, as the virus can persist viable in the air for hours [31]. Transmission of the virus through aerosols is affected by many factors, such as the physical parameters of the particles, properties of the virus and environmental factors [32]. It has been observed that the aerosols generated in the clinic are kept in the air for 30 minutes and that the procedures that produce the most contamination are those where ultrasound is used [33] and the turbine [34].

In these cases, ventilation is essential to produce a renewal of the air. Ventilation consists of providing outside air to an enclosed space and is a key factor in the elimination of virus-laden air, since it reduces the concentration of the virus and thus reduces the possibility of contagion [35]. It can be done through natural methods, such as opening windows (which has proved effective in the current pandemic [36]) or mechanical methods such as air conditioning and can be complemented by air filtration and disinfection systems.

If natural methods are used, an estimate of the external flow rate must be made in each case as it depends largely on specific local conditions (such as the size of openings and weather conditions). If the temperature in the clinic is unpleasant because it is too low, additional heating methods should be used. In addition, air recirculation should be avoided, as well as overcrowding in the room [35]. Filtration of contaminated air can also be useful, there are different methods, the most used being HEPA [37]. HEPA is an acronym for "High Efficiency Particulate Air Filter" which can remove at least 99.97% of any airborne particles with a size of 0.3 micron (μm), the most penetrating particle size. Particles that are larger or smaller are trapped with even greater efficiency [38]. If filtration systems are used, the manufacturer's maintenance recommendations must be followed.

Different methods have been used to disinfect the air in the current pandemic, including ultraviolet radiation and ozone. Ultraviolet (UV) germicidal radiation can damage microbial DNA and RNA, prevent the reproduction of infectious organisms and reduce the harmful effects they cause [39]. Ultraviolet germicidal irradiation (UVGI) uses UVC radiation to inactivate microorganisms by causing DNA damage and preventing replication. It has been noted that UVC can inactivate coronaviruses [40]. Ozone is a natural gas and an effective environmental sanitation system that provides highly reactive free radicals capable of oxidising bacteria, viruses and organic and inorganic compounds [41].

If there is no natural or artificial ventilation, wait half an hour for the aerosols to settle and then clean the surfaces.

## 3. Applications of distance dentistry

Although there is a need to reduce face-to-face visits to decrease the risk of infection, dentists must ensure continuity of care and "teleodontology" or "teledentistry" (TD) is a solution of choice [42]. In periods of pandemic, in many medical specialties as well as in dentistry, teleconsultation can be an effective alternative to office visits in many oral diseases, (as shown in **Figure 2**) while in a normal setting, this system could be used as a complement.

In the case of patients with COVID-19, or those who suspect they may be infected, TD can assist in remote assessment (triage) and continuity of care. For people who are not infected with the virus, particularly those at higher risk of being affected, TD can provide rapid access to care [43].

Teledentistry (TD) could be described as the combination of telecommunications and dentistry that involves the exchange of clinical information and images over remote distances for dental consultation, diagnosis and treatment planning. There are two main types of teleconsultation: real-time or synchronous and store-and-forward or asynchronous.

Real-time consultation requires a video conference in which the dentist and patient can see, hear and communicate with each other despite being in different locations. The benefit of the real-time consultation format is that information is transferred immediately, so patients and dentists are able to interact with each other regarding dental health issues.

The store-and-forward format enables a patient to store data in a local database that is subsequently forwarded to the dentist. In this system the patient's relevant information and images are collected and stored before being reviewed by the dentist at a later stage. After reviewing the information, the dentist is able to present their diagnosis and subsequent treatment plan. This methodology has several advantages over real time telemedicine systems; the most important being the fact that it is not necessary for the patient and the consultant to coincide in time and space, and furthermore, this system makes it possible for the technological and organisational difficulties that are commonplace during consultations via videoconference to be avoided. It also allows for a greater number of patients to be evaluated per session, and it is also cost-effective as it makes use of already-existing elements, such as e-mail and the upcoming digitalisation of radiology in the hospital.

There is a growing interest in adopting telemedicine systems given that these contribute to the reduction of inequalities in health care [44]. In general, TD can be a useful tool in practically all fields of dentistry, especially during a pandemic in which social distancing is of the utmost importance, given that it saves time for both the patients and the health-care practitioner and it is also more cost-effective.

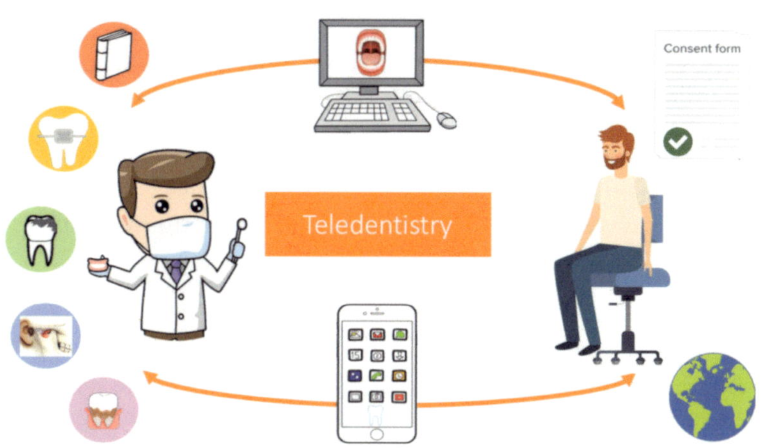


**Figure 2.**
*Teleconsultation in dentistry.*

| | |
|---|---|
| Oral Medicine | Diagnosis, treatment, follow-up |
| Maxillofacial | Diagnosis, referrals, follow-up |
| Orthodontics | Diagnosis, emergencies, follow-up |
| Traumatology | Diagnosis, follow-up |
| Periodontics | Diagnosis (mucositis, periimplantitis, tartar detection, mobility...) |
| Caries | Diagnosis (detection) |
| Endodontics | Diagnosis, recognition of root canal, follow-up |
| Paediatrics | Diagnosis (caries, anomalies, fluorosis, MIH...) |
| Prosthodontics | CAD-CAM, diagnosis, treatment plan, follow-up, urgencies |
| Gerodontology | Diagnosis, follow-up |
| Education | Professionals and students (training and updating) |
| | Patients (Instruction) |

**Table 2.**
*Main uses of teledentistry.*

| PROS | CONS |
|---|---|
| It saves time<br>There is a financial saving<br>It reduces inequalities (geographical barriers)<br>It improves communication between professionals<br>It reduces patient anxiety | It requires access to a software, hardware and the necessary skills to use it<br>People may feel uneasy about using technology<br>Certain clinical tests such as palpation or radiographs cannot be performed<br>Privacy related problems may exist |

**Table 3.**
*Advantages and disadvantages of using teledentistry.*

Although visits to the dental surgery are still necessary for many procedures, TD opens new horizons for the diagnosis, treatment and follow-up of many patients, as we can see in **Table 2**.

In almost all of the fields, referrals by teleconsultation are considered very useful in reducing other unnecessary referrals. Several studies have shown that telemedicine consultations are as reliable as those performed by traditional methods [45].

Teleconsultation offers many advantages, including it can reduce a patient's dental anxiety, which can be important for people who have an irrational fear of dentists, for children and for patients with special needs. Although it also has limitations (**Table 3**), its use is widespread and there are a growing number of applications for mobile phones and videoconferencing programmes being developed for this purpose. In general, the perceptions of professionals and patients are positive, although in many cases they receive limited training about this technology.

## 4. Education

This pandemic has also led to changes in education all over the world due to the social distancing measures. The impact of the COVID-19 pandemic greatly affected dental education, with smart technology showing certain benefits in the learning process [46]. The training of future health science professionals is changing thanks to this digital age. Mariño et al. discovered that the field in which TD was used most was education [47]. It can be an excellent tool for dentistry students, keeping dentists continuously updated.

E-learning offers advantages for students such as eliminating travel time and encouraging student-teacher interactions. Online education connects students and teachers geographically, making the university more universal and accessible [28, 48]. Some disadvantages of online courses for the student may include a sense of isolation and difficulty in adjusting, and may also lead to misperceptions and misunderstandings between students and teachers [49]. Although these virtual tools were previously available, their use and exploitation in the Covid-19 crisis has changed substantially. Recent studies confirm that training based on digital tools can improve the learning and clinical decision-making skills of dental students [50–53] especially in the pre-clinical setting [54]. According to Mardani et al. [55], in a study among dental students divided into virtual (intervention) and face-to-face (control) training, the mean clinical decision-making score in the intervention group was higher than the control group ($p < 0.001$), indicating that the application of virtual patient-based training can enhance students′ skills.

In a previous study carried out by the group studied the perceptions of teachers in Galicia, Spain with regards to online teaching, it was observed that prior to the Covid-19 crisis, 49.2% of teachers did not use any of the available online tools, but as a result of this health crisis their usage has increased [56]. However, the synchronous method is seldom used.

It can also be used for teaching patients. The effectiveness of a mobile phone app in educating mothers of children aged below 6 years of age about oral hygiene has also been studied, and it was discovered that using this app significantly improves the knowledge of mothers towards their child's oral health [57].

## 5. Health and economic impact

In Beijing, China, 2,537 participants evaluated how the pandemic influenced the use of emergency dental services and noted that the distribution of dental problems has varied significantly. Oral infections increased from 51.0% before COVID-19 to 71.9% during COVID-19, and injuries decreased from 14.2% to 10.5%. Meanwhile, non-urgent cases decreased to three tenths of pre-COVID-19 cases [58].

Costs of dental care may increase in the future for a number of reasons, including the need for additional resources such as personal protective equipment, changes in dental practice and the fact that the number of patients we will be able to see each day will decrease due to the measures taken. There may also be an increased demand for electronic consultations in the near future [59].

A study of 400 dentists in Galicia, Spain to determine the economic and health impact of SARS-CoV-2 found that the economic impact appeared to be greater for male participants than for female participants ($OR = 3,121$, $p < 0.001$). These losses appear to have contributed to the requests for financial support, with 29.5% of respondents who requested financial support recording losses of more than 15,000 euros. The number of patients treated was reduced, although it was noted that more urgent patients were seen per week in the public sector than in private clinics. In terms of health, only four professionals tested positive [60].

To date, we have not found any other document that addresses the economic impact of COVID-19 in dentistry, however, the impact on patient loss and income from SARS CoV-1 in Taiwan has been studied between 2000 and 2003. Significant reductions in dental care (16.7%) have been observed, so fears of COVID-19 significantly affected people's care-seeking behaviour and this fear compromised their accessibility to quality care [61].

Anxiety and fear of becoming infected with COVID-19 among dentists has also been studied in a cross-sectional study with 669 participants from different countries around the world. More than two-thirds were found to be frightened by the effects of the virus and 90% were aware of recent changes in treatment protocols. Dentists around the world, despite their high level of knowledge, are in a state of fear while working due to the impact of the virus [62]. A multi-country study found that in general, most dentists had good knowledge and practice scores with respect to SARS-CoV-2 [63]. As fear among the population to visit dentists after the outbreak of COVID-19 could decrease the demand for conservative dental treatment and increase emergency treatment [59].

## 6. Conclusions

The SARS-CoV-2 virus outbreak has had many immediate complications for dentistry, some of which may have more long-term repercussions in the clinic. COVID-19 forces oral health care personnel to understand the implications of the outbreak in their clinical setting and to be aware of possible changes and updates to protocols. New approaches such as teleconsultation could be very useful. Teledentistry will help to assist patients without the need for contact, reducing consultation time and costs. Modern forms of online information-based education have also seen increased use during the current pandemic. Negative oral health and economic impacts have been observed in the dental sector, however more global studies are needed to examine the health and economic impact that the virus is having on both public and private dental clinics.

## Conflict of interest

The authors declared that there is no conflict of interest.

## Author details

Alba Pérez González[1], Cintia Chamorro Petronacci[2], Karem L. Ortega[3], Eva M. Otero Rey[4] and Mario Pérez-Sayáns[1,2]*

1 Faculty of Medicine and Dentistry, Oral Medicine, Oral Surgery and Implantology Unit (MedOralRes), Universidade de Santiago de Compostela, Spain

2 Instituto de Investigación Sanitaria de Santiago de Compostela (IDIS), Spain

3 Department of Stomatology, School of Dentistry, University of Sao Paulo, Sao Paulo, Brazil

4 Restorative Dentistry and Endodontology Unit, Faculty of Medicine and Dentistry, Universidade de Santiago de Compostela, Spain

*Address all correspondence to: marioperezsayans@usc.es

## References

[1] Peng X, Xu X, Li Y, Cheng L, Zhou X, Ren B. Transmission routes of 2019-nCoV and controls in dental practice. International Journal of Oral Science 2020 -03-03;12(1):1-6.

[2] Wang N, Shang J, Jiang S, Du L. Subunit vaccines against emerging pathogenic human coronaviruses. Front Microbiol 2020;11.

[3] Brandão TB, Gueiros LA, Melo TS, Prado-Ribeiro AC, Nesrallah, Ana Cristina Froelich Alo, Prado GVB, et al. Oral lesions in patients with SARS-CoV-2 infection: could the oral cavity be a target organ? Oral Surg Oral Med Oral Pathol Oral Radiol 2021 -02;131(2):e45-e51.

[4] Cruz Tapia RO, Peraza Labrador AJ, Guimaraes DM, Matos Valdez LH. Oral mucosal lesions in patients with SARS-CoV-2 infection. Report of four cases. Are they a true sign of COVID-19 disease? Spec Care Dentist 2020 -11;40(6):555-560.

[5] Huang N, Pérez P, Kato T, Mikami Y, Okuda K, Gilmore RC, et al. SARS-CoV-2 infection of the oral cavity and saliva. Nat Med 2021 -03-25.

[6] Xu J, Li Y, Gan F, Du Y, Yao Y. Salivary Glands: Potential Reservoirs for COVID-19 Asymptomatic Infection. J Dent Res 2020;99(8):989-989.

[7] Dziedzic A, Wojtyczka R. The impact of coronavirus infectious disease 19 (COVID-19) on oral health. Oral Dis 2020.

[8] Qu X, Zhou XD. [Psychological intervention for patients with oral disease during the pandemic period of COVID-19]. Zhonghua Kou Qiang Yi Xue Za Zhi 2020;55(4):235-240.

[9] Fallahi HR, Keyhan SO, Zandian D, Kim S, Cheshmi B. Being a front-line dentist during the Covid-19 pandemic: A literature review. Maxillofacial Plastic and Reconstructive Surgery 2020 Dec;42(1):12.

[10] Giudice A, Barone S, Muraca D, Averta F, Diodati F, Antonelli A, et al. Can Teledentistry Improve the Monitoring of Patients during the Covid-19 Dissemination? A Descriptive Pilot Study. Int J Environ Res Public Health 2020;17(10).

[11] The Australian Dental Association. 2020; Available at: https://www.ada.org.au/Covid-19-Portal/Cards/Dental-Profesionals/Practice-Policies/ADA-Guidelines-for-Teledentistry. Accessed Aug 29, 2020.

[12] Your 5 Moments for Hand Hygiene Dental Care. 2012; Available at: https://www.who.int/gpsc/information_centre/es/. Accessed Nov 8, 2020.

[13] Nejatidanesh F, Khosravi Z, Goroohi H, Badrian H, Savabi O. Risk of Contamination of Different Areas of Dentist's Face During Dental Practices. Int J Prev Med 2013 -5;4(5):611-615.

[14] Baghizadeh Fini M. What dentists need to know about COVID-19. Oral Oncol 2020 06;105:104741.

[15] Checchi V, Bellini P, Bencivenni D, Consolo U. COVID-19 dentistry-related aspects: A literature overview. Int Dent J 2020 Jul 05,.

[16] Comparison of FFP2, KN95, and N95 Filtering Facepiece Respirator Classes. 3M Science. Revision 4. Techn Bull 2020 May:1-3.

[17] CDC. Implementing Filtering Facepiece Respirator (FFR) Reuse, Including Reuse after Decontamination, When There Are Known Shortages of N95 Respirators. 2020; Available at: https://www.cdc.gov/

coronavirus/2019-ncov/hcp/ppe-strategy/decontamination-reuse-respirators.html. Accessed Nov 7, 2020.

[18] Strategies for Optimizing the Supply of N95 Respirators. 2020; Available at: https://www.cdc.gov/coronavirus/2019-ncov/hcp/n95-other-respirators.html. Accessed Nov 7, 2020.

[19] Lu C, Liu X, Jia Z. 2019-nCoV transmission through the ocular surface must not be ignored. The lancet (British edition) 2020;395(10224):e39.

[20] Ortega KL, Rech BdO, Costa ALF, Sayans MP, Braz-Silva PH. Is 0.5% hydrogen peroxide effective against SARS-CoV-2? Oral Diseases 2020;n/a(n/a).

[21] K.L. Ortega, B.O. Rech, G.L.C. El Haje, C.B. Gallo, M. Pérez-Sayáns, P.H. Braz-Silva. Do hydrogen peroxide mouthwashes have a virucidal effect? A systematic review . 2020;0(0).

[22] Eggers M. Infectious disease management and control with povidone iodine. Infectious Diseases and Therapy 2019 Dec;8(4):581-593.

[23] Kampf G, Todt D, Pfaender S, Steinmann E. Persistence of coronaviruses on inanimate surfaces and their inactivation with biocidal agents. The Journal of hospital infection 2020;104(3):246-251.

[24] Yoon JG, Yoon J, Song JY, Yoon SY, Lim CS, Seong H, et al. Clinical Significance of a High SARS-CoV-2 Viral Load in the Saliva. Journal of Korean medical science 2020 May 25,;35(20):e195.

[25] Vergara-Buenaventura A, Castro-Ruiz C. Use of mouthwashes against COVID-19 in dentistry. Br J Oral Maxillofac Surg 2020 -10;58(8):924-927.

[26] Villani FA, Aiuto R, Paglia L, Re D. COVID-19 and Dentistry: Prevention in Dental Practice, a Literature Review. Int J Environ Res Public Health 2020 06 26,;17(12).

[27] Samaranayake LP, Reid J, Evans D. The efficacy of rubber dam isolation in reducing atmospheric bacterial contamination. ASDC J Dent Child 1989 Nov-Dec;56(6):442-444.

[28] Samaranayake LP, Peiris M. Severe acute respiratory syndrome and dentistry: A retrospective view. J Am Dent Assoc 2004 Sep;135(9):1292-1302.

[29] Meng L, Hua F, Bian Z. Coronavirus Disease 2019 (COVID-19): Emerging and Future Challenges for Dental and Oral Medicine. Journal of Dental Research 2020 05;99(5):481-487.

[30] Kampf G, Todt D, Pfaender S, Steinmann E. Corrigendum to "Persistence of coronaviruses on inanimate surfaces and their inactivation with biocidal agents" [J Hosp Infect 104 (2020) 246-251]. J Hosp Infect 2020 Jun 17,.

[31] van Doremalen N, Bushmaker T, Morris DH, Holbrook MG, Gamble A, Williamson BN, et al. Aerosol and Surface Stability of SARS-CoV-2 as Compared with SARS-CoV-1. New England Journal of Medicine 2020 April 16,;382(16):1564-1567.

[32] Zhang Y, Leung NHL, Cowling BJ, Yang Z. Role of viral bioaerosols in nosocomial infections and measures for prevention and control. Journal of aerosol science 1970;117:200-211.

[33] Veena HR, Mahantesha S, Joseph PA, Patil SR, Patil SH. Dissemination of aerosol and splatter during ultrasonic scaling: A pilot study. Journal of infection and public health 2015 May;8(3):260-265.

[34] Allison JR, Currie CC, Edwards DC, Bowes C, Coulter J, Pickering K, et al. Evaluating aerosol and splatter

following dental procedures: Addressing new challenges for oral health care and rehabilitation. Journal of Oral Rehabilitation ;n/a(n/a).

[35] Morawska L, Tang JW, Bahnfleth W, Bluyssen PM, Boerstra A, Buonanno G, et al. Environment international. Environment international 1978;142:105832.

[36] Howard-Reed C, Wallace LA, Ott WR. The effect of opening windows on air change rates in two homes. J Air Waste Manag Assoc 2002 Feb;52(2):147-159.

[37] Ge Z, Yang L, Xia J, Fu X, Zhang Y. Possible aerosol transmission of COVID-19 and special precautions in dentistry. Journal of Zhejiang University. B. Science 2020 May;21(5):361-368.

[38] US EPA O. What Is a HEPA Filter? 2019; Available at: https://www.epa.gov/indoor-air-quality-iaq/what-hepa-filter-1. Accessed Nov 6, 2020.

[39] Qureshi Z, Yassin MH. Role of ultraviolet (UV) disinfection in infection control and environmental cleaning. Infectious Disorders Drug Targets 2013 Jun;13(3):191-195.

[40] Hamzavi IH, Lyons AB, Kohli I, Narla S, Parks-Miller A, Gelfand JM, et al. Ultraviolet germicidal irradiation: Possible method for respirator disinfection to facilitate reuse during the COVID-19 pandemic. J Am Acad Dermatol 2020 -6;82(6):1511-1512.

[41] Martinelli M, Giovannangeli F, Rotunno S, Trombetta CM, Montomoli E. Water and air ozone treatment as an alternativesanitizing technology. J Prev Med Hyg 2017 -3;58(1):E48-E52.

[42] Maret D, Peters OA, Vaysse F, Vigarios E. Integration of telemedicine into the public health response to COVID-19 must include dentists. International Endodontic Journal 2020;53(6):880-881.

[43] Smith AC, Thomas E, Snoswell CL, Haydon H, Mehrotra A, Clemensen J, et al. Telehealth for global emergencies: Implications for coronavirus disease 2019 (COVID-19). J Telemed Telecare 2020 June 1,;26(5):309-313.

[44] Bhanushali P, Katge F, Deshpande S, Chimata VK, Shetty S, Pradhan D. COVID-19: Changing Trends and Its Impact on Future of Dentistry. International journal of dentistry 2020 May 29,;2020:1-6.

[45] Alabdullah JH, Daniel SJ. A systematic review on the validity of Teledentistry. Telemed J E Health 2018;24(8):639-648.

[46] Chang T, Hong G, Paganelli C, Phantumvanit P, Chang W, Shieh Y, et al. Innovation of dental education during COVID-19 pandemic. Journal of Dental Sciences 2020 Aug 19,.

[47] Mariño R, Ghanim A. Teledentistry: A systematic review of the literature. J Telemed Telecare 2013;19(4):179-183.

[48] Bigony L. Can you go the distance? Attending the virtual classroom. Orthopedic Nursing 2010 Nov-Dec;29(6):390-392.

[49] Swartzwelder K, Clements P, Holt K, Childs G. Confronting Incivility in the Online Classroom. Journal of Christian Nursing: A Quarterly Publication of Nurses Christian Fellowship 2019 Apr/Jun;36(2):104-111.

[50] Thilakumara IP, Jayasinghe RM, Rasnayaka SK, Jayasinghe VP, Abeysundara S. Effectiveness of procedural video versus live demonstrations in teaching laboratory techniques to dental students. Journal of Dental Education 2018 Aug;82(8): 898-904.

[51] Abdul-Razzak S. Evaluation of the first year of Dental Health Partnerships: a web-based distance learning partnership between UK dental educators and students from low-resource countries. British Dental Journal 2018 08 10,;225(3):252-256.

[52] Chen Y, Hsue S, Lin D, Wang W, Chen J, Lin C, et al. An application of virtual microscopy in the teaching of an oral and maxillofacial pathology laboratory course. Oral Surgery, Oral Medicine, Oral Pathology, Oral Radiology, and Endodontics 2008 Mar;105(3):342-347.

[53] Broudo M, Walsh C. MEDICOL: Online learning in medicine and dentistry. Academic Medicine: Journal of the Association of American Medical Colleges 2002 Sep;77(9):926-927.

[54] Towers A, Field J, Stokes C, Maddock S, Martin N. A scoping review of the use and application of virtual reality in pre-clinical dental education. British Dental Journal 2019 03;226(5):358-366.

[55] Mardani M, Cheraghian S, Naeeni SK, Zarifsanaiey N. Effectiveness of virtual patients in teaching clinical decision-making skills to dental students. Journal of Dental Education 2020 May;84(5):615-623.

[56] Sayáns MP, Petronacci CMC, Reboiras D, Gándara P, Torreira MG. Percepción por los docentes de la Facultad de Medicina y Odontología de la USC sobre la docencia virtual y sincrónica tras la crisis del Covid-19. Rev Esp Edu Med 2020 /10/19;1(2):53-64.

[57] AlKlayb SA, Assery MK, AlQahtani A, AlAnazi M, Pani SC. Comparison of the effectiveness of a Mobile phone-based education program in educating mothers as Oral health providers in two regions of Saudi Arabia. J Int Soc Prev Community Dent 2017;7(3):110-115.

[58] Guo H, Zhou Y, Liu X, Tan J. The impact of the COVID-19 epidemic on the utilization of emergency dental services. Journal of Dental Sciences 2020 March 16.

[59] Barabari P, Moharamzadeh K. Novel Coronavirus (COVID-19) and Dentistry–A Comprehensive Review of Literature. Dent J (Basel) 2020 -5-21;8(2).

[60] Chamorro-Petronacci C, Martin Carreras-Presas C, Sanz-Marchena A, A Rodríguez-Fernández M, María Suárez-Quintanilla J, Rivas-Mundiña B, et al. Assessment of the Economic and Health-Care Impact of COVID-19 (SARS-CoV-2) on Public and Private Dental Surgeries in Spain: A Pilot Study. Int J Environ Res Public Health 2020 -7;17(14).

[61] Chang H, Huang N, Lee C, Hsu Y, Hsieh C, Chou Y. The Impact of the SARS Epidemic on the Utilization of Medical Services: SARS and the Fear of SARS. American Journal of Public Health 2004 Apr 1,;94(4):562-564.

[62] Ahmed MA, Jouhar R, Ahmed N, Adnan S, Aftab M, Zafar MS, et al. Fear and Practice Modifications among Dentists to Combat Novel Coronavirus Disease (COVID-19) Outbreak. International Journal of Environmental Research and Public Health 2020 04 19,;17(8).

[63] Kamate SK, Sharma S, Thakar S, Srivastava D, Sengupta K, Hadi AJ, et al. Assessing knowledge, attitudes and practices of dental practitioners regarding the COVID-19 pandemic: A multinational study. Dental and Medical Problems 2020 Jan-Mar;57(1):11-17.

Chapter 10

# COVID-19, Telehealth and Access to Care

*Charles M. Lepkowsky*

## Abstract

Telehealth has become increasingly prominent during the COVID-19 pandemic, highlighting limitations in access to care for older adults less fluent in information technology (IT). Although the 20 percent disparity in IT use between younger and older adult cohorts remains unchanged over several decades, insurers, institutional and independent providers of health care have made increasing use of IT for patient communication. Data demonstrate an age-related decline in the frequency of IT use for accessing health care. Restrictions on reimbursement for the use of the telephone for accessing health care during the COVID-19 pandemic are discussed as a barrier to access to care. Recommendations are made for assessment of media most available to older adults for accessing health care, as well as providing funding to support increased access to care.

**Keywords:** COVID-19, older adults, access to health care, information technology (IT), FACETS

## 1. Introduction

The COVID-19 virus (SARS-CoV-2) was first identified in December of 2019 [1]. COVID-19 spread rapidly, and by the end of January 2020, the World Health Organization (WHO) had officially labeled the COVID-19 outbreak a pandemic [2]. At risk populations were soon identified, including older adults [3–6]. In an effort to contain the growth of the contagion, in early 2020 shelter in place practices were adopted in many countries, forcing the closure of routine businesses including schools, restaurants, and outpatient healthcare facilities [7–11]. Patient care rapidly shifted to virtual contact using telehealth platforms including internet-based videoconferencing software [12]. In the United States (US), the Center for Medicare and Medicaid Services (CMS) made changes liberalizing standards allowing reimbursement for videoconferencing telehealth, increasing access to care [13, 14]. However, the rapid shift to telehealth brought to the forefront an access to care issue that had been simmering for some time: compared with younger age cohorts, most adults over the age of 65 make limited use of information technology (IT) [15–18]. The intersection of the rapid growth of telehealth, age-related declines in IT utilization, and access to care is a growing area of concern for the health care systems with strong implications for the future of healthcare delivery.

## 2. COVID-19: background and description

In December of 2019, a new coronavirus was identified in Wuhan, China. Based on symptom presentation, it was called SARS-CoV-2, and based on the date of identification was later called COVID-19. COCVID-19 spread rapidly. On January 30, 2020 the World Health Organization (WHO) officially declared COVID-19 a public health emergency of international concern, assigning it the status of a pandemic [2]. The first identified symptoms of COVID-19 included fever, cough, fatigue, dyspnea, sore throat, headache, conjunctivitis and gastrointestinal issues. Loss of the senses of smell and taste were soon added to the symptom list. More severe reactions included acute respiratory failure and death [10]. Disproportionate severe acute respiratory symptoms appeared in patients with cardiovascular comorbidities [19–21], which were eventually understood as a consequence of SARS-CoV-2 infecting the host using the angiotensin converting enzyme 2 (ACE2) receptor [22], which is expressed in several organs, including the lung, heart, kidney, and intestine, as well as endothelial cells [23]. It was found that SARS-CoV-2 can directly infect engineered human blood vessel organoids in vitro, and vascular derangements in COVID-19 might reflect endothelial cell involvement by the virus [22].

### 2.1 COVID-19: epidemiology and treatment

COVID-19 transmission appears to occur primarily from direct person to person contact, but infection can also occur through contact with contaminated environmental surfaces. Hand hygiene, wearing personal protective equipment (especially masks covering the nose and mouth) and maintaining social distance (of at least six feet) were soon recommended. COVID-19 testing rapidly evolved using nasal swab, tracheal aspirate or bronchoalveolar lavage samples [11]. A variety of interventions have been employed, but as of the time of this writing, there are no clinically approved vaccines or specific therapeutic drugs available for COVID-19, and quarantine is the only intervention that appears to be effective in decreasing the contagion rate [7–11]. COVID-19 is currently treated with available antiviral drugs, and in severe cases, supportive care including oxygen and mechanical ventilation [24, 25].

The genetic structure, pathogenic mechanism, and clinical characteristics of COVID-19 have been studied extensively [26, 27]. Vaccination against COVID-19 is widely believed to be the most promising path to resolution of the pandemic [28]. Having proven effective against similar coronaviruses SARS-CoV and MERS-CoV, monoclonal antibody vaccination is being pursued by a number of laboratories [29–33].

### 2.2 COVID-19: psychological impact

In addition to the physical threat posed by COVID-19, the pandemic has also had a significant worldwide psychological impact. During the initial stage of the CoViD-19 pandemic, acute psychological reactions were observed among the general population, healthcare workers, clinical populations, and other at risk groups [34–36]. Psychological triage has long been recognized as an essential care component before, during and after emergencies and disasters [12, 37]. Care delivery during the COVID-19 pandemic has been complicated by efforts to shelter in place and minimize personal interactions, leading to a rapid increase in the utilization of telehealth [12].

As the duration of the pandemic grew, increased autonomic arousal in response to fear of contagion soon translated to chronic stress, with consequent elevation in adrenaline and cortisol production, activation of the amygdala, and consequent suppression of activity in the pre-frontal lobe, impairing judgment and impulse control [38–41]. Stress resulting from the effects of the disease itself was multiplied by extended periods of social isolation, further complicated by what has been called an "infodemic:" around the clock news about the pandemic, distributed not only by news media, but also by social media. The widespread use of social media also provided a platform for unprecedented expression of racism, stigmatization, and xenophobia. The intense psychological impact of these combined factors has produced acute panic, anxiety, obsessive behaviors, hoarding, paranoia, and depression, and post-traumatic stress disorder (PTSD) [42].

Populations especially at risk for chronic stress related to COVID-19 include frontline healthcare workers who are at higher risk than other for contracting the disease, and are prone to burnout, anxiety, fear of transmitting infection, feelings of incompatibility, depression, increased substance-dependence, and PTSD. Along with psychiatric patients and marginalized communities, children isolated by school closures and parents responsible for additional child care during school hours, as well as assisting children with distance learning have also been identified as at-risk populations for chronic stress. The psychosocial needs of older adults have been significantly affected by the pandemic [42].

### 2.3 COVID-19 and older adults

Older adults have been identified as a high risk population for severe or fatal responses to COVID-19 [43, 44]. Older adults demonstrate higher peaks of viral load in response to COVID-19, and are in the highest risk group for comorbidities including hypertension, cardiovascular disease, diabetes, chronic respiratory disease, and chronic kidney disease, all of which demonstrate more severe reactions to COVID-19 and higher rates of fatality [3–6]. Increasing the risks associated with COVID-19 for older adults, many patients with hypertension, diabetes, and chronic kidney disease are prescribed medications containing angiotensin-converting enzyme (ACE) inhibitors and angiotensin II receptor blockers. These medications upregulate the ACE-2 receptor, which (as discussed above) is the specific receptor used by the SARS-CoV-2 virus to enter host cells [3, 22, 23].

## 3. COVID-19 and telehealth

The unprecedented social, economic and healthcare challenges presented by COVID-19 include the significant strain on medical center resources, and the need to deliver healthcare at a distance. Telemedicine is a growing methodology that makes possible timely healthcare delivery while minimizing exposure to protect medical practitioners and patients. The combination of these factors quickly led to the rapid adoption of telehealth during the COVID-19 pandemic [45]. Following system-wide expansion of virtual urgent care staff at a large health system at the epicenter of the COVID-19 outbreak in the United States, in a six week period between March 2nd and April 14th 2020 telemedicine visits for urgent healthcare delivery increased 683 percent. The majority of urgent care visits shifted to telemedicine (56.2%), and the utilization of telemedicine was found to be highest among patients 20 to 44 years of age [46]. U.S. healthcare organizations report consistent expansion of telehealth adoption during the 3 phases of the U.S.

COVID-19 pandemic: (1) stay-at-home outpatient care, (2) initial COVID-19 hospital surge, and (3) post-pandemic recovery [47].

A retrospective observational cohort study found an 8729 percent increase in telehealth visit utilization between March 4 and March 31, 2020 during the COVID-19 pandemic compared to the same period the previous year (2019), with patients reporting higher satisfaction for telehealth visits than in-person visits. The authors of the study concluded that patient satisfaction with telemedicine is high and is not a barrier toward a paradigm shift away from traditional in-person clinic visits [48]. A literature review of 35 research studies published from 2019 to May 2020 demonstrated the effectiveness of telemedicine as a healthcare delivery platform. The authors of the literature review concluded that the effectiveness of virtual healthcare delivery suggests increased integration of digital technologies into healthcare in the near future [49].

## 3.1 Disparities in IT utilization

Significant disparities in IT utilization have long been associated with numerous variables, including ethnicity, age, and socioeconomic status (SES) [15, 17]. People with intellectual and developmental disabilities also utilize IT at a significantly lower rate than the general population [50], despite organized efforts to engage young adults with intellectual disability with social media and other IT [51]. Disparities in IT utilization and access have been described as the digital divide [52], digital inequality [53, 54], and digital diversity [55].

In addition to variables including ethnicity, disability, and SES, everyone is affected by the process of aging. In the United States, the number of adults over the age of 65 is expected to more than double from 46.5 million today to over 98 million (nearly 25% of the population) by the year 2060 [56, 57]. People over the age of 65 utilize health care at a significantly higher rate than members of younger age cohorts: 136% of the under 65 group's use of Emergency Department admissions, 263% for inpatient discharges, and 241% for outpatient office visits [58]. Median health care costs for people over the age of 65 are 167% the costs for people 64 and younger [59]. Although older adults' IT use has increased during the last twenty years, it continues to trail behind that of younger age cohorts by at least 20% [15–17], as shown in **Table 1.**

The current disparity in IT utilization between age groups remains consistent with that reported over a decade ago by the U.S. Census Bureau and Bureau of Labor Statistics [15, 18, 55, 60, 61].

## 3.2 Default utilization of IT by insurers: potential barriers to care

Paradoxically, in the face of a substantial and growing body of research data demonstrate disparities in IT utilization between groups associated with numerous variables including age, SES, ethnicity, disability, and educational experience [62],

| Age in years | Access to home high speed internet |
|---|---|
| 18–34 | 79.2% |
| 35–44 | 83.2% |
| 45–64 | 79.1% |
| 65 and older | 59.2% |

**Table 1.**
*IT access and utilization by age: Data from U.S. Census Bureau, 2016.*

over the past decade Medicare and private insurers have increasingly defaulted to the use of IT (websites, MyChart, text messaging) for communication with patients [63–65]. Similarly, hospitals, regional health centers, university teaching hospitals, and local medical clinics have done so [66, 67], in the absence of any data indicating that the populations they serve have fluency with IT [18].

Based on research data demonstrating disparities in IT utilization [15–18, 50–54], the default use of IT for communication with all patients may create a barrier to care for some patient populations. The potential consequence is that patient populations most in need of health care (including older adults) will find it most difficult to access [18, 55, 60, 61]. For older adults, CMS tracks potential access to care issues including economic disparity [68], but it has not addressed IT fluency among older adults [15–18, 55, 60, 61, 69].

## 4. Communication with patients and outcomes: assessment of IT utilization by patient populations

Effective treatment and good outcome rely upon effective communication with patients. Better communication with patients produces better health outcomes and increased ratings of satisfaction by patients and providers of care [70, 71]. Paradoxically, over the past decade health care organizations have defaulted to the use of IT for patient communication, in the absence of any data supporting patient utilization of IT for the purpose of communication with health care providers. With one exception [18, 60, 69, 72], health care protocols, especially for working with older adults, have not included frequency of internet or IT utilization as a specific area of assessment or treatment [18, 55, 60, 61, 69, 72–74]. In fact, the American Psychological Association's (APA's) 21 Guidelines for psychologists working with older adults [75] do not specifically include familiarity with the assessment and treatment of technology challenges or barriers for older adults as a guideline [18, 55, 60, 61, 69].

In general, IT has not been included as area of assessment or treatment in healthcare protocols [18, 55, 60, 61, 69, 72, 74]. Most of the research exploring IT utilization has come from the IT sector [76–88]. Most IT assessment instruments assess the person's perception of their own proficiency with various technologies [89–95]. These instruments and studies assess factors determining a person's decision to use specific technologies, or self-perceived proficiency in using specific technologies, but none of them assesses the person's frequency of actual IT use or perhaps more importantly, the person's frequency of different kinds of IT use, information necessary for individualized treatment planning using media that allows effective communication with the specific patient to facilitate better treatment outcomes [18, 55, 60, 61, 69]. The Functional Assessment of Currently Employed Technology Scale (FACETS, Appendix 1) [18, 69] was designed specifically to meet those previously unaddressed needs.

### 4.1 The Functional Assessment of Currently Employed Technology Scale (FACETS): description, reliability and validity

The Functional Assessment of Currently Employed Technology Scale (FACETS) is a 10-item questionnaire that can be completed in one to three minutes. It asks two questions in each of 5 functional IT domains: Home, Social, E-commerce, Health Care, and Technical [18, 60, 69]. For each question there are 6 optional answers, characterizing the respondent's frequency of use for the specific type of IT referenced in the question. Higher scores are associated with more frequent utilization of IT. A subtotal score for each functional domain is derived from summating the scores for the two questions in that domain. The combined total of the subtotal scores from each of the functional domains yields an overall FACETS score. Higher utilization of IT across domains produces a higher overall FACETS score. High reliability and validity have been found for FACETS, including multiple group factor analysis, McDonald's omega, Cronbach's alpha coefficient, and confidence intervals for alpha and omega [69].

### 4.2 FACETS outcome research

FACETS outcome research has been conducted with populations of varied age, ethnicity, socio-economic status, household income, and educational level. Respondents who had been diagnosed with, or demonstrated any symptoms of, any neurocognitive disorder, including Alzheimer's Disease, Neurocognitive Disorder with Lewy Bodies, or Vascular Neurocognitive Disease were screened and excluded from research samples. Among other variables, age groups were used to assess potential differences in IT utilization between age groups. Age groups were established based on age per decade, except those younger than 30 and those older than or equal to 80, each of whom formed their own group. The age groups were defined as 18 to 29, 30 to 39, 40 to 49, 50 to 59, 60 to 69, 70 to 79, and 80 or older. The seven age groups are summarized in **Table 2**.

FACETS outcomes indicate that the strongest effect on IT utilization is for differences in age. Older respondents consistently score lower in each of the five FACETS functional domains, and although almost all respondents report access to a computer (93.3%) and access to the internet (93.5%), the age effect is consistent with previous data indicating lower internet and IT utilization with increasing age [15, 17, 18]. FACETS outcome data also indicate that the decline in IT utilization associated with increasing age advances differently for each domain, suggesting that IT use is not a homogenous category. The frequency of IT utilization in the Home domain showed the weakest correlation with age, while frequency of IT utilization in the Health Care domain showed the highest association with age. **Figure 1** shows the differing patterns of decline in frequency of use for the five domains.

Although the frequency of IT utilization declines with age in all domains, the Health Care domain shows the steepest decline, which also occurs earlier than declines in the other domains. Although previous research indicated that the 20% discrepancy in IT utilization between younger age cohorts and people aged over 65 has not changed since 1985 [16], FACETS data indicate that discrepancies in the frequency of IT utilization continue to increase with greater age beyond the age of

| Group | Age in years |
|---|---|
| 1 | 18 to 29 |
| 2 | 30 to 39 |
| 3 | 40 to 49 |
| 4 | 50 to 59 |
| 5 | 60 to 69 |
| 6 | 70 to 79 |
| 7 | 80 or older |

**Table 2.**
*FACETS age group cutoff points [18].*

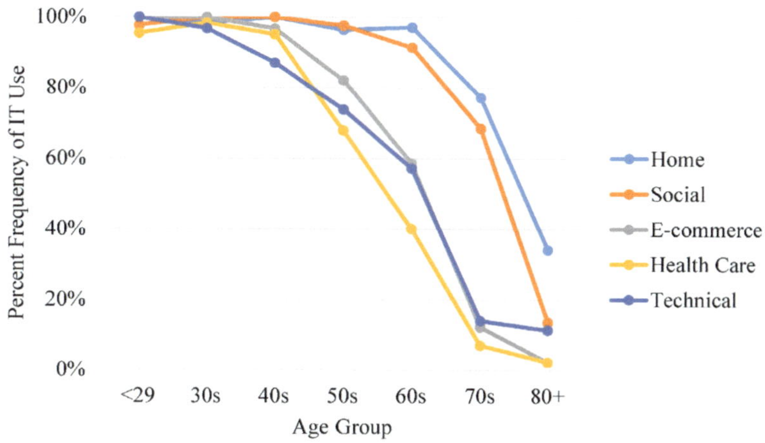


**Figure 1.**
*Frequency of IT use for each FACETS domain by age group [18].*

| Domain | Age under 29 | Age 30 to 39 | Age 40 to 49 | Age 50 to 59 | Age 60 to 69 | Age 70 to 79 | Age over 80 |
|---|---|---|---|---|---|---|---|
| Health Care | 95 | 98 | 95 | 68 | 40 | 7 | 2 |

**Table 3.**
*% IT utilization of health care by age [18].*

65. This is a significant finding, suggesting that people over 65 years of age are not a homogenous population [18].

Specifically, the frequency of IT utilization for communicating with doctors, clinics and insurers declines most rapidly with age. In comparison with cohorts up to age 40, the frequency of IT utilization for communication with insurers and health care providers declined 28% by age 50, 58% by age 60, 93% by age 70, and 98% by age 80. The demonstrated decline in IT utilization with increasing age is consistent with earlier research [15–17], but importantly provides more detailed information about the age at which the rate of decline is greatest, and about preferences regarding IT utilization for communicating with health care providers at different ages [18].

## 5. IT and access to health care

Older adults use IT less than younger age cohorts specifically for accessing health care. While 95–98% of people under the age of 50 prefer to use IT to communicate with health care providers and insurers, only 7% of people over the age of 70 and only 2% of people over the age of 80 do so [18]. These data are shown in **Table 3**.

The decline in the use of IT for accessing health care with increasing age is more dramatically apparent when viewed graphically, as in **Figure 2**.

For example, even though they state that are capable of doing so, adults in age group 4 (50–59) prefer not to use IT to communicate with insurers or doctors. The distinction between the respondent's self-perceived ability to use IT as oppose to their willingness to use it is especially important in the context of health care, and has not previously been addressed. FACETS scores for members of older age groups (aged 70 to 79, and those over 80) whose health care utilization is highest [58, 59]

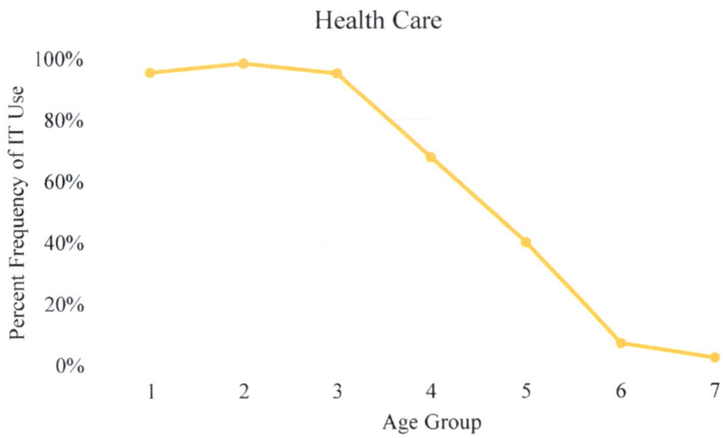


**Figure 2.**
*% frequency of IT use for accessing health care by age group [18].*

indicate that they almost never utilize IT for communication with insurers or doctors [18].

### 5.1 Insurers and IT

The FACETS outcome research data demonstrate that the default use of IT media (videoconferencing, websites, MyChart, text messaging) by insurers, health care agencies or providers for communicating with older adult patients is ineffective, making health care least accessible to the population with the greatest health care needs, older adults [58, 59]. The FACETS outcome research data also suggest that the default use of IT by Medicare, private insurers, and providers of health care for communicating with their patient populations might create a barrier to care and communication, which in turn might lead to poor health outcomes and lower satisfaction ratings by patients and providers of care [70, 71].

Despite these data, Medicare and private insurers continue to make increasing use of websites for communication with patients [63–65, 69]. This trend is shared by hospitals, regional health centers, university teaching hospitals, and local medical clinics [66, 67]. This is somewhat alarming, in the absence of any data indicating that the populations they serve have fluency using the internet or with IT [60, 74].

### 5.2 Looking forward: IT and younger age cohorts

One of the arguments employed in defense of the increasing use of IT media by Medicare, insurers and health care providers is that younger age cohorts are more IT fluent and in time, those lacking IT fluency will no longer be part of the population. The data demonstrate that this is a flawed premise. For example, the highest internet users in the 1985 U.S. Census Bureau study (age 30–35) are now in the low internet user category in the U.S. Census Bureau 2016 findings (now aged 63–68).

This finding appears paradoxical, and invites investigation and speculation. Data from FACETS outcome research suggest that the high IT users of 1985 did not stop using the internet as they aged, but rather, that adoption of new IT platforms including those for accessing the internet is lower among increasingly older cohorts. The lower rate of new IT adoption with age might reflect reduced neuroplasticity with increasing age [96–98], or detachment from newly introduced technologies after retirement, and/or lack of access to and/or training in the use of novel IT.

Perhaps more importantly, these findings suggests that high IT utilization is tied less to a specific individual consistently over time than it is tied to a person's age at the time novel IT is introduced. Younger people appear to adopt new IT & use it more consistently than older people, even if the older people were high IT users when they were young. This is especially relevant in the context of introducing new or evolving IT for communicating with patient populations. The FACETS outcome research data indicate that older adults continue frequent use of IT that is familiar, likely adopted prior to age 40 or 50, while people over the age of 70 demonstrate much lower utilization of IT introduced after they were in mid-life. Late-life introduction of novel IT appears to dramatically decrease the likelihood that it will be utilized. In the context of access to care, the introduction of novel IT by Medicare and health care providers for patient communication with populations over the age of 70 is likely to represent a future barrier to care even for people who currently belong to younger age cohorts [18].

### 5.3 Insurers, IT and other age-related issues

It is important to recall that no symptoms or diagnosis of neurocognitive disorder had been observed in any of the participants in the study, including but not limited to Vascular Neurocognitive Disease, Neurocognitive Disorder with Lewy Bodies, or Alzheimer's Disease. In 2015 the global number of people diagnosed with neurocognitive disease was 46.8 million, and 50 million in 2017. It is expected that by 2030, the number of people with neurocognitive disease will exceed 75 million, and by 2050 it will exceed 131.5 million [99–101]. The progressive organic deterioration characteristic of neurocognitive disease correlates with decreasing episodic memory [102, 103], making it even more challenging for older adults with neurocognitive illness to learn how to utilize new IT in order to communicate with health care providers or insurers. The use of IT for communicating with patients in this population may be neither practical nor realistic, and potentially creates a barrier to access to care [18].

## 6. COVID-19, CMS, IT and access to care

Along with people who have serious underlying health conditions, older adults belong to the cohort most at risk for serious illness reactions to COVID-19, for whom shelter in place is most strongly recommended. People over age 70 have been encouraged not to leave their homes to purchase groceries or perform other routine tasks, but only to leave their homes in the case of a physical emergency [104].

In the context of shelter in place measures to reduce exposure to COVID-19, between February and April of 2020 the Center for Medicare and Medicaid Services (CMS) made a number of policy changes intended to make telehealth more accessible to older adults. These include non-enforcement of policies limiting the patient's location to approved rural facilities, and the HIPAA compliance of the audio-visual platforms used for telehealth communications [13, 105]. While these measures increased access to care to Medicare subscribers with IT fluency, they failed to address access to care for Medicare subscribers who lack IT fluency. As the data demonstrate, 93% of people over the age of 70 and 98% of people over the age of 80 lack IT fluency and do not use the internet to communicate with health care providers, but instead rely entirely on face-to-face or telephone interactions with health care providers [18].

### 6.1 Advocacy for access to care for older adults during shelter in place

Beginning in March 2020, the American Psychological Association (APA) made repeated appeals to CMS to allow reimbursement for the use of telephonic psychotherapy services during shelter in place [106]. On April 30, 2020, after a series of refusals, CMS agreed to provide reimbursement for the use of routine psychotherapy CPT codes for service provided using the telephone [107, 108]. Although the Medicare policy change is temporary, it makes health care accessible to 95.5% of Medicare subscribers over the age of 70. The policy change was intended to expire when the status of COVID-19 was reduced from a national state of emergency, but legislation is being considered that might make the changes partially or wholly permanent [74].

### 6.2 Advocacy for making CMS changes permanent

During shelter in place due to COVID-19, the public was encouraged to utilize virtual communications, especially videoconferencing, for access to health care. A growing body of research demonstrates the effectiveness of telemedicine [48, 109–113]. While this is a viable alternative for younger age cohorts, research data demonstrate that older adults make very limited use of, and/or have very limited access to IT for the purpose communicating with health care providers. While the discrepancy in internet and IT use between younger age cohorts and people aged over 65 is generally about 20% [16], mean utilization of IT (internet, web-based interaction) for access to health care by people over the age of 70 is only about 4.5% [18]. In other words, during shelter in place, 95.5% of people over the age of 70 relied exclusively on telephonic contact for access to health care. This finding is of special concern because older adults belong to the cohort most at risk for serious illness reactions to COVID-19 [104]. Limiting reimbursement for telephonic health care represents a barrier to care for older adults [74].

While CMS's decision to reimburse telephonic psychotherapy [108] is an important acknowledgement of the potential barriers to health care IT represents for older adults and makes health care accessible to an average of 95.5% of Medicare subscribers over the age of 70 [18], the change is temporary and will expire when the COVID-19 pandemic has been resolved [114]. Making reimbursement for telephonic psychotherapy services a permanent policy will facilitate better communication with patients, leading to better treatment outcomes [70, 71]. To facilitate better communication between patients and health care providers, routine assessment of IT utilization might be conducted a part of the standardized initial intake evaluation with older adults and other populations, in order to determine the most effective means through which they can access health care. FACETS is a valid and reliable instrument for assessing which media people use for accessing health care [18, 69]. Instruments like FACETS can be employed in order to determine the most effective means through which patients can access health care. Such assessment is especially important for older adults and other populations with limited IT fluency and/or access to IT or high-speed internet.

## 7. Conclusions

Although people over the age of 65 account for only 9% of the world's population, they account for 30 to 40 percent of COVID-19 cases and 80 percent of COVID-19 deaths [114]. Despite these statistics, people over the age of 65 have been excluded from more than half of COVID-19 trials seeking effective treatments, and from all of the vaccine trials [114]. These data speak to the healthcare system's tendency to overlook the needs of older adults. Hospitals, community health clinics, government-funded health agencies and private practices might also conduct similar assessments to build a larger data base that informs decisions about which media are most effective for communicating with older adult patients. A larger broad-based sample might also provide valuable information about the ways in which older adults access social contact, financial management, and other business functions. At the time of this writing, the COVID-19 pandemic remains unresolved. However, it is increasingly apparent that older adults rely heavily upon telephonic access to health care, emphasizing the importance of permanent changes that liberalize CMS telehealth policy.

## Conflict of interest

No conflict of interest is declared by the author.

## Declarations

This work received no specific grant from any funding agency in the public, commercial, or not-for-profit sectors. The sole author, Charles M. Lepkowsky, PhD, wrote this chapter in accordance with the Ethical Principles of the American Psychological Association. Accordingly, patient identifiers were intentionally minimized. The author accepts responsibility for the conception and design of the chapter, acquisition, analysis, and interpretation of data, drafting, writing, editing and final approval of the version published. The author is accountable for ensuring that any questions regarding the accuracy or integrity of all parts of the chapter were thoroughly investigated and resolved.

## Appendix 1: Functional Assessment of Currently Employed Technology Scale (FACETS)

**Age:** ______ ◯ Male/◯ Female ◯ Hispanic ◯ African American ◯ Asian ◯ Other

**Household Income:** ◯ < $25,000 ◯ < $50,000 ◯ < $100,000 ◯ < $150,000 ◯ > $150,000.

**Degree:** ◯ N/A ◯ High School ◯ Some college ◯ AA ◯ Bachelor's ◯ Post graduate.

**Access to a computer at home?** ◯ Yes/◯ No **Access to internet at home?** ◯ Yes/◯ No.

**Instructions**: Check the response that most accurately completes each

| | | | | | | | |
|---|---|---|---|---|---|---|---|
| **A.** | **Home Domain** | | | | | | |
| 1. | I send email... | ◯ **Never** | ◯ **A few times a year** | ◯ **A few times a month** | ◯ **Once a week** | ◯ **A few times a week** | ◯ **Daily** |
| 2. | I find, open & close files in my computer... | ◯ **Never** | ◯ **A few times a year** | ◯ **A few times a month** | ◯ **Once a week** | ◯ **A few times a week** | ◯ **Daily** |

| | | | | | | |
|---|---|---|---|---|---|---|
| **A. Home Domain** | | | | | | |
| Home Domain Subtotal | | | | | | |
| B. Social Domain | | | | | | |
| 3. I send text messages using a smart phone ... | ○ **Never** | ○ **A few times a year** | ○ **A few times a month** | ○ **Once a week** | ○ **A few times a week** | ○ **Daily** |
| 4. I post on social media (e.g., facebook, twitter) ... | ○ **Never** | ○ **A few times a year** | ○ **A few times a month** | ○ **Once a week** | ○ **A few times a week** | ○ **Daily** |
| Social Domain Subtotal | | | | | | |
| C. E-Commerce Domain | | | | | | |
| 5. I manage my banking and credit card accounts online ... | ○ **Never** | ○ **Tried, but it did not work** | ○ **Got help but did not work** | ○ **Only with help** | ○ **Can but prefer not to** | ○ **Prefer to** |
| 6. I pay bills and make purchases via the internet ... | ○ **Never** | ○ **Tried, but it did not work** | ○ **Got help but did not work** | ○ **Only with help** | ○ **Can but prefer not to** | ○ **Prefer to** |
| E-Commerce Domain Subtotal | | | | | | |
| D. Health Care Domain | | | | | | |
| 7. I communicate with my doctor or clinic online ... | ○ **Never** | ○ **Tried, but it did not work** | ○ **Got help but did not work** | ○ **Only with help** | ○ **Can but prefer not to** | ○ **Prefer to** |
| 8. I communicate with my health insurance company online ... | ○ **Never** | ○ **Tried, but it did not work** | ○ **Got help but did not work** | ○ **Only with help** | ○ **Can but prefer not to** | ○ **Prefer to** |
| Health Care Domain Subtotal | | | | | | |
| E. Technical Domain | | | | | | |
| 9. I have installed components (monitors, speakers, mice) ... | ○ **Never** | ○ **Tried, but it did not work** | ○ **Got help but did not work** | ○ **Only with help** | ○ **Myself, with difficulty** | ○ **Myself easily** |
| 10. I have reset a modem or router in my home ... | ○ **Never** | ○ **Tried, but it did not work** | ○ **Got help but did not work** | ○ **Only with help** | ○ **Myself, with difficulty** | ○ **Myself easily** |
| Technical Domain Subtotal | | | | | | |
| **Total FACETS Score** | | | | | | |

*DOI: http://dx.doi.org/10.5772/intechopen.99300*

## Author details

Charles M. Lepkowsky
Independent Practice, Solvang, CA, USA

*Address all correspondence to: clepkowsky@gmail.com

## References

[1] Kannan S, Shaik Syed Ali P, Sheeza A, Hemalatha K. COVID-19 (Novel Coronavirus 2019) - recent trends. Eur Rev Med Pharmacol Sci. 2020 Feb;24(4): 2006-2011. DOI: 10.26355/eurrev_202002_20378. PMID: 32141569.

[2] Guo YR, Cao QD, Hong ZS, Tan YY, Chen SD, Jin HJ, Tan KS, Wang DY, Yan Y. The origin, transmission and clinical therapies on coronavirus disease 2019 (COVID-19) outbreak - an update on the status. Mil Med Res. 2020 Mar 13; 7(1):11. DOI: 10.1186/s40779-020-00240-0. PMID: 32169119; PMCID: PMC7068984. https://pubmed.ncbi.nlm.nih.gov/32169119/

[3] Shahid Z, Kalayanamitra R, McClafferty B, Kepko D, Ramgobin D, Patel R, Aggarwal CS, Vunnam R, Sahu N, Bhatt D, Jones K, Golamari R, Jain R. COVID-19 and older adults: What we know. J Am Geriatr Soc. 2020 May;68(5):926-929. DOI: 10.1111/jgs.16472. Epub 2020 Apr 20. PMID: 32255507; PMCID: PMC7262251. https://pubmed.ncbi.nlm.nih.gov/32255507/

[4] Fried LP, Tangen CM, Walston J, Newman AB, Hirsch C, Gottdiener J, Seeman T, Tracy R, Kop WJ, Burke G, McBurnie MA, Cardiovascular Health Study Collaborative Research Group. Frailty in older adults: evidence for a phenotype. J Gerontol A Biol Sci Med Sci 2001;56:M146–156.

[5] Nickel CH, Rueegg M, Pargger H, Bingisser R. Age, comorbidity, frailty status: effects on disposition and resource allocation during the COVID-19 pandemic. Swiss Med Wkly 2020; 150:w20269.

[6] Vellas C, Delobel P, de Souto Barreto P, Izopet J. COVID-19, Virology and geroscience: A perspective. J Nutr Health Aging. 2020;24(7):685-691. DOI: 10.1007/s12603-020-1416-2. PMID: 32744561; PMCID: PMC7301052

[7] Heinrich MA, Martina B, Prakash.2020. Nanomedicine strategies to target coronavirus. J.Nano Today. 2020 Dec;35:100961. DOI: 10.1016/j.nantod.2020.100961.

[8] Ahn DG, Shin HJ, Kim MH, Lee S, Kim HS, Myoung J, Kim BT, Kim SJ. Current status of epidemiology, diagnosis, therapeutics, and vaccines for novel Coronavirus disease 2019 (COVID-19). J Microbiol Biotechnol. 2020 Mar 28;30(3):313-324. DOI: 10.4014/jmb.2003.03011. PMID: 32238757.

[9] Harapan H, Itoh N, Yufika A, Winardi W, Keam S, Te H, Megawati D, Hayati Z, Wagner AL, Mudatsir M. Coronavirus disease 2019 (COVID-19): A literature review. J Infect Public Health. 2020 May;13(5):667-673. DOI: 10.1016/j.jiph.2020.03.019. Epub 2020 Apr 8. PMID: 32340833; PMCID: PMC7142680.

[10] Li H, Liu SM, Yu XH, Tang SL, Tang CK. Coronavirus disease 2019 (COVID-19): current status and uture perspectives. Int J Antimicrob Agents. 2020 May;55(5):105951. DOI: 10.1016/j.ijantimicag.2020.105951. Epub 2020 Mar 29. PMID: 32234466; PMCID: PMC7139247.

[11] Pascarella G, Strumia A, Piliego C, Bruno F, Del Buono R, Costa F, Scarlata S, Agrò FE. COVID-19 diagnosis and management: a comprehensive review. J Intern Med. 2020 Aug;288(2):192-206. DOI: 10.1111/joim.13091. Epub 2020 May 13. PMID: 32348588; PMCID: PMC7267177.

[12] Talevi D, Socci V, Carai M, Carnaghi G, Faleri S, Trebbi E, di Bernardo A, Capelli F, Pacitti F. Mental health outcomes of the CoViD-19 pandemic. Riv Psichiatr. 2020 May-Jun; 55(3):137-144. DOI: 10.1708/3382.33569. PMID: 32489190.

[13] Center for Medicare and Medicaid Services. 2020a. Additional background: Sweeping regulatory changes to help U.S. healthcare system address COVID-19 patient surge. Retrieved from: https://www.cms.gov/newsroom/fact-sheets/additional-backgroundsweeping-regulatory-changes-help-us-healthcare-system-address-covid-19-patient

[14] Center for Medicare and Medicaid Services. 2020b. Billing for professional telehealth distant site services during the public health emergency — Revised. Retrieved from: https://www.cms.gov/outreach-and-educationoutreachff sprovpartprogprovider-partnership-email-archive/2020-04-03-mlnc-se#_Toc36815181

[15] U.S. Census Bureau. 2016. Measuring America: A digital nation. Retrieved from: https://www.census.gov/content/dam/Census/library/visualizations/2016/comm/digital_nation.pdf

[16] Anderson & Perrin A. Tech adoption climbs among older adults. 2017. Pew Research Center: Internet & Technology. Retrieved from: http://www.pewinternet.org/2017/05/17/tech-adoption-climbs-among-older-adults/

[17] Hunsaker A & Hargittai E. A review of internet use among older adults. New Media & Society. 2008. Retrieved from: https://doi.org/10.1177/1461444818787348

[18] Lepkowsky CM & Arndt S. The Internet: Barrier to Health Care for Older Adults? Practice Innovations. 2019;4(2), 124-132. DOI: https://doi.org/10.1037/pri0000089

[19] Mehra MR, Desai SS, Kuy S, Henry TD, Patel AN. Cardiovascular disease, drug therapy, and mortality in Covid-19. N Engl J Med. 2020; DOI: https://doi.org/10.1056/NEJMoa2007621.

[20] Zhou F, Yu T, Du R, Fan G, Liu Y, Liu Z, Xiang J, Wang Y, Song B, Gu X, Guan L, Wei Y, Li H, Wu X, Xu J, Tu S, Zhang Y, Chen H, Cao B. Clinical course and risk factors for mortality of adult inpatients with COVID-19 in Wuhan, China: a retrospective cohort study. Lancet. 2020 Mar 28;395(10229): 1054-1062. doi: 10.1016/S0140-6736(20)30566-3. Epub 2020 Mar 11. Erratum in: Lancet. 2020 Mar 28;395(10229):1038. Erratum in: Lancet. 2020 Mar 28;395(10229):1038. PMID: 32171076; PMCID: PMC7270627.

[21] Horton R. Offline: COVID-19-bewilderment and candour. Lancet. 2020 Apr 11;395(10231):1178. doi: 10.1016/S0140-6736(20)30850-3. PMID: 32278372; PMCID: PMC7146680.

[22] Varga, Z, Flammer, AJ, Steiger, P, Habaerecker M, Andermatt, R, Zinkernagel. AS, Mehra, MR, Schuepbach, RA, Ruschitzka, F & Moch, H. 2020. Endothelial cell infection and endotheliitis in COVID-19. The Lancet 395(10234), 1417-1418. DOI:https://doi.org/10.1016/S0140-6736(20)30937-5

[23] Ferrario CM, Jessup J, Chappell MC, Averill DB, Brosnihan KB, Tallant EA, Diz DI, Gallagher PE. Effect of angiotensin-converting enzyme inhibition and angiotensin II receptor blockers on cardiac angiotensin-converting enzyme 2. Circulation. 2005 May 24;111(20):2605-10. DOI: 10.1161/CIRCULATIONAHA.104.510461. Epub 2005 May 16. PMID: 15897343.

[24] Santos IA, Grosche VR, Bergamini FRG, Sabino-Silva R, Jardim ACG. 2020. Antivirals against coronaviruses: Candidate drugs for SARS-CoV-2 treatment? Front Microbiol. 2020 Aug 13;11:1818. DOI: 10.3389/fmicb.2020.01818. eCollection 2020.PMID: 32903349

[25] Esakandari H, Nabi-Afjadi M, Fakkari-Afjadi J, Farahmandian N, Miresmaeili SM, Bahreini E. A comprehensive review of COVID-19

characteristics. Biol Proced Online. 2020 Aug 4;22:19. DOI: 10.1186/s12575-020-00128-2. PMID: 32774178; PMCID: PMC7402395.

[26] Wan Y, Shang J, Graham R, Baric RS, Li F. 2020. Receptor recognition by the novel Coronavirus from Wuhan: an analysis based on decade-long structural studies of SARS Coronavirus.. J Virol. 2020 Mar 17;94 (7):e00127-20. DOI: 10.1128/JVI.00127-20. Print 2020 Mar 17.PMID: 31996437

[27] Zhu C, Sun B, Zhang X, Zhang B. 2020. Research progress of genetic structure, pathogenic mechanism, clinical characteristics, and potential treatments of Coronavirus disease 2019. Front Pharmacol. 2020 Aug 27;11:1327. DOI: 10.3389/fphar.2020.01327. eCollection 2020.PMID: 32973534

[28] Jiang S, Hillyer C, Du L. 2020. Neutralizing antibodies against SARS-CoV-2 and other human Coronaviruses. Trends Immunol. 2020 May;41(5): 355-359. DOI: 10.1016/j.it.2020.03.007. Epub 2020 Apr 2.PMID: 32249063

[29] AminJafari A, Ghasemi S. 2020. The possible of immunotherapy for COVID-19: A systematic review. Int Immunopharmacol. 2020 Jun;83: 106455. DOI: 10.1016/j.intimp.2020.106455. PMID: 32272396

[30] Rabaan AA, Al-Ahmed SH, Sah R, Tiwari R, Yatoo MI, Patel SK, Pathak M, Malik YS, Dhama K, Singh KP, Bonilla-Aldana DK, Haque S, Martinez-Pulgarin DF, Rodriguez-Morales AJ, Leblebicioglu H. 2020. SARS-CoV-2/COVID-19 and advances in developing potential therapeutics and vaccines to counter this emerging pandemic. Ann Clin Microbiol Antimicrob. 2020 Sep 2; 19(1):40. DOI: 10.1186/s12941-020-00384-w.PMID: 32878641

[31] Owji H, Negahdaripour M, Hajighahramani N. 2020. Immunotherapeutic approaches to curtail COVID-19. Int Immunopharmacol. 2020 Aug 21;88:106924. DOI: 10.1016/j.intimp.2020.106924. Online ahead of print.PMID: 32877828

[32] Shanmugaraj B, Siriwattananon K, Wangkanont K, Phoolcharoen W. Perspectives on monoclonal antibody therapy as potential therapeutic intervention for Coronavirus disease-19 (COVID-19). Asian Pac J Allergy Immunol. 2020 Mar;38(1):10-18. DOI: 10.12932/AP-200220-0773. PMID: 32134278.

[33] Zhou G, Zhao Q. 2020. Perspectives on therapeutic neutralizing antibodies against the Novel Coronavirus SARS-CoV-2. Int J Biol Sci. 2020 Mar 15;16 (10):1718-1723. DOI: 10.7150/ijbs.45123

[34] Blake H, Bermingham F, Johnson G, Tabner A. Mitigating the psychological impact of COVID-19 on healthcare workers: A digital learning package. Int J Environ Res Public Health. 2020 Apr 26; 17(9):2997. DOI: 10.3390/ijerph17092997. PMID: 32357424; PMCID: PMC7246821.

[35] Alessi J, de Oliveira GB, Franco DW, Brino do Amaral B, Becker AS, Knijnik CP, Kobe GL, de Carvalho TR, Telo GH, Schaan BD, Telo GH. Mental health in the era of COVID-19: prevalence of psychiatric disorders in a cohort of patients with type 1 and type 2 diabetes during the social distancing. Diabetol Metab Syndr. 2020 Aug 31;12: 76. DOI: 10.1186/s13098-020-00584-6. PMID: 32879637; PMCID: PMC7457442.

[36] Wesemann U, Hadjamu N, Willmund G, Dolff S, Vonderlin N, Wakili R, Vogel J, Rassaf T, Siebermair J. Influence of COVID-19 on general stress and posttraumatic stress symptoms among hospitalized high-risk patients. Psychol Med. 2020 Aug 14:1-2. DOI: 10.1017/S0033291720003165. Epub ahead of print. PMID: 32794442; PMCID: PMC7453354.

[37] Jakovljevic M, Bjedov S, Jaksic N, Jakovljevic I. COVID-19 Pandemia and public and global mental health from the perspective of global health security. Psychiatr Danub. 2020 Spring;32(1): 6-14. DOI: 10.24869/psyd.2020.6. PMID: 32303023.

[38] McGonagle, K.A., Kessler, R.C. Chronic stress, acute stress, and depressive symptoms. Am J CommunPsychol 18, 681–706 (1990). DOI: https://doi.org/10.1007/BF00931237

[39] Mariotti A. The effects of chronic stress on health: new insights into the molecular mechanisms of brain-body communication. Future Sci OA. 2015;1 (3):FSO23. Published 2015 Nov 1. DOI: 10.4155/fso.15.21

[40] McEwen BS. Neurobiological and Systemic Effects of Chronic Stress. Chronic Stress (Thousand Oaks). 2017 Jan-Dec;1:2470547017692328. DOI: 10.1177/2470547017692328. Epub 2017 Apr 10. PMID: 28856337; PMCID: PMC5573220.

[41] Vyas A, Mitra R, Shankaranarayana Rao BS, Chattarji S. Chronic stress induces contrasting patterns of dendritic remodeling in hippocampal and amygdaloid neurons. J Neurosci. 2002 Aug 1;22(15):6810-8. DOI: 10.1523/JNEUROSCI.22-15-06810.2002. PMID: 12151561; PMCID: PMC6758130.

[42] Dubey S, Biswas P, Ghosh R, Chatterjee S, Dubey MJ, Chatterjee S, Lahiri D, Lavie CJ. Psychosocial impact of COVID-19. Diabetes Metab Syndr. 2020 Sep-Oct;14(5):779-788. DOI: 10.1016/j.dsx.2020.05.035. Epub 2020 May 27. PMID: 32526627; PMCID: PMC7255207.

[43] Nikolich-Zugich J, Knox KS, Rios CT, Natt B, Bhattacharya D, Fain MJ. SARS-CoV-2 and COVID-19 in older adults: what we may expect regarding pathogenesis, immune responses, and outcomes. Geroscience. 2020 Apr;42(2):505-514. DOI: 10.1007/s11357-020-00186-0. Epub 2020 Apr 10. Erratum in: Geroscience. 2020 May 3;: PMID: 32274617; PMCID: PMC7145538.

[44] Nanda A, Vura NVRK, Gravenstein S. COVID-19 in older adults. Aging Clin Exp Res. 2020 Jul;32(7): 1199-1202. DOI: 10.1007/s40520-020-01581-5. Epub 2020 May 10. PMID: 32390064; PMCID: PMC7211267.

[45] Peden CJ, Mohan S, Pagán V. Telemedicine and COVID-19: an Observational Study of Rapid Scale Up in a US Academic Medical System. J Gen Intern Med. 2020 Sep;35(9):2823-2825. DOI: 10.1007/s11606-020-05917-9. Epub 2020 Jun 4. PMID: 32500329; PMCID: PMC7272134.

[46] Mann DM, Chen J, Chunara R, Testa PA, Nov O. COVID-19 transforms health care through telemedicine: Evidence from the field. J Am Med Inform Assoc. 2020 Jul 1;27(7): 1132-1135. DOI: 10.1093/jamia/ocaa072. PMID: 32324855; PMCID: PMC7188161.

[47] Wosik J, Fudim M, Cameron B, Gellad ZF, Cho A, Phinney D, Curtis S, Roman M, Poon EG, Ferranti J, Katz JN, Tcheng J. Telehealth transformation: COVID-19 and the rise of virtual care. J Am Med Inform Assoc. 2020 Jun 1;27 (6):957-962. DOI: 10.1093/jamia/ocaa067. PMID: 32311034; PMCID: PMC7188147.

[48] Ramaswamy A, Yu M, Drangsholt S, Ng E, Culligan PJ, Schlegel PN, Hu JC. Patient satisfaction with telemedicine during the COVID-19 Pandemic: Retrospective cohort study. J Med Internet Res. 2020 Sep 9;22(9): e20786. DOI: 10.2196/20786. PMID: 32810841.

[49] Bokolo Anthony Jnr. Use of telemedicine and virtual care for remote treatment in response to COVID-19 pandemic. J Med Syst. 2020 Jun 15;44

(7):132. DOI: 10.1007/s10916-020-01596-5. PMID: 32542571; PMCID: PMC7294764.

[50] Dobransky K & Hargittai E. The disability divide in internet access and use. Information, Communication & Society. 2006;9(3), 313-334. DOI: https://doi.org/10.1080/13691180600751298

[51] Davies DK, Stock SE, King LR, Brown RB, Wehmeyer ML & Shogren KA. An interface to support independent use of facebook by people with intellectual disability. Intellectual and Developmental Disabilities. 2015;53 (1), 30-41. DOI: https://doi.org/10.1352/1934-9556-53.1.30

[52] Hoffman DL & Novak TP. The growing digital divide: Implications for an open research agenda. In B. Kahin & E. Brynjolffson (Eds.), Understanding the Digital Economy: Data, Tools and Research. 2000. Cambridge: MIT Press. Retrieved from: https://www.researchgate.net/publication/240313230_The_Growing_Digital_Divide_Implications_for_an_Open_Research_Agenda

[53] DiMaggio P & Hargittai E. From the "Digital divide" to digital inequality: Studying internet use as penetration increases. Princeton, NJ: Center for Arts and Cultural Policy Studies, University Working Paper 15. 2001; Retrieved from: https://culturalpolicy.princeton.edu/sites/culturalpolicy/files/wp15_dimaggio_hargittai.pdf

[54] DiMaggio P, Hargittai E, Celeste C & Shafer S. Digital inequality: From unequal access to differentiated use. In: K. Neckerman (Ed.), Social Inequality. 2004. (pp. 355–400). New York: Russell Sage Foundation.

[55] Lepkowsky CM. (Technological Diversity: A Cost-Saving, Person-Centered Alternative to Systemic Technocentrism and Technological Provider Bias. Psychology Behav Med Open Access J. 2017;1(1):1-7. http://ologyjournals.com/pbmoaj/pbmoaj_00001.pdf

[56] U.S. Department of Health and Human Services, Centers for Disease Control and Prevention. 2016. Retrieved from: https://www.cdc.gov/aging/pdf/cognitive_impairment/cogimp_poilicy_final.pdf

[57] U.S. Census Bureau. 2015. Projections of the size and composition of the U.S. population: 2014 to 2060. Retrieved from: https://pdfs.semanticscholar.org/09c9/ad858a60f9be2d6966ebd0bc267af5a76321.pdf

[58] Hayes SL, Salzberg CA, McCarthy D, Radley D C, Abrams MK, Shah T & Anderson G. High-need, high-cost patients: Who are they and how do they use health care? A population-based comparison of demographics, health care use, and expenditures. The Commonwealth Fund. 2016. Retrieved from: https://www.commonwealthfund.org/publications/issue-briefs/2016/aug/high-need-high-cost-patients-who-are-they-and-how-do-they-use

[59] Center for Medicare and Medicaid Services. 2014. Health Expenditures by age and gender. Retrieved from: https://www.cms.gov/Research-Statistics-Data-and-Systems/Statistics-Trends-and-Reports/NationalHealthExpendData/Age-and-Gender.html

[60] Lepkowsky CM. Functional Assessment of Comfort Employing Technology Scale (FACETS): A brief intake instrument to facilitate treatment planning and communication with patients. Psychology Behav Med Open Access 2017; J 1(1):9-13. http://ologyjournals.com/pbmoaj/pbmoaj_00002.pdf

[61] Lepkowsky CM. A multiple domain collaborative care model for independent practice psychologists working with older adults. Practice Innovations. 2017;2(4), 173–194. DOI: https://doi.org/10.1037/pri0000052

[62] Hunsaker A, Hargittai E. A review of Internet use among older adults. New Media & Society. 2018;20(10): 3937-3954. DOI:10.1177/ 1461444818787348

[63] Blue Cross Blue Shield. 2018. Welcome to Blue Cross Blue Shield. 2018. Retrieved from https://www.bcbs.com/

[64] Medicare. 2018. Medicare.gov, the official U.S. Government site for Medicare. Retrieved from https://www.medicare.gov/

[65] United Healthcare. 2018. Welcome to United healthcare online. Retrieved from: https://www.unitedhealthcareonline.com/b2c/CmaAction.do?viewKey=PreLoginMain&forwardToken=PreLoginMain

[66] Cleveland Clinic. 2018. MyChart. Retrieved from: https://my.clevelandclinic.org/online-services/mychart

[67] Duke University. Duke MyChart. 2018. (online). Retrieved from: https://www.dukemychart.org/home/

[68] Center for Medicare Advocacy. 2015. CMS report finds access to care problems for low-income Medicare beneficiaries. Retrieved from: http://www.medicareadvocacy.org/cms-report-finds-access-to-care-problems-for-low-income-medicare-beneficiaries/

[69] Lepkowsky CM & Arndt S. Functional Assessment of Currently Employed Technology Scale (FACETS): Reliability and validity. International Journal of Medical Science and Clinical Invention. 2018;5(9), 064-4068. DOI: https://doi.org/10.18535/ijmsci/v5i9.07

[70] Zolnierek KB & Dimatteo MR. Physician communication and patient adherence to treatment: A meta-analysis. Medical Care. 2009;47, 826–834. DOI: https://doi.org/10.1097/MLR.0b013e31819a5acc

[71] Vermeir P, Vandijck D, Degroote S, Peleman R, Verhaeghe R, Mortier E, Hallaert G, Van Daele S., Buylaert W, Vogelaers D. Communication in healthcare: a narrative review of the literature and practical recommendations. Int J Clin Pract. 2015; 69(11), 1257-1267. DOI: https://doi.org/10.1111/ijcp.12686.

[72] Lepkowsky CM. Functional Assessment of Currently Employed Technology Scale (FACETS) 4.0: Update on a Brief Intake Instrument to Facilitate Treatment Planning and Communication with Patients. International Journal of Medical Science and Clinical Invention. 2020; 7(5), 4802-4809. DOI: https://doi.org/10.18535/ijmsci/v7i05.03

[73] Hill R, Betts LR, Gardner SE. Older adults' experiences and perceptions of digital technology: (Dis)empowerment, wellbeing, and inclusion. Computers in Human Behavior. 2015;48:415-423. DOI: 10.1016/j.chb.2015.01.062

[74] Lepkowsky CM. Telehealth Reimbursement Allows Access to Mental Health Care During COVID-19. American Journal of Geriatric Psychiatry. 2020;28(8) 898-899. DOI: https://doi.org/10.1016/j.jagp.2020.05.008

[75] American Psychological Association. (2014). Guidelines for psychological practice with older adults. Retrieved from: http://www.apa.org/practice/guidelines/older-adults.aspx

[76] Davis FD. Perceived usefulness, perceived ease of use, and user acceptance of information technology. MIS Quarterly. 1989;13(3):319–340. DOI: 10.2307/249008

[77] Smither JA, Braun CC. Technology and older adults: factors affecting the adoption of automatic teller machines. The Journal of General Psychology. 1994;121(4):381-389. DOI: 10.1080/00221309.1994.9921212

[78] Chappell N L, Zimmer Z. Receptivity to new technology among older adults. Disability and Rehabilitation. 1999;21(5-6):222-230. DOI: 10.1080/096382899297648

[79] Morris M G, Venkatesh V. Age differences in technology adoption decisions: Implications for a changing workforce. Personnel Psychology. 2000; 53(2):375–403. doi:10.1111/ j.1744-6570.2000.tb00206.x

[80] White J, Weatherall A. A grounded theory analysis of older adults and information technology. Educational Gerontology. 2000;26(4), 371-386. http://dx.doi.org/10.1080/ 036012700407857

[81] Venkatesh V, Davis FD. A theoretical extension of the technology acceptance model: Four longitudinal field studies. Management Science. 2000;46(2):186–204. doi:10.1287/ mnsc.46.2.186.11926

[82] Venkatesh, V. Determinants of perceived ease of use: Integrating control, intrinsic motivation, and emotion into the technology acceptance model. Information systems research. 2000;11(4):342–365.

[83] Zajicek, M. Interface design for older adults. Published in: Proceedings of the 2001 EC/NSF workshop on Universal accessibility of ubiquitous computing: providing for the elderly, 60 – 65. 2001. New York, NY, Association for Computing Machinery. http://dl. acm.org/citation.cfm?id=564543

[84] Venkatesh V, Morris MG, Davis GB, DavisFD. User acceptance of information technology: Toward a unified view. MIS Quarterly. 2003;27 (3):425–478.

[85] Selwyn N. The information aged: A qualitative study of older adults' use of information and communications technology. Journal of Aging Studies. 2004;18(4):369–384. doi: 10.1016/j. jaging.2004.06.008

[86] Melenhorst A, Rogers W, Bouwhuis D. Older adults' motivated choice for technological innovation: Evidence for benefit-driven selectivity. Psychology and Aging. 2006;21(1): 190-195. http://dx.doi.org/10.1037/ 0882-7974.21.1.190

[87] Carpenter B, Buday S. Computer use among older adults in a naturally occurring retirement community. Computers in Human Behavior. 2007;23 (6):3012–3024. doi: 10.1016/j. chb.2006.08.015

[88] Venkatesh V, Thong J, Xu X. Consumer acceptance and use of information technology: Extending the Unified Theory of Acceptance and Use of Technology. MIS Quarterly. 2012;36 (1):157-178. https://papers.ssrn.com/ sol3/papers.cfm?abstract_id=2002388).

[89] Caldwell B. Comfort with technology in MFT self-assessment. 2015 AAMFT Annual Conference | Session 508: How technology will radically change family therapy's future. 2015. Internet. Available from: https://cdn.shopify.com/s/files/1/ 0809/6573/files/508-_Comfort_with_ technology_in_MFT_survey.pdf.

[90] Christensen R, Knezek G. The Technology Proficiency Self-Assessment Questionnaire (TPSA). 2015. Internet. Available from https://www.researchgate. net/publication/291411935_The_Tech nology_Proficiency_Self-Assessment_ Questionnaire_TPSA.

[91] Christensen R, Knezek G. Validating the Technology Proficiency Self-Assessment Questionnaire for 21st century learning (TPSA C-21). Journal of Digital Learning in Teacher Education. 2017;33(1):20-31. doi: 10.1080/21532974.2016.1242391

[92] University of the State of New York at Albany. Technology Integration

Self-Assessment. 2017. Internet. Available from http://www.acces.nysed.gov/common/acces/files/aepp/EDITTISASurvey12_04_2012.pdf

[93] Florida Gulf Coast University. Technology Skills Self-Assessment. 2017. Internet. Available from https://survey.fgcu.edu/Survey.aspx?s=311d40c08e234f9181d7f97e6623fbcc.

[94] Kerr B. Technology Skills Self-Assessment Survey. 2017. Internet. Available from http://mtweb.mtsu.edu/bkerr/Technology_Skills_Self-Assessment_Survey.asp.

[95] Nimrod G. Technostress: measuring a new threat to well-being in later life. Aging Ment Health. 2017;31:1-8. doi: 10.1080/13607863.2017.1334037).

[96] Cabeza R, Grady CL, Nyberg L, McIntosh AR, Tulving E, Kapur S, Jennings JM,Houle S & Craik FI. Age-related differences in neural activity during memory encoding and retrieval: a positron emission tomography study. Journal of Neuroscience. 1997;17(1), 391-400. PMID: 8987764

[97] Burke SN & Barnes CA. Neural plasticity in the ageing brain. National Review of Neuroscience. 2006;7(1), 30-40. doi: 10.1038/nrn1809

[98] Goha JO & Park DC. Neuroplasticity and cognitive aging: The scaffolding theory of aging and cognition. Restorative Neurological Neuroscience. 2009;27(5), 391–403. doi: 10.3233/RNN-2009-0493

[99] Hebert LE, Weuve J, Scherr PA & Evans DA. Alzheimer disease in the United States (2010–2050) estimated using the 2010 census. Neurology. 2013; 80(19), 1778–1783. doi: 10.1212/WNL.0b013e31828726f5

[100] Kowal S, Dall T, Chakrabarti R, Storm M & Jain A. The current and projected economic burden of Parkinson's disease in the United States. Movement Disorders. 2013;28(3), 311-318. doi: 10.1002/mds.25292

[101] Alzheimer's Disease International. World Alzheimer report 2015: The global impact of dementia: An analysis of prevalence, incidence, cost and trends. 2016. Retrieved from: https://www.alz.co.uk/research/WorldAlzheimerReport2015.pdf

[102] Moradi E, Hallikainen I, Hänninen T, Tohka J & Alzheimer's Disease Neuroimaging Initiative. Rey's Auditory Verbal Learning Test scores can be predicted from whole brain MRI in Alzheimer's disease. Neuroimage Clinical. 2016;18;13:415-427. DOI: 10.1016/j.nicl.2016.12.011

[103] Gillaspy S. 2020. Re: [APAPRACTICELIST] BREAKING NEWS – Billing Update.

[104] Center for Disease Control and Prevention. 2020. Coronavirus disease 2019 (COVID-19): People who are at higher risk for severe illness. Retrieved from: https://www.cdc.gov/coronavirus/2019-ncov/need-extra-precautions/people-at-higher-risk.html

[105] American Psychological Association. 2020. Temporary changes to federal Medicare telehealth policies. Retrieved from: https://www.apaservices.org/practice/reimbursement/government/medicare-telehealth-temporary-changes

[106] U.S. Census Bureau. 2003. Computer and internet use in the United States: Retrieved from: https://www.census.gov/prod/2005pubs/p23-208.pdf

[107] Skillings J. 2020. Billing Update: New phone-only billing codes. Retrieved from: https://www.apaservices.org/practice/clinic/covid-19-audio-only-phone-service-codes

[108] American Psychological Association Services, Inc. 2020. Phone only telehealth services for Medicare during COVID-19. Retrieved from: https://www.apaservices.org/practice/clinic/covid-19-telehealth-phone-only

[109] Farrugia G, Plutowski RW. Innovation lessons from the COVID-19 pandemic. Mayo Clin Proc. 2020 Aug;95 (8):1574-1577. DOI: 10.1016/j.mayocp.2020.05.024. Epub 2020 Jun 6. PMID: 32753130; PMCID: PMC7275154.

[110] Julien HM, Eberly LA, Adusumalli S. Telemedicine and the forgotten America. Circulation. 2020 Jul 28;142(4):312-314. DOI: 10.1161/CIRCULATIONAHA.120.048535. Epub 2020 Jun 11. PMID: 32525712; PMCID: PMC7382527.

[111] Smith AC, Thomas E, Snoswell CL, Haydon H, Mehrotra A, Clemensen J, Caffery LJ. Telehealth for global emergencies: Implications for coronavirus disease 2019 (COVID-19). J Telemed Telecare. 2020 Jun;26(5): 309-313. DOI: 10.1177/1357633X20916567. Epub 2020 Mar 20. PMID: 32196391; PMCID: MC7140977.

[112] Shah ED, Amann ST, Karlitz JJ. The Time Is Now: A guide to sustainable telemedicine during COVID-19 and beyond. Am J Gastroenterol. 2020 Sep; 115(9):1371-1375. DOI: 10.14309/ajg.0000000000000767. PMID: 32694293; PMCID: PMC7382421.

[113] Cubo E, Hassan A, Bloem BR, Mari Z; MDS-telemedicine study group. implementation of telemedicine for urgent and ongoing healthcare for patients with Parkinson's Disease during the COVID-19 pandemic: New Expectations for the Future. J Parkinsons Dis. 2020;10(3):911-913. DOI: 10.3233/JPD-202108. PMID: 32417800.

[114] Inouye SK, Helfand B, Webb M, Gartanis S, Fuller L & Kwon C-S. Older persons underrepresented in COVID-19 treatment and vaccine trials. JAMA. 2020; prepublication. Available online from: https://www.hebrewseniorlife.org/news/study-finds-older-persons-underrepresented-covid-19-treatment-and-vaccine-trials

Chapter 11

# Mobile Clinics in the United States and the COVID-19 Pandemic: A Response Strategy Model

*Sharon Attipoe-Dorcoo and Rigoberto Delgado*

## Abstract

Mobile health clinics are critical avenues for reaching under-resourced populations. There are over 2,000 mobile clinics serving 7 million individuals annually. Costs per patient are low compared to stationary clinics. Further, they play a critical role in reducing healthcare access disparities by ensuring healthcare is delivered at the doorstep of patients. However, this model of healthcare delivery is a tool that is rarely considered for dealing with emergencies such as a pandemic. The case of the COVID-19 pandemic illustrates several potential areas where mobile clinic programs can play a critical role. Apart from the role mobile clinics have played in improving COVID-19 testing for under-resourced populations, and the current efforts in expanding their use in vaccinations, there are other proposed initiatives that should be explored. Establishing a comprehensive approach to incorporate mobile clinics in our entire health system, would not only be effective for addressing health outcomes of under-resourced patient populations, but will also contribute to the success of a national pandemic response. Mobile healthcare clinics are a vital part of equitable national healthcare solutions, and it is time to recognize their broader potential, and include them in preparation efforts for current and future health crises.

**Keywords:** mobile clinics, pandemic, COVID-19, under-resourced, community, healthcare

## 1. Introduction

In this chapter, we discuss mobile clinics and their importance in healthcare delivery especially during health emergencies such as a pandemic. The COVID-19 pandemic has highlighted the need for creating channels for reaching under-resourced populations in a fast and effective manner. We present the case that mobile clinics, properly equipped, could deliver services to rural and urban communities alike. However, creating an integrated system of mobile clinics is necessary to successfully and sustainably achieve the opportunities which are described in this chapter. We start by providing a thorough description of mobile clinics, highlight cases of selected programs in Southern states of the United States, and finally discuss examples and initiatives to strategically integrate mobile clinics in our healthcare delivery systems to efficiently respond in emergencies.

## 2. Role of Mobile clinics in health delivery systems

Mobile clinics are vehicles customized with medical equipment to provide health services in communities for different health populations. They are staffed with health professionals to increase health access to populations and enforce disease prevention, as well as improve access to chronic health management at reduced costs [1]. Mobile clinics have also been used to increase healthcare staff and provide specialty equipment such as orthoses and prostheses to disabled patients in Sao Paulo [2]. In situations such as flooding when building facilities were destroyed or individuals were unable to access stationary healthcare facilities, mobile clinics were alternatives to providing adequate medical services as was in the case in Malaysia [3]. These examples illustrate how mobile clinics can provide the healthcare needs of populations similarly to stationary healthcare facilities, and addresses geographical barriers by bringing the care to patients. Additionally, a study on patient satisfaction for preventive services in Saudi Arabia showed that patients were satisfied with the working hours and human resources of the mobile clinics 95% of the time, while in northern Nigeria, [4] there were positive perceptions of mobile clinics by providers, community leaders and patients [5].

Mobile health clinics have been used in the United States to provide healthcare services to the uninsured or individuals lacking geographic access to health [6]. They continue to be longstanding community-based service delivery models that fill gaps in healthcare delivery safety-nets and reach under-resourced populations in both urban and rural areas [1]. Their effectiveness could potentially increase should they be used together with other forms of healthcare services delivery for coordinated health management. There are about 2,000 mobile clinics in the United States serving 7 million at-risk people annually [5, 7]. The mobile clinic model is an efficient avenue for healthcare delivery ($36 saved from mobile clinic services compared to emergency visits for every $1 invested in the mobile clinic) [8]. "They work in some places where the economics make sense, and where the technology can survive the bumpy roads" [9].

## 3. Geographic distribution of Mobile clinic programs in the United States

A self-reported survey was sent to representatives of mobile clinics who were either clinic managers, providers, or directors in Texas, Florida, North Carolina,

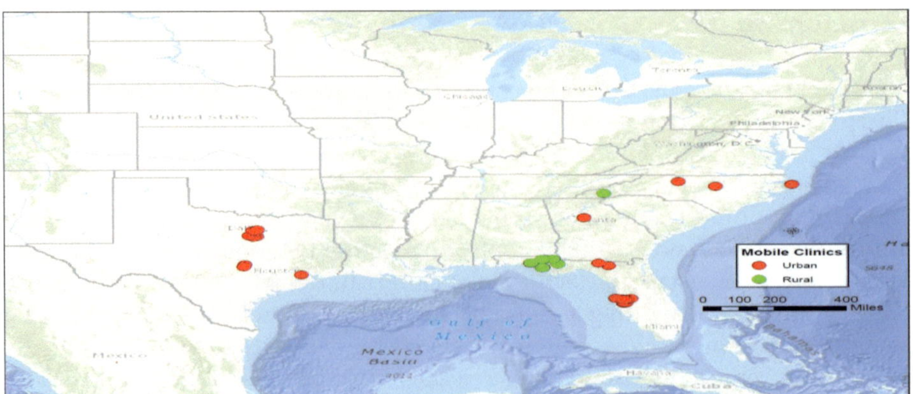


**Figure 1.**
*National map with Mobile clinics in TX, FL, NC, GA.*

and Georgia [10]. There were a total of 49 mobile clinics that were operated by 15 organizations across all four states. **Figure 1** illustrates the overall distribution of the mobile clinics across the states in the surveyed programs. Florida had six rural

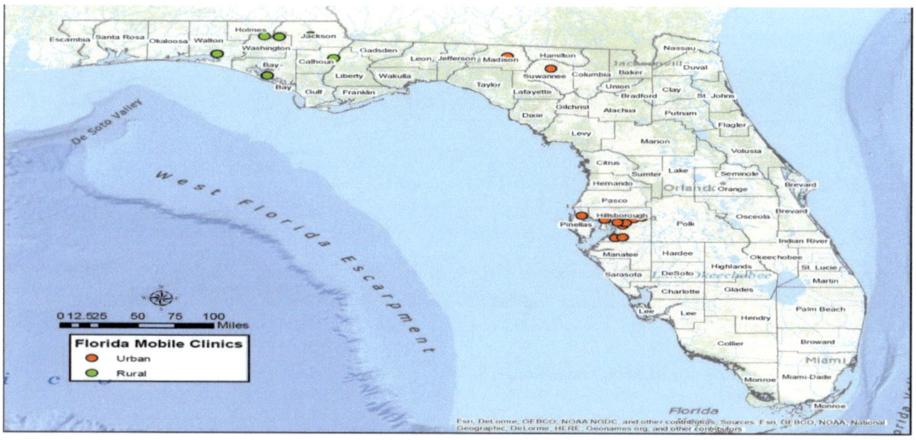


**Figure 2.**
*Map of FL with Mobile clinics in urban and rural locations.*

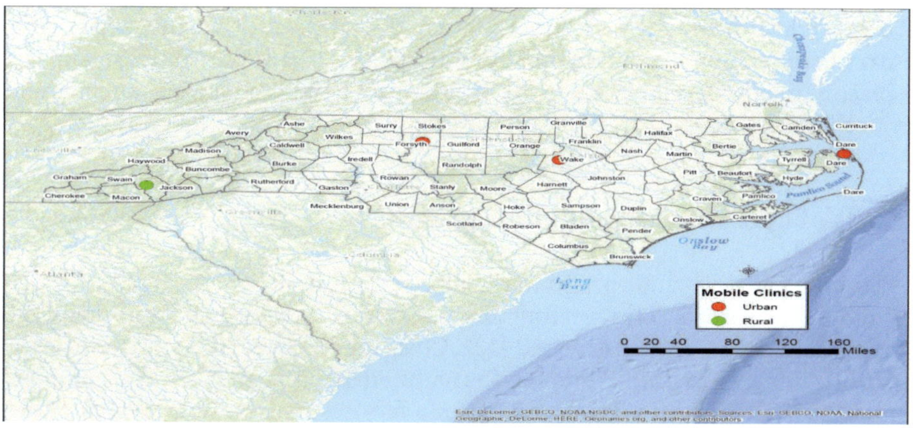


**Figure 3.**
*Map of NC with Mobile clinics in urban and rural locations.*

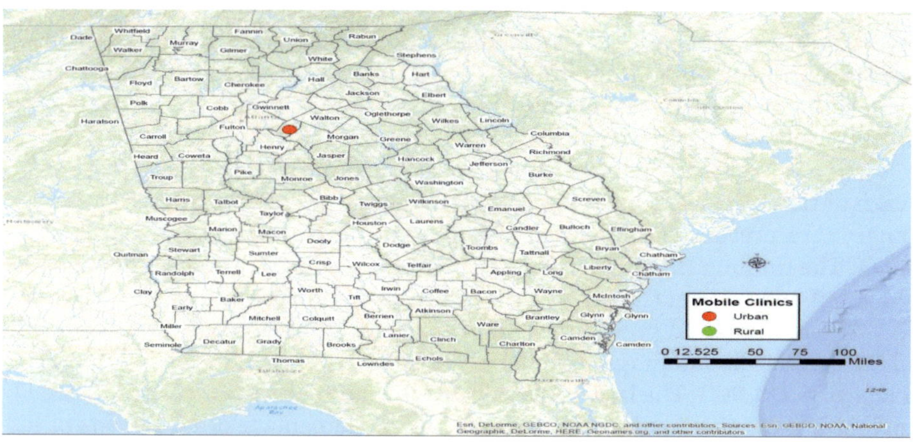


**Figure 4.**
*Map of GA with Mobile clinics in urban location.*

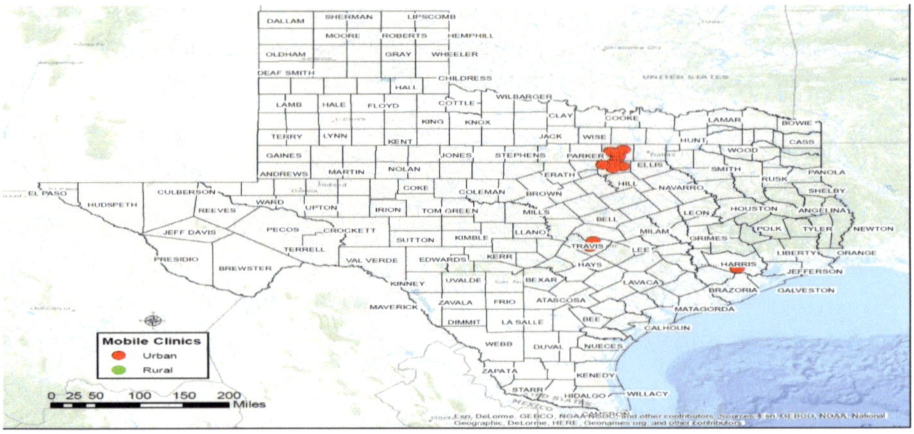


**Figure 5.**
*Map of TX with Mobile clinics in urban location.*

and 12 urban locations (**Figure 2**); North Carolina had three urban and one rural (**Figure 3**); Georgia and Texas had all clinics in urban locations, **Figure 4** and **Figure 5** respectively. Reasons provided by the mobile clinic representatives as to how they choose their respective locations varied across the different states and the types of healthcare delivery strata (dental, dental/preventive, preventive care, primary care/preventive, and mammography/primary care/preventive). Some of the reasons mentioned included using results from hotspot mapping, and community needs assessments [10].

## 4. Costs of operating Mobile clinic programs

Planning a mobile clinic program requires several stakeholders in both the private and public sectors [11] therefore the costs and complexities of running mobile clinics should not be underestimated [12]. Costs include recurrent costs (variable costs of running the mobile clinic such as maintenance, repair, fuel, and compensation for the healthcare providers who provide services in the mobile clinics), as well as capital costs such as the acquisition costs of equipment, and vehicle [13]. Brazil, for example, has a sustainable 8-year mobile clinic program integrating the community, government, and private sectors [14] as a way to ensure the sustainability of the program. Mobile clinic outreach programs can be complex and expensive; however, these complexities can be mediated by public policy or resource planning [15]. Acquiring mobile clinics and delivering healthcare services is therefore an effort that needs careful planning and assessment, as well as consideration of outcomes and how performance would be evaluated [16].

A survey [10] based on the accounting documentation of the mobile clinics in each of the stratified service types: dental, dental/preventive, preventive care, primary care/preventive, and mammography/primary care/preventive was conducted. The findings highlighted in a recent publication [17] showed the highest averages of annual operating costs for dental and dental/preventive services ranging ($2.3–$2.5 million) and preventive and primary care/preventive between $479,000 and $822,000. Mammography/primary care/preventive had the lowest annual average of $300,000. The largest overall cost line item was labor costs, followed by depreciation and then maintenance costs. Largest percentage of labor costs of more than 90% of total costs was in preventive and primary care/preventive. Dental and dental/preventive labor costs represented 80%, while mammography/primary care/

preventive had 65%. The highest percentage for depreciation costs was for mammography/primary care/preventive with (25%), followed by dental and dental/preventive (13%), and preventive and primary care/preventive services at 5% [17]. The variation in depreciation costs was attributable to the differences in the type of capital equipment used by each of the stratified service types. For example, mammography's 25% likely corresponded to the expensive screening equipment. The percent of total costs attributable to maintenance was 10% for mammography/primary care/preventive, followed by dental and dental/preventive with 7%, and preventive and primary care/preventive at 3% [17].

The estimated cost per patient visit was analyzed using the reported annual patient visits from survey responses. Average annual operating cost per patient visit ranged from $243 in preventive services to $65 for mammography/primary care/preventive delivery services. While the cost per patient visit for dental services ($123) was considerably lower than dental/preventive services ($225), preventive services had an average cost per patient visit of $243, suggesting an overall high cost for prevention programs [17].

## 5. Role of Mobile clinic programs in healthcare disparities

The COVID-19 pandemic has exacerbated existing limitations of our health systems when confronted with the unexpected emergence of major diseases and highlighted the prevailing disparities in the healthcare delivery system. Populations affected in such situations tend to be the poor [18]. Mobile healthcare delivery programs play an important role in effectively supporting under-resourced populations during pandemics, and do so in a cost-effective manner [1]. Harvard Medical School's Family Van is an excellent example, offering blood pressure screenings, and other chronic disease management services [19]. These screenings decrease the risk of heart disease and stroke, and other chronic conditions which if left untreated can result in negative health outcomes and further increase health disparities.

Mobile clinics are adaptive and have the capability to help address emergencies in both an innovative and timely fashion [20]. As long-standing community-based healthcare delivery avenues, they play a critical role in addressing healthcare access barriers that exacerbate healthcare disparities. For example, representatives from a clinic in North Carolina highlighted challenges around equitable access to healthcare that the population of farmworkers they serve, face. "The idea of having those responsible for meeting the economic need of providing food for individuals in the nation, have difficulty with accessing healthcare, is unimaginable". The ways in which the mobile clinic has proven resourceful to the farmworkers is by providing healthcare at minimal costs, and partnering with stationary clinics to ensure a continuum of care [10].

## 6. Decision tool for Mobile clinics deployment

Results from the survey conducted by Attipoe-Dorcoo et al. [10], also indicated that counties in North Carolina and Florida experienced varying degrees of additive effects from the provision of primary and preventive care via mobile clinic providers. Mobile clinics in these counties were influential in delivering critical primary and preventive healthcare services to under-resourced populations. A mobile clinic primary care service index was constructed taking into account miles traveled by the mobile clinic, speed of the mobile clinic, number of primary care providers per mobile clinic program, number of primary care providers available in a primary care service area (PCSA), and the total population in a PCSA [21]. The index provides a valuable unit of measure to enable program managers of primary care mobile clinics to allocate their resources accordingly based on either a goal to extend their level of influence, which can be a metric to share with funders, or identify other potential areas of need to establish influence. Geographic areas with the greatest need can be identified via the lowest index, and resources can be allocated either as additional providers or mobile clinics to ensure the health needs of populations are met [21].

The findings from Attipoe-Dorcoo et al. [10] also highlighted that only one mobile clinic organization was identified in three counties in North Carolina and a similar situation was observed for rural counties in Florida as well. Anecdotally mobile clinic representatives constantly advocate for more mobile clinic access in rural areas, however, the challenges of implementing such efforts are yet to be overcome nationally. The index could be a tool that is leveraged to help provide the needed geographic metric needed in operational decision-making to ensure efficient allocation of resources [21].

## 7. Examples and opportunities for improved pandemic responses with Mobile clinics

A recently published commentary shared the findings of a webinar co-hosted by the Harvard Medical School's Family Van together with the Mobile Healthcare Association to gain an understanding of the current state of efforts by the clinics, discuss best practices, and exchange ideas [20]. Several mobile clinics in the United States offered services to different populations during the early stages of the COVID-19 pandemic, and still continue to do so. Examples highlighted in the commentary include the Parkland Health and Hospital System, which had staging areas at COVID-19 testing sites, or triage locations in the parking lots near hospital emergency departments. Another was a federally qualified health clinic in Austin, Texas, conducting outdoor testing. Nurses at the clinic triaged patients in their vehicles and not the mobile van, and then patients drove around to a doctor to get tested. Finally, Cincinnati Children's used the mobile clinic to test employees using an algorithm for employees to call a centralized number for a referral [20]. Mobile clinics are an essential aspect of our healthcare delivery system with innovative and adaptable approaches to problem-solving. Mobile clinic programs repurposed their operations to serve other dire needs of their patient populations, and communities. For example, the Harvard Medical School's Family Van hosted call-in hours, contacted clients directly, and distributed handouts put together with the COVID-19 Health Literacy Project [22]. The vans for the Vision to Learn program were used to take food and household supplies to seniors in East Los Angeles in a partnership with the Weingart East Los Angeles YMCA, University of Southern California Keck School of Medicine, Adventist Health White Memorial, and the American Heart Association. Other programs also used their vans to distribute food, and supplies to families in public housing [20].

In order to efficiently leverage the adaptable and community-based approach to healthcare delivery that mobile clinics provide, especially as an avenue to improve pandemic responses, there is a need to consider moving beyond the grant-based model of funding to create sustainable mobile clinic programs [20]. We need to be asking health policy questions about how we can leverage innovation in mobile healthcare delivery to help enhance efforts to narrow the widening gap in disparities that have resulted from this pandemic. For example, mobile clinics can be used in case management approaches similar to the model used by Uber Technologies, where mobile clinics can be requested on-demand to address localized and contextualized needs in areas where there are increases in reported cases of health conditions during a pandemic.

Additionally, as part of the National Emergency Preparedness Strategy, mobile clinics can play a pivotal role in the deployment of health resources to areas with the direst need. The model can serve to provide trained medical professionals, the use of the actual vehicles for triage and isolation units, temporary housing, and sourcing additional medical equipment. Integrating mobile health clinics in our national healthcare delivery systems in a comprehensive way will create an existing structure of collaboration with stationary facilities, and an innovative infrastructure that aims to address the underlying disparities in healthcare access and geographic barriers to care. With the evidence around costs, their geographical influence, and populations served, healthcare policies and funding models that support mobile clinic programs and their integration in our healthcare delivery systems will ensure improved responses during pandemics and other health crises.

National funding programs that expand the use of technology can also provide the opportunity to establish close collaborative involvement with other stakeholders in the healthcare system. As the nation grapples with logistical challenges and other gaps in current vaccination efforts, more critical attention needs to be given to the long-standing community model of healthcare delivery with mobile clinics, and their capability to refer and navigate patients in a comprehensive real-time manner. This will not only support the success of current efforts in response to combating the COVID-19 pandemic but other potential future pandemics in an equitable fashion.

## 8. Conclusions

Mobile clinics are both effective and efficient in ensuring populations have access to equitable healthcare. They have been shown to be a sound complement to stationary clinics. In order to better leverage, their critical role in addressing health disparities that have dramatically worsened throughout the COVID-19 pandemic, significant shifts in healthcare reimbursement policies will need to occur. With national efforts to combat health disparities by addressing social determinants of health, there is now more than ever the need to consider cohesive funding for mobile health clinics, as well as a comprehensive approach to incorporating mobile clinics in our entire health system. These efforts will not only be effective for improving health outcomes of under-resourced populations but will also play a role in contributing to the success of the current national pandemic response, and future health crises.

## Acknowledgements

The authors acknowledge the Mobile Healthcare Association, and the Mobile Health Map, a program of Harvard Medical School's Family Van for their contributions with access and insights into mobile health programs.

## Author details

Sharon Attipoe-Dorcoo[1*] and Rigoberto Delgado[2]

1 Tersha, LLC, Alpharetta, GA, USA

2 Healthcare Management and Health Economics, Department of Economics and Finance, The University of Texas at El Paso, TX, USA

*Address all correspondence to: sharon.dorcoo@tershallc.com

## References

[1] Hill, C. F., Powers, B. W., Jain, S. H., Bennet, J., Vavasis, A., & Oriol, N. E. (2014). Mobile health clinics in the era of reform. American Journal of Managed Care, 20(3), 261-264.

[2] Battistella, L. R., Juca, S. S. H., Tateishi, M., Oshiro, M. S., Yamanaka, E. I., Lima, E., & Ramos, V. D. (2015). Lucy Montoro rehabilitation network mobile unit: An alternative public healthcare policy. Disability & Rehabilitation Assistive Technology, 10(4), 309-315.

[3] Ahmad, R., Mohamad, Z., Mohd Noh, A. Y., Mohamad, N., Saharudin, M., Hamzah, S. C., Kamauzaman Tuan, T. H. (2008). Health major incident: The experiences of mobile medical team during major flood. Malaysian Journal of Medical Sciences, 15(2), 47-51.

[4] Aljasir, B., & Alghamdi, M. S. (2010). Patient satisfaction with mobile clinic services in a remote rural area of Saudi Arabia. Eastern Mediterranean Health Journal = La Revue DeSanté De La Méditerranée Orientale = Al-Majallah Al-Ṣiḥḥīyah Li-Sharq Al-Mutawassiṭ, 16(10), 1085.

[5] Peters, G., Doctor, H., Afenyadu, G., Findley, S., & Ager, A. (2014). Mobile clinic services to serve rural populations in Katsina State, Nigeria: Perceptions of services and patterns of utilization. Health Policy & Planning, 29(5), 642-649.

[6] Campos, Mendes M., & Olmstead-Rose, L. (2012). Mobile Health Clinics Increasing Access to Care in Central and Eastern Contra Costa County. Final Report Prepared for East and Central County Health Access Action Team.

[7] Malone NC, Williams MM, Fawzi MC, Bennet J, Hill C, Katz JN, Oriol NE (2020). Mobile health clinics in the United States. International Journal for Equity in Health, 19 (20) https://doi.org/10.1186/s12939-020-1135-7.

[8] Oriol, N. E., Cote, P. J., Vavasis, A. P., Bennet, J., Delorenzo, D., Blanc, P., & Kohane, I. (2009). Calculating the return on investment of mobile healthcare. BMC Medicine, 7(1), 27-27. doi: 10.1186/1741-7015-7-27.

[9] Sisler, J. (2013). Roll, roll, roll me away. CMAJ: Canadian Medical Association Journal, 185(3), E145. doi:10.1503/cmaj.l09-4367.

[10] Attipoe-Dorcoo S et al. (2018). An Overview of Costs, Utilization, Geographical Distribution & Influence of Mobile Clinics in Rural Healthcare Delivery in the United States. (Doctoral dissertation, The University of Texas School of Public Health).

[11] Brunner, Bettina, Andrew Carmona, Alphonse Kouakou, Ibrahima Dolo, Chloé Revuz, Thierry Uwamahoro, Leslie Miles, and Sessi Kotchofa. (2014). The Private Health Sector in West Africa: Six Macro-Level Assessments. Bethesda, MD: Strengthening Health Outcomes through the Private Sector Project, Abt Associates Inc.

[12] Douglass, J. M. (2005). Mobile Dental Vans. Journal of public health dentistry, 65(2), 110-113.

[13] Arevalo, O., Chattopadhyay, A., Lester, H., & Skelton, J. (2010). Mobile dental operations: capital budgeting and long-term viability. Journal of public health dentistry. 70(1), 28-34.

[14] Centro De Integracao De Educacao E Saude. (2016). Mobile Medical Center. Retrieved from http://www.projetocies.org.br/medical-center-mobile.php. Accessed April 12, 2016.

[15] Lien, C., Raimo, J., Abramowitz, J., Khanijo, S., Kritharis, A., Mason, C., ... & Carney, M. T. (2014). Community Healthcare Delivery Post-Hurricane Sandy: Lessons from a Mobile Health Unit. Journal of community health, 39(3), 599-605.

[16] Muolavie, D., Busby, A., Peterson, J., & Stullenbarger, E. (2000). Thinking about a mobile health unit to deliver services? Things to consider before buying. Australian Journal of Rural Health, 8(1), 6-16.

[17] Attipoe-Dorcoo, S., Delgado, R., Lai, D., Gupta, A., & Linder, S. (2020). Analysis of Annual Costs of Mobile Clinics in the Southern United States. Journal of Primary Care & Community Health, 11, 2150132720980623.

[18] Blake Farmer, Nashville Public Radio. Long-Standing Racial And Income Disparities Seen Creeping Into COVID-19. Accessed on April 6, 2020. Available at: https://khn.org/news/covid-19-treatment-racial-income-health-disparities.

[19] The Family Van. Accessed January 28, 2021. Available at: http://www.familyvan.org.

[20] Attipoe-Dorcoo, S., Delgado, R., Gupta, A., Bennet, J., Oriol, N. E., & Jain, S. H. (2020). Mobile health clinic model in the COVID-19 pandemic: lessons learned and opportunities for policy changes and innovation. International Journal for Equity in Health, 19(1), 1-5.

[21] Attipoe-Dorcoo, S., Delgado, R., Lai, D., Gupta, A., & Linder, S. (2021). Geographical Influence of Mobile Clinics in the Southern United States. Applied Spatial Analysis and Policy, 14(1), 81-87.

[22] Covid19 Health Literacy Project. Accessed April 5, 2020. Available at: https://covid19healthliteracyproject.com.

Chapter 12

# Practice Changing Innovations for Emergency Care during the COVID-19 Pandemic in Resource Limited Settings

*Tej Prakash Sinha, Brunda RL, Sakshi Yadav and Sanjeev Bhoi*

## Abstract

COVID-19 has affected millions worldwide. To combat the infectious pandemic in resource limited settings, healthcare workers and techies have come up with multiple innovations. Nations with scarcity of resources have resorted to innovative strategies involving optimal utilization and repurposing of available commodities to overcome the demand–supply mismatch. Emergency rooms overburdened with diseased population are resorting to local innovative ideas to overcome obstacles in COVID-19 patient care. Point of care testing strategies in emergency rooms, sampling booths to reduce Personal Protective Equipment (PPE) use, disinfection strategies such as tunnel disinfection and local production of sanitizers, face masks/shields, aerosol containment chambers, novel triage protocols, telehealth care strategies reaching out to remote population and utilizing point for care ultrasound for resuscitation are few of the novel innovations which have benefitted medical fraternity and patient care in testing times. Medical innovations have emerged as the positive outcome of otherwise devastating COVID-19 pandemic. These practice changing innovations could also prove beneficial in future infectious pandemics.

**Keywords:** COVID-19, innovations, emergency care, resource limited settings, demand–supply mismatch

## 1. Introduction

COVID-19 pandemic has affected millions worldwide. Most developing countries being densely populated, has witnessed swarming number of cases. To combat the infectious pandemic in the resource constraint settings healthcare workers and techies have come up with multiple innovations [1]. Government has also played a role by implementing policies of universal masking, physical distancing, lockdowns, ban on mass gatherings, testing, tracing and isolating suspected and positive cases [2]. Challenges faced by developing economies have been distinct in comparison to those faced by developed nations during the pandemic situation. The COVID-19 pandemic has had devastating impact on already fragile developing nation economies. To cater to demand–supply mismatches, countries have resorted to innovative ideas with available resources. Emergency care deemed a crucial component of healthcare systems, has been affected enormously. Emergency department has been operating as frontline portal of entry for patients with undifferentiated symptoms into the healthcare setup. Innovations to facilitate emergency care, to reduce burden over healthcare systems, to ensure standard care for all emergency patients by bridging economic and knowledge gaps are being implemented in majority of developing nations.

## 2. Emergency care during COVID-19

Emergency services in most parts of the world have been overwhelmed with patients since the onset of COVID-19 pandemic.

- Need for reorganization of emergency setup: The highly infectious COVID-19 disease warrants strict infection control and prevention measures. Need for areas to cater to COVID-19 positive and suspected patients away from non-COVID-19 patients has forced emergency rooms to reorganize their existing setups.

- Triage: Emergency Room (ER) triage to detect suspected patients early and care for them in designated areas is of paramount importance to prevent spread. This has led to new triage tools such point of care ultrasound based triage in emergency rooms to supplement clinical history and examination in detecting cases quickly. Studies have demonstrated high sensitivity but low specificity in comparison with CT scan to detect COVID-19 related lung pathology [3]. Point of care ultrasound being easily available, portable, quick to perform even in resource limited settings with unavailability of CT scan, has been found helpful in quick ER triage.

- Aggressive symptom screening: As ER is the first point of contact for most patients presenting with severe and undifferentiated symptoms, a need for aggressive symptom screening, manpower training to detect/screen patients, need for judicious resource allocation has aroused.

- Isolation of patients: ER caters to both COVID-19 positive and negative patients thus allowing risk of cross-contamination. Infection prevention measures such as distancing, masking patients, creation of isolation rooms with adequate air exchange has become the new norm. Separate rooms for doffing and donning of Personal Protective Equipment (PPE) are also necessary. All these measures have been challenging to fulfill promptly in emergency setups of resource limited settings.

- Increased need for manpower, PPE, infrastructure: Increasing patient number has translated to increased demands for manpower and essential equipment thus overwhelming the economies [4]. Working hours have undergone modification to ensure healthcare professionals with PPE work 4–6 hours shifts, thus increasing the manpower demand.

## 3. Challenges faced by hospital setups

- Lack of infrastructure: This is one of the major challenge faced by hospitals due to this pandemic. Many hospitals in developing countries lack the preparedness to handle a sudden outbreak of a pandemic like this and provide for the health needs for every individual of the large population.

- Shortage of beds: Admission of new patients has become difficult because of the burden of the existing patients which are already admitted for treatment. Expanding capacity and creating space for new patients has therefore become a major challenge.

- Ventilators: Apart from the shortage of beds and doctors, hospitals are also facing the shortage of medical equipment like ventilators due to which many of them are not able to treat patients efficiently.

- PPE for healthcare staff: Due to a sudden increase in the demand of the testing kits and PPEs in this outbreak, the supply chains have faced many issues which have also depleted the reserves of the PPEs of the hospitals.

- Difficulty in maintaining adequate number of staff: There is a sudden rise in the requirement of manpower especially during this crisis because these are the people who are required to take the charge of running and managing the hospitals while the doctors and the nurses take up the forefront role of treating the patients. Along with testing and treating the patients for COVID-19, it is essential to keep the hospital staff safe from contracting the virus and getting infected which might lead to the shortage of staff even more.

- Safety and hazardous waste management: Proper and safe disposition of used PPE, masks and wastes from COVID positive patients is also one of the major challenge

- Downfall in the revenue generation for the hospitals: Due to the pandemic, there is a decrease in the patient visits to the hospitals because people try to avoid going to hospitals due to the fear of contracting the virus. Many hospitals had to cancel or postpone the surgeries of their previous patients because they are under the pressure to free up bed space for COVID-19 patients. This has also led to many people losing their jobs or salary cuts in some cases because hospitals are not able to pay them their salaries [5].

## 4. Practice changing innovations

Few simple yet effective solutions have evolved to help developing countries tackle the pandemic.

### 4.1 Innovative testing strategies

Sampling patients to diagnose cases of COVID-19 is considered aerosol generating procedure by itself, thus requiring healthcare personnel (HCP) in full Personal Protective Equipment (PPE) to be recruited. In resource limited settings with scarcity of PPE, the concept of sampling booths has emerged. These are booths similar to telephone booths which are being used widely to sample patients in Delhi, Kerala and other states [6]. An innovative modification of the traditional kiosk called by the name "COVSACK" was made functional at ESI hospital in Hyderabad. The main differences from traditional kiosk being that COVSACK has the suspected patient inside the kiosk instead of the HCP. HCP is positioned outside the kiosk. Kiosk is also equipped with self-disinfection capability. As HCP is positioned outside the kiosk and at theoretically reduced risk of aerosol exposure, the need for PPE is also reduced [7]. Few models with dual chamber booths have also been proposed and tried [8]. South Korea has devised an innovative model of "Drive Through" COVID-19 testing of patients [9].

Testing using RT-PCR has been the standard but with a drawback of prolonged downtime to obtain results especially in emergency settings. Over ten rapid antibody based kits for quick point of care testing have been devised, approved by Indian Council of Medical Research (ICMR) and validated for clinical use [10]. With easy availability this has led to increased rates of testing along with quicker results particularly in life threatening conditions.

A paper strip based COVID-19 detection test named "Feluda" has been devised by research team at the CSIR-Institute of Genomics and Integrative Biology in India and has been approved by Drug Controller General Of India (DCGI). Feluda is based on Clustered Regularly Interspaced Short Palindromic Repeats-cas 9 (CRISPR-cas 9) technology. The test has been performed on over 2000 patients reporting a sensitivity of 96% and a specificity of 98% which is very similar to the gold standard RT-PCR [11]. With quicker results feluda could help reduce number of patients waiting for over 12 hrs before interventions and definitive management procedures at emergency rooms.

### 4.2 Innovative infection control and prevention strategies

Care of COVID-19 patients revolves around several logistic issues such as availability of oxygen ports and ventilators in resource constraint settings. Innovative methods of oxygen splitting and ventilator splitting to benefit multiple patients using a single device have been proposed and utilized in few parts of the country with success [12, 13]. Critically ill patients mandate interventions such as intubation which is aerosol generation procedure requiring measures to ensure HCP safety. Novel aerosol containment chambers have been designed with modifications and used in India [14, 15]. These plastic or acrylic boxes have openings to allow HCP insert his hands and maneuver as per need.

Innovative negative pressure isolation tents called "Care cube" have been functional in United States to care for COVID-19 patient population [16]. These tents being low-cost models, similar designs can be adapted in resource limited settings for infection control and prevention. Overcrowded ER with lack of free space to set up new isolation areas can resort to such negative pressure tents to cater to COVID-19 positive patients.

### 4.3 Innovative airway management strategies

Companies like AgVa solutions, Big Band Boom Solutions, Aerobiosys, etc. are building cost-effective portable ventilators. They are also lending a helping hand in ramping up the production and supply of ventilators to the hospitals.

InnAccel Bangalore, a Stanford India Biodesign based medical devices setup, has come to the fore with SAANS Pro, a non-invasive breathing support system that was developed to serve as an alternative for ventilators in low resource settings. The device has been designed to function with limited or no oxygen supply, with an added benefit of being portable. This can be used in ambulances to transport patients and in rural tertiary care centers where ventilators are in short supply [17].

The Gradian CCV (Comprehensive Care Ventilator) supports critically-ill patients in settings with unreliable supplies of power and oxygen, including temporary field hospitals being set up to manage COVID-19 patients in many countries.

The ventilator can run for 21 hours on battery power, and its portability features enable single-ventilator use throughout critical care, including patient transport. Simulation-based training is a critical component of Gradian's model, with teams of clinicians and bio-medical technicians providing remote and on-site training to healthcare providers. Gradian has placed ventilators in Nepal, Sierra Leone, Kenya, and several other countries, conducted several remote trainings with clinicians, and is continuing to work with more health systems to build capacity for COVID response and other critical care needs [18].

RespirAID is a portable breathing support system developed by Biodesign Innovation Labs with an aim to meet the shortage of ventilators in Indian hospitals and globally. It uses a ventilation strategy called Intermittent Positive airway pressure that can moderate essential respiratory parameters. This makes it suitable for patients who are at severe risk of lung collapse [17].

### 4.4 Telemedicine innovations to combat COVID-19

Digital healthcare has been a boon in testing times of COVID-19 pandemic. Telemedicine has been used widely for obtaining consultations and care via virtual pathway. Many healthcare setups across the country have switched to telemedicine based patient care. From obtaining appointments before presenting at a healthcare facility thereby reducing overcrowding to obtaining consultations and treatment for minor ailments, telemedicine has facilitated patient care in a simple and user-friendly manner. Telehealth care to a certain extent has helped in maintaining the continuum of care of chronically ill patients unable to visit healthcare setups amid COVID-19 case surges and lockdowns. Telemedicine has been a virtually perfect way to deploy HCP for patient care in remote parts of the country [19, 20].

Prior to the pandemic, the growth of telemedicine has been very slow. The apprehension among the medical practitioners regarding the legality of providing virtual healthcare has been a major contributory factor for the lack of exponential growth of telemedicine. All it required was a little help from the virus, to take telemedicine from sidelines to the centre stage.

With hospital beds and isolation centers stretched more than ever, healthcare organizations are helping patients better manage their care at home when it's deemed safe to discharge them. It can prevent costly and life-threatening readmissions by catching problems before they arise. Patients with mild symptoms receive a telehealth kit that includes a laptop with preloaded apps through which they can monitor their signs and communicate twice daily with a nurse by phone or virtual visit.

### 4.5 Technological innovations to combat COVID-19

#### *4.5.1 Online COVID-19 screening tools*

Artificial Intelligence (AI) Highway provides pre-screening and triage tools that are based on risk-assessment scores for Covid-19, linked to symptoms, contact history and more.

#### *4.5.2 Robots on duty*

With pandemic continuing, many countries have come up with the idea of using robots to help the medical staff which limits the risk to their lives. The major duties of these robots are autonomous delivery of food, medicine and other consumables inside the isolation wards. They also disinfect the used items and allow patients to communicate with physicians and relatives [21].

### *4.5.3 3D-printed medical equipment*

With the increasing number of COVID cases, the nation is scrambling to address the shortage of Ventilators, Personal Protective Equipment (PPE) and other medical devices. Amid this crisis, Indian research institutions and companies have started hinging on 3D-printing techniques as a quick fix. Medical equipment such as ventilators, face shields, oxygen masks, parts of virus test kits and other protective gear to deal with the pandemic are produced in large numbers with the help of this modern technology to address the shortage. 3D-printed ear guards for hospital staff to help alleviate the pain caused by wearing face masks for too long [22] and 3D-printed ventilator valves for dealing with COVID-19 [23].

### *4.5.4 Artificial intelligence*

The use of AI in healthcare is not a new concept and has been around for long. Researchers and data scientists around the world are looking to use Artificial Intelligence as a way of addressing the challenges posed by the coronavirus. Several hospitals have started using AI software- which learns from experience- to help with diagnosis and assessments. Recently, a group of scientists made use of Artificial Intelligence to identify an underlying genomic signature for 29 different DNA sequences of the novel coronavirus, providing an important tool for vaccine and drug developers.

Indian based Internet of Things (IoT) startup called HELYXON uses AI-enabled devices for better management of the pandemic by constantly monitoring the vital parameters of patients or suspects. 98.6 Fever Watch is another innovation which is useful particularly for unwell children in whom continuous monitoring of temperature is a vital parameter in disease management. It connects to hospitals systems or personal systems and keeps transferring patient information to a central dashboard.

Qure.ai has deployed new solutions that automatically read and interpret chest X-Ray scans for COVID-19 in seconds. This tool quantifies how much of the patient's lungs have been affected, enabling the clinicians to monitor disease progression more effectively.

Bengaluru start-up Predible Health is using AI-based radiology solutions to pre-screen COVID-19 patients with the help of a tool LungIQ, which can measure percentage of lung damage in patients through CT scans & help doctors understand how badly a patient is affected and if he needs a ventilator or not.

Aggressive contact tracing:

Using mobile apps, security camera footage, facial recognition technology, bank card records, and global positioning system (GPS) data from vehicles and mobile phones to provide real-time data and detailed timelines of people's travel. Acrylosorb- an instrument to collect body fluids and to dispose of it safely, an isolation pod that restricts COVID-19 patients from having contact with others.

### *4.5.5 Contact tracing apps*

Contact tracing applications enable users who have come in contact with COVID-19 positive patients to be notified, traced and suitably supported. The Aarogya Setu was initially conceived as a sophisticated tracking tool to map out epidemic hotspots. But along with that it is capable of exchanging short-distance Bluetooth signals when individuals are in proximity to each other. The application records these encounters and stores them in their respective mobile phones. If an individual is diagnosed with COVID-19, government accesses the data to identify contacts of the infected person. South Korea implemented tools for aggressive contact tracing, using security camera footage, facial recognition technology, bank card records, and global positioning system (GPS) data from vehicles and mobile phones to provide real-time data and detailed timelines of people's travel. By identifying and isolating infections early, South Korea maintained among the lowest per-capita mortality rates in the world [24].

Through "Corona Watch" application, the location of corona affected patients can be tracked and their movement history of last 14 days can be recorded. A containment watch app has also been developed to undertake survey in containment zones and ensure the provision of essential services.

#### *4.5.6 Drone technology*

Drones are being used for delivery of blood, medicines, PPE and other essential medical supplies in many countries [25].

## 5. Proposed innovations

World economic forum has described five ways collective intelligence could prove beneficial to help combat coronavirus in developing countries. Similar strategies could be the way forward to deal with the infectious pandemic.

### 5.1 Mapping medical supply demands

Awareness regarding the needs and necessities of the nation is of paramount importance. Developing countries may not be able to compete with richer economies to procure resources and supplies such as masks, ventilators and other essential commodities. It has thus been proposed for frontline workers to use applications such as "Frontline SMS" to report shortage of key equipment on a common website. The reported data can be uploaded on a map showing shortage locations. This will allow local manufacturers, humanitarian agencies, government organizations and businessmen to respond and help in crisis areas. Similar technology is already in use since over a decade in Africa to map essential medicine supplies.

### 5.2 Localized production of supplies

When traditional logistics fail to cater to overwhelming crisis situations, organizations such as "Field Ready" have proven beneficial to procure essential supplies and equipment for care in crisis zones. "Field ready" is already functional in countries such as Nepal to cater to local demands and to improvise healthcare. Its utility can be extended to cater to COVID-19 pandemic. Governing bodies can utilize local marketplace and manufactures to fulfill essential supply demands. During COVID-19 lockdown situations, local 3D printing vendors can be allowed to operate as "essential infrastructure" thus helping economies become self-reliant.

### 5.3 Resource and asset identification

Identification of available assests is important. Emergency care has been burdened by increasing load of COVID-19 positive patients. Stable patients and those fit for home isolation might hoard in emergency care facilities as emergency is readily accessible and these patients might be dwellers of overcrowded households with no opportunity to isolate themselves at their residence. In such scenarios identification and repurposing of areas such as schools, stadiums into mass quarantine centers could prove helpful.

### 5.4 Smarter surge response

Most countries face shortage of healthcare workers to cater to rapidly expanding patient population. Training and education activities to deploy community health workers for screening and symptom assessment could prove beneficial [26]. This would also reduce the burden of patients with minor symptoms presenting at hospital triage facilities. In India, ASHA (Accredited Social Health Activists) and anganwadi workers are being trained on infection prevention measures, infection control, initial patient assessment, care and other COVID-19 related topics [27]. Such initiatives can be implemented in other developing countries with gross shortage of healthcare staff.

### 5.5 Medical education

Mobilizing collective intelligence of frontline healthcare professionals across the world can help medical staff in developing countries gain relevant and essential knowledge quickly. Praekelt.org in South Africa has introduced Health-Alert, a WhatsApp-based helpline disseminating accurate, timely COVID-19 information, with automated answers to frequently asked questions, relieving call centre traffic. Machine learning and its ability to understand natural language enable automatic triage advice and large volume conversations. Insights from real-time data support effective systems-level COVID- 19decision-making [18]. Telemedicine and internet based communications could serve as portals for percolation of knowledge among peers.

## 6. Future perspectives

COVID-19 pandemic has taught many useful lessons to the world. Handling the chaos, judiciously utilizing the available humanitarian supplies, re-purposing resources to meet demands and striving to cater to masses affected has been the prime focus during this pandemic. Every sphere of life has been hampered by COVID-19 and left developing economies struggling. Health for all being the goal of every existing nation, emergency care during the pandemic has been hampered. To prevent and attenuate similar stressful scenarios in future, there is need for:

- Mitigation and emergency preparedness for future infectious pandemics: Infectious pandemic such as COVID-19 are public health emergencies. Applying the concepts of emergency management, such as use of Emergency Operation Centers (EOCs) and Incident Management Systems (IMS) could help public health systems protect populations impacted by health emergencies. State and national programmes to device a uniform "Emergency Management Plan" (EMP) as per CDC (Centre for Disease Control) advice for preparedness and response during pandemics is need of the hour [28]. With EMP in place nations will be aware of their resources, demands and shortcomings. During an infectious outbreak there will be reduced chaos with easier and earlier recruitment of humanitarian supplies as per the response strategy of emergency management plan.

*DOI: http://dx.doi.org/10.5772/intechopen.98293*

- COVID-capable/Pandemic resilient healthcare system: Existing healthcare systems need to transform into pandemic resilient healthcare setups considering the current day scenario of ever increasing disease burden. Rather than focusing on building COVID-19 patient care setups, the emphasis should now be on making the existing healthcare setups to become self-reliant to care for COVID-19 patient population. Repurposing humanitarian supplies and infrastructure to achieve this could prove useful.

## 7. Conclusion

COVID-19 has had devastating effects on health and economy of the country, but COVID-19 has also forced innovative minds to emerge with novel ideas for combating the infectious pandemic and helping mankind. Thus COVID-19 era has witnessed a bundle of innovations with majority of them aiming to balance demand supply discrepancy.

## Acknowledgements

None.

## Funding

None.

## Conflict of interest

The authors declare no conflict of interest.

## Acronyms and abbreviations

| | |
|---|---|
| PPE | Personal Protective Equipment |
| ER | Emergency Room |
| HCP | Healthcare personnel |
| ICMR | Indian Council of Medical Research |
| DCGI | Drug Controller General Of India |
| AI | Artificial Intelligence |
| IoT | Internet of Things |
| EOC | Emergency Operation Centers |
| IMS | Incident Management Systems |
| EMP | Emergency Management Plan |

## Author details

Tej Prakash Sinha*, Brunda RL, Sakshi Yadav and Sanjeev Bhoi
Department of Emergency Medicine, All India Institute of Medical Sciences, New Delhi, India

*Address all correspondence to: drsinha123@gmail.com

## References

[1] Mathew JL, Mathew TL. Invention, Innovation, and Imitation in India—Necessity Arising from the COVID-19 Pandemic. Annals of the National Academy of Medical Sciences (India). 21.06.2020. 2020 Jun 8;56(02):077-86.

[2] Chowdhury R, Luhar S, Khan N, Choudhury SR, Matin I, Franco OH. Long-term strategies to control COVID-19 in low and middle-income countries: an options overview of community-based, non-pharmacological interventions. European Journal of Epidemiology [Internet]. 2020 Aug 1;35(8):743-748. Available from: https://doi.org/10.1007/s10654-020-00660-1

[3] Narinx N, Smismans A, Symons R, Frans J, Demeyere A, Gillis M. Feasibility of using point-of-care lung ultrasound for early triage of COVID-19 patients in the emergency room. Emerg Radiol [Internet]. 2020/09/10 ed. 2020 Dec;27(6):663-70. Available from: https://pubmed.ncbi.nlm.nih.gov/32910323

[4] Freund Y. The challenge of emergency medicine facing the COVID-19 outbreak. European Journal of Emergency Medicine [Internet]. 2020;27(3). Available from: https://journals.lww.com/euro-emergencymed/Fulltext/2020/06000/The_challenge_of_emergency_medicine_facing_the.1.aspx

[5] https://innohealthmagazine.com/2020/covid19/innovation-for-hospitalsduring-covid-19/.

[6] Sruthi (2020) India's 1st walk-in COVID-19 test kiosks become functional in Kerala. https://www.biotecnika.org/2020/04/first-walk-in-covid-19-test-booth-functional-in-kerala/. Accessed 10 Apr 2020.

[7] Joshi JR. COVSACK: an innovative portable isolated and safe COVID-19 sample collection kiosk with automatic disinfection. Transactions of the Indian National Academy of Engineering [Internet]. 2020 Jun 1;5(2):269-275. Available from: https://doi.org/10.1007/s41403-020-00139-1

[8] Nair SS, Prajapati AK, Venkatesan RB, Vayalappil MC, Kishore A. Design and Evaluation of Chitra Swab Collection Booths for Health Professionals in COVID-19 Pandemic. Transactions of the Indian National Academy of Engineering [Internet]. 2020 Aug 31; Available from: https://doi.org/10.1007/s41403-020-00167-x

[9] Lee D, Lee J. Testing on the move: South Korea's rapid response to the COVID-19 pandemic. Transportation Research Interdisciplinary Perspectives [Internet]. 2020/04/21 ed. 2020 May;5:100111-100111. Available from: https://www.ncbi.nlm.nih.gov/pmc/articles/PMC7172645/

[10] Guidance on Rapid Antibody Kits for COVID-19. Available at: https://www.icmr.gov.in/pdf/covid/kits/Antibody_based_tests_14052020.pdf. Accessed May 18, 2020.

[11] Rajalakshmi N. Explained: How Does India's Feluda COVID-19 Test Work? 2020 Oct 28; Available from: https://science.thewire.in/the-sciences/explained-feluda-covid-19-test-india-crispr-technology/

[12] Tamil Nadu: Ventilator Splitters Being 3D Printed in Case of Shortage for Covid-19 Patients. Available at: https://www.indiatoday.in/india/story/tamil-nadu-ventilator-splitters-being-3d-printed-in-case-of-shortage-for-covid-19-patients-1668167-2020-04-17. Accessed May 17, 2020.

[13] Badve A. Coronavirus India: Nagpur's Dr Anand Sancheti Develops Ventilator Splitters. Avilable at: https://

www.sakaltimes.com/coronavirus-maharashtra/coronavirus-india-nagpur's-dr-anand-sancheti-develops-ventilator-splitters. Accessed May 17, 2020.

[14] Railways New Innovative Device, 'Intubation Boxes', to Aid the Medical Fraternity In Our Fight Against COVID-19. Available at: https://news.fresherslive.com/articles/railway-s-new-innovative-device-intubation-boxes-to-aid-the-medical-fraternity-in-our-fight-against-covid-19-126438. Accessed May 18, 2020.

[15] Singh B. IIT Guwahati Students Design Low-Cost Intubation Box to Help Doctors in Covid-19 Fight. Available at: https://economictimes.indiatimes.com/industry/healthcare/biotech/healthcare/iit-guwahati-students-design-low-cost-intubation-box-to-help-doctors-in-covid-19-fight/articleshow/75475246.cms?from=mdr. Accessed May 18, 2020.

[16] Harrison K. Innovative infection isolation tent humanises treatment for COVID-19 patients. 2020 Jul 29; Available from: https://newsroom.unsw.edu.au/news/art-architecture-design/innovative-infection-isolation-tent-humanises-treatment-covid-19

[17] https://indiabioscience.org/columns/indian-scenario/innovations-to-make-india-self-reliant-in-tackling-covid-19.

[18] Global health innovators mobilize to help developing countries combat COVID-19 | EurekAlert! Science News: https://www.eurekalert.org/pub_releases/2020-04/tca-imt042120.php.

[19] Keri VC, R.L B, Sinha TP, Wig N, Bhoi S. Tele-healthcare to combat COVID-19 pandemic in developing countries: A proposed single centre and integrated national level model. The International Journal of Health Planning and Management [Internet]. 2020 Aug 3 [cited 2020 Oct 16];n/a(n/a). Available from: https://doi.org/10.1002/hpm.3036

[20] Sh. R Ramanan(Additional Secretary and Mission Director, Himanshu Agrawal(Young Professional, AIM, NITI Aayog)AIM, NITI Aayog), Naman Agrawal(Innovation Lead, AIM, NITI Aayog). Telemedicine: A Blessing In Disguise In Time Of COVID-19. 2020.

[21] Rl B, Keri V, Sinha T, Bhoi S. Re-purposing humanoid robots for patient care in COVID-19 pandemic. The International Journal of Health Planning and Management. 2020 Sep 1;

[22] Barnes S. Boy scout 3D prints 'ear guards' to help relieve hospital workers' pain caused by facemasks. https://mymodernmet.com/3d-printed-ear-guards/.

[23] Peters J. Volunteers produce 3D-printed valves for life-saving coronavirus treatments.https://www.theverge.com/2020/3/17/21184308/coronavirus-italy-medical-3d-print-valves-treatments.

[24] Digital Healthcare Innovating During Pandemic| VMware Radius: https://www.vmware.com/radius/impact/digital-healthcare-pandemic/.

[25] How Delivery Drones Are Being Used to Tackle COVID-19 (Updated) [Internet]. We Robotics- The power of Local. 2020. Available from: https://blog.werobotics.org/2020/04/25/cargo-drones-covid-19/

[26] Peach kathy, Gray I. Five ways collective intelligence can help beat coronavirus in developing countries [Internet]. 2020. Available from: https://theconversation.com/five-ways-collective-intelligence-can-help-beat-coronavirus-in-developing-countries-136548

[27] Ganesh M. It's Time ASHAs And Anganwadi Workers Are Given Recognition As Healthcare Employees.

2020 May 28; Available from: https://www.outlookindia.com/website/story/opinion-its-time-ashas-and-anganwadi-workers-are-given-recognition-as-healthcare-employees/353769

[28] Bryant JL, Sosin DM, Wiedrich TW, Redd SC. Emergency Operations Centers and Incident Management Structure. In: CDC Field Epidemiology manual. 4th ed. Oxford University press 2019;

Section 5

# Impact of COVID-19 on Socioeconomic and Psychosocial Life and Status

Chapter 13

# Origin and Impact of COVID-19 on Socioeconomic Status

*Gaffar Sarwar Zaman and Mesfer Al Shahrani*

## Abstract

The coronavirus pandemic, known as COVID-19, is an evolving pandemic caused by a coronavirus, the SARS-CoV-2. The virus was first detected in Wuhan, China, in December 2019. In January 2020, the World Health Organization (WHO) notified this upsurge as an international emergency concerning public health. It was declared a pandemic later in March 2020. By May 12, 2021, 160,363,284 cases had been registered, and 3,332,762 deaths have been reported, caused by COVID-19, characterized as a horrific pandemic in the history of humankind. Scientists have reached a consensus about the origin of COVID-19, a zoonotic virus arising from bats or other animals in a natural habitat. The economic impact of this outbreak has left far-reaching repercussions on world business transactions, along with bond, commodity, and stock markets. One of the crucial incidents that popped up was the oil price war among OPEC countries. It caused plummeting oil prices and the collapse of stock markets globally in March 2020, as the OPEC agreement failed. However, COVID-19 plays a crucial role in the economic recession. The monetary deficit impact on the travel and trade industries is likely to be huge, in billions of pounds, increasing daily. Other sectors have also suffered significantly.

**Keywords:** pandemic, COVID-19, zoonotic virus, economic impact, economic recession

## 1. Introduction

### 1.1 Historical background

Coronavirus (CoV) was tracked down in the 1960s. The Coronavirus Study Group, patronized by the International Committee on Taxonomy of Viruses (ICTV), applied the principle of comparative genomics to further evaluate and segregate the reproductive proteins on open reading frames to identify the variables that convert CoV at varying cluster ranks. CoVs are linked to diseases of different magnitudes. SARS (in 2002–2003) and MERS (in 2012) were the most severe types causing far-reaching pandemics.

Recently, people worldwide have been hugely impacted by COVID-19; it holds the fifth rank as a pandemic since its inception following the 1918 Spanish flu. Since late December 2019, there were possible warning signs followed by the flare-up because of unusual pneumonia incidences in the Chinese city of Wuhan. The symptoms of this complex disease in patients suffering from fever, malaise, dry cough, and dyspnea have been identified as viral pneumonia [1, 2], termed by the press, in the first instance, as Wuhan pneumonia, because of its association with its symptoms. A comprehensive analysis of the entire genomes has concluded that the outbreak has been caused by the novel coronavirus that has earned the 7th rank as a member of the coronavirus family that infects human beings [3]. The WHO temporarily used terminology for this latest virus as 2019-nCoV on January 12, 2020; soon after, this infectious ailment was officially named COVID-19 on February 12, 2020. Based on phylogeny, taxonomy, and established practices, a subsequent designation for this virus has been considered SARS-CoV-2 by the ICTV [4]. Eventually, the people-to-people transmission of COVID-19 in Hong Kong was identified in the clinical data [5]. As COVID-19 first cropped up in a Chinese city, it gradually developed in four months and swiftly flared up to other parts as a worldwide emergency. Finally, on March 11, 2020, the WHO evaluated COVID-19 as a pandemic, followed by the 1918 Spanish flu, 1957 Asian flu, 1968 Hong Kong flu, and 2009 Pandemic flu. All these pandemics exterminated about 55.5 million people collectively (**Figure 1**) [6–9].

## 2. Structure of COVID-19

Coronaviruses (CoVs) are affiliated with the Coronaviridae family, constituting a group of enveloped, positive-sense, single-stranded RNA viruses [10, 11]. They are named "CoVs" because of their crown-like structure under an electronic microscope [12–15]. Coronaviruses emerge from the Coronaviridae family, of the order of nidovirales. It was called the "coronavirus" due to the crown-like spikes on its periphery. Coronaviruses comprise a single-stranded RNA that is a tiny nucleic particle (65–125 nm in diameter) (**Figure 1**).

Four subcategories of coronaviruses—(a) alpha, (b) beta, (c) gamma, and (d) delta coronavirus—exist. These viruses were considered the agents of infections only in animals until an upsurge of SARS-CoV was identified in Guangdong, China,

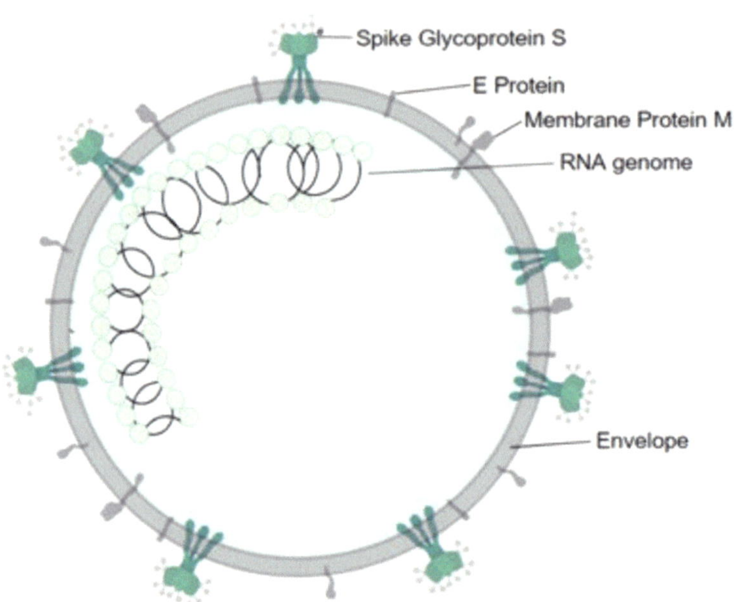


**Figure 1.**
*Construction of respiratory syndrome that generates coronavirus in humans. [This file is licensed under the Creative Commons Attribution-Share Alike 4.0 International license; https://en.wikipedia.org/wiki/COVID-19].*

in 2002 [14]. MERS-CoV, another pathogenic coronavirus, caused an endemic in the Middle East countries within ten years [15]. Around December 2019, Wuhan, a burgeoning business point of China, had experienced a flare-up of an unusual coronavirus, causing deaths of an estimated eighteen hundred people and infecting seventy thousand citizens in a fortnight of the outbreak. A formal notification announced that this virus was a member of the beta-type coronaviruses.

According to the ICTV, the main reason for COVID-19 is SARS-CoV-2; Chinese researchers have labeled this extraordinary virus as 2019-nCov or Wuhan coronavirus [16–18]. Statistically, 8098 individuals were infected by SRAS-CoV (2003), causing several deaths; the mortality rate reached 9% in 26 countries, whereas the novel coronavirus (2019) affected 120,000 individuals. In 109 nations, the infection caused a huge human loss, leaving a 2.9% mortality rate when this paper was published. Regarding communicability, SARS-CoV-2 is more intense than SRAS-CoV. The fundamental basis of the transmission was genetic rearrangements of the spike protein in the receptor-binding domain (RBD) of SARS-CoV-2, expected to have developed its transferability. In this review article, the source of human coronaviruses has been discussed as precisely as possible. The correlated infectivity and biological characteristics of MERS and SARS have been discussed with exceptional attention on COVID-19.

## 3. The virus (COVID-19)

From a pneumonia patient with an unidentified etiology, three specimens of bronchoalveolar washing were extracted on December 30, 2019, in Wuhan Jinyintan Hospital. However, close observation was established regarding this etiology due to the SARS outbreak that flared up in 2000–2003. The polymerase chain reaction (PCR) (reverse transcription-polymerase chain reaction RT-PCR) assessment of these specimens was positive for the entire beta coronaviruses. For the procurement of the whole genome sequences of the virus, Illumina and nanopore sequencing were used only to establish that the characteristics of the virus are identical to those of the coronavirus family. It was also proven that the virus belonged to the Beta-coronavirus 2 B lineage, designated by bioinformatics analyses. Arrangement of genome size of the COVID-19 virus and existing Beta-coronavirus depicted the nearest interrelation with the strains of Bat-Cov RaTG13 with 96% similarity. Virus segregation was carried out by commonly used cell lines—such as Vero E6, Huh-7, and human airway epithelial cells; simultaneously, cytopathic effects (CPE) were put in surveillance for 96 hours after vaccination. Typical crown-shaped flecks were observed under a transmission electron microscope (TEM) with negative staining. Sera extracted from convalescent patients have the potential to neutralize the cellular infection of the isolated virus completely. Interstitial hyperplasia-induced multifocal pneumonia was isolated from ACE2 Rhesus monkeys and mice intranasally challenged with the same virus. One hundred and four strains of the virus were separated from COVID-19 patients in different locations. The observation started at the end of December 2019 and lasted until mid-February 2020 for genome arrangement analysis; it exhibited 99.9 percent homogeneity lacking transformation (**Figure 1**).

At the outset of the outbreak, the WHO announced the name of the interim virus as 2019-nCoV for COVID-19. For histological examination, post-mortem samples were collected from the liver, lungs, and heart of a 50-year-old male. The analysis made it clear that there was bilateral alveolar disruption with cellular fibromyxiod exudation. The lung is the organ where a desquamation of pneumocytes and a hyaline membrane is formed, indicating acute respiratory distress syndrome

[ARDS]. These tissues in the lungs also exhibited cellular and fibromyxoid excretion, pneumocyte exfoliation, and lung congestion. In addition to both lungs, the domination of lymphocytes was also detected in interstitial mononuclear inflammatory infiltrates. Polynuclear syncytial cells with unusually expanded pneumocytes featuring stretched nuclei, prominent nucleoli, acidic and basic granular cytoplasm were deciphered within alveolus areas with an exhibition of cytopathic effects, leaving no evidence of intranuclear inclusions.

## 4. Most likely ecological pool and source of coronavirus

It is important to be acquainted with its origin and transmission to develop preventive measures and to inhibit the spread of infection. As far as the occurrence of SARS-CoV, surveyors primarily concentrate on palm civets and raccoon dogs as the main storehouse of infection. Only the specimens excluded from the civets demonstrated positive outcomes for viral RNA identification in the food market, suggesting that the secondary host might be the civet palm [19]. In 2001, the samples obtained from sound people of Hong Kong were isolated, and the molecular analyses were conducted; the result showed 2.5 percent of antibodies developed against SARS-coronavirus. This implied that SARS-coronavirus might have circulated in humans before giving rise to the outbreak in 2003 [20]. Subsequently, Rhinolophus bats were also discovered to develop antibodies against SARS-CoV, suggesting that bats were a source for viral reproduction [21]. For the first time, MERS-coronavirus evolved in the Kingdom of Saudi Arabia in 2012 [22]. MERS-coronavirus, known as beta-coronavirus, had camels as a primary host for the zoonotic disease [23]. In a recent study, MERS-coronavirus is believed to be spotted in Perimyotisbats and Pipistrellus [24], implying that bats are the virus' primary source and transmission mode [25, 26]. At the outset, a group of researchers believed that snakes were the probable origin; however, genomic analysis for similarity measures explains that novel coronaviruses and SARS viruses support the assertion that snakes were not the central storehouse, however, bats were [27, 28]. Further analyses of homologous rearrangement showed that SARS-CoV (CoVZXC21) generated receptor binding and the prim of the spike glycoprotein of novel coronaviruses (as shown in **Figure 1**). The construction of respiratory syndrome generating human coronavirus CoVZC45 is an unknown Beta-CoV [29].

## 5. Transmission of COVID-19

It is universally acknowledged that people-to-people transmission of SARS-CoV-2 occurs in the community, family settings, and health care. Substantial dissemination methods involve droplets from the respiratory duct and indirectly through fomites and aerosols. Some circumstantial evidence shows that PCR and culture are two important laboratory tests used to separate the virus from saliva and identify its feces [30–33]. It has also been observed that the virus appears differently in both blood and urine [34, 35]. If the COVID-19 is mild, the virus shedding in respiratory samples remains for a long period in the case of children; the virus having RNA is obtained in higher magnitude (83.3%) in feces with lasting shedding for a fortnight, whereas it lasts for more than one month in children [27]. Diverse research suggests that the spread of the virus can be seen during incubation on the day or the day before the signs are set forth and spread from very mild asymptomatic infections [36–40]. From the day of his admission, positive samples were collected from the nasopharynx of a half-year-old baby with a high viral load;

these specimens were positive for several days [41]. Therefore, multiple instances may remain undetected and pose a sustainable challenge for virus transmission [42]. The replication number (Ro) is usually considered to be in the range of 2.0 and 2.8 [37–40]; in case higher multiplication numbers are recommended, the serial interlude remains within a span of 5 to 7 days [43–45]. The mean incubation period is between 4.75 and 7 days [46, 47], ranging from 3 to 14 days. Information about the virus load is increasing simultaneously with an increase in our understanding of the virus. In another instance, patients with higher viral loads were identified; the viral droplets in the nose were higher than those in the throat. The intensity of viral droplets was alike in the case of a single symptomatic patient and an asymptomatic patient [32]. On another occasion, for a comprehensive study, the assessment of the virus load was conducted in a pair of patients with a series of samples collected from swabs, throat, urine, stool, and sputum over consecutive days from admission to hospitalization. The viral loads peaked with 104 to107 copies/mL at approximately 5 to 6 days after the onset of symptoms. Similar samples of viral droplets from other patients were examined by the writers, who found the viral loads to be nearly 1011 copies/mL in the throat sample, but the sputum samples had a median of 7.99 × 194, 7.52 ×105. Additionally, the virus was examined using RT-PCR in feces from 9 out of 17 established studies [24]. An examination of nine pregnant women infected with the virus did not provide substantial proof of ureteral transmission to the fetus [48].

As a positive-stranded RNA virus, SARS-CoV-2 was discovered, which is said to belong to the genus beta coronavirus, having a crown-like spike composed of glycoproteins enveloping the surface (**Figure 2**) [18]. There are six categories of coronaviruses found in human beings along with SARS-CoV-2; they are MERS-CoV, HCoV-HKU1, HCoV-OC43, HCoV-229E, SARS-CoV, and HCoV-NL63 [22]. Evaluation of phylogenetics demonstrated that ARS-CoV-2 was nearly related to SARS, with 88–89% similarity; it is also deemed to be derived from bat-SL-CoVZXC21 (unique identifier: MG772934.1) and bat-SL-CoVZC45 (unique identifier: MG772933.1); however, it has a comparatively distant relationship with SARS-CoV and MERS-CoV being 79% and 50% similar, respectively [23–25]. SARS-CoV-2 is covered with a wrapper; it is circular, elliptic, and often

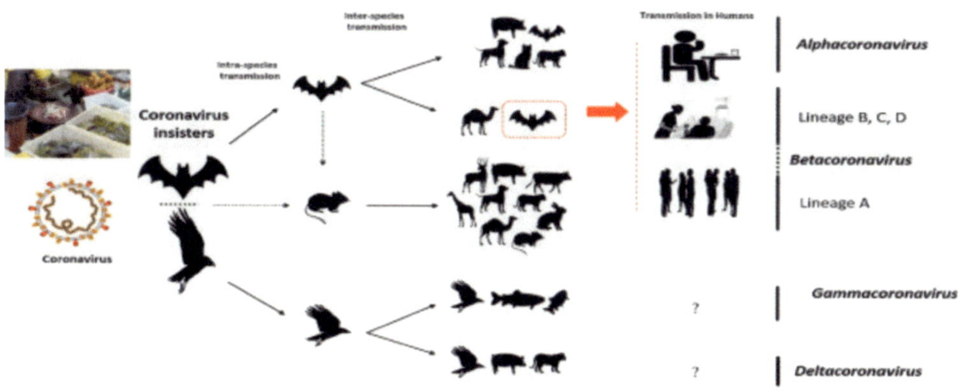


**Figure 2.**
*The main stockpile and medium of transmission of coronaviruses (presumed stocks of SARS-CoV-2 are circled red); the alpha and beta members of coronaviruses have the potential to afflict human beings; the devouring of animals, infected with the virus as an origin of food, is the prime reason of virus spreading from beasts to human beings. Owing to being in contact with a virus-infected person, finally, the virus spread to sound individuals. Arrow with dotted black lines demonstrates the likelihood of virus spread from the bat, whereas the arrow with solid black lines represents the accurate transferal. Reference: [49]. This is an open access article under the CC BY-NC-ND license (http://creativecommons.org/licenses/by-nc-nd/4.0/).*

polymorphic elements have a radius ranging between 30 nm and 70 nm [26]. The phylogenetic reports and additional research on entire genome sequencing have shown that COVID-19 is inconsistent with SARS-CoV. It can thus be considered the latest beta-coronavirus damaging human organs [27]. The genesis of the 2019-nCoV has been mysterious ever since, but the rising surge is deemed to be connected to the Seafood Market of Huanan in South China [28]. Researchers have been striving to discover the sources in animals to do away with the spread of this novel coronavirus, but none are certain until now. The maximum number of hosts is consistent with the prospective sources of the 2019-nCoV that it belongs to seafood, pangolins, or even bats [3, 4, 26]. The immediate work is to track down the transitory source instrumental in transmitting the coronavirus to human beings. Therefore, determining the source of the virus must bear the potential to help discover the zoonotic transmission method [26]. SARS-CoV-2 demonstrates the risk of high pathogenicity and communicability [29]. It is likely to be transferred from one person to another by the viral loads of infected persons who are directly in contact with the surfaces already contaminated by the respiratory droplets through sneezing, coughing, and physical contact with infected patients [29]. According to several reports, symptomatic individuals are the most recurring sources of COVID-19 escalation [27]. Furthermore, there are opinions that asymptomatic individuals can also transmit the virus as intensely as symptomatic individuals. Besides, more studies are required to understand and explain the durability of infectiveness, the procedures of transmission, and the incubation period of the virus. As HCoV-19 is the latest phenomenon among human beings, much effort is needed to be acquainted with the sources of this virus. Based on a twisted explanation or inappropriate delineation of the early released and restricted amount of data on the HCoV-19 genome, different suppositions or hypotheses are prevalent in that HCoV-19 was artificially produced in mysterious circumstances [50, 51] Specifically, the installation of a polybasic (furin) at the cleavage site of the spike protein was discovered in beta-coronaviruses for the first time (48). Based on the comprehension and information collected from the MERS-CoV and SARS-CoV outbreaks, SARS (Bat-CoVRaTG13) in *Rhinolophus* affinis was successfully detected and separated; it was 95% similar to HCoV-19. It could be propounded that the COVID-19 virus possibly belongs to bats with a higher degree of conviction [52]. Additionally, phenylacetic acid amide on the cleavage region of S1 and S2 has recently been observed in the coronavirus genetic arrangement detected in a different *Rhinolophus malayanus* [52]. These outcomes imply that there are nearly two bat types: *Rhinolophus malayanus* and *Rhinolophus* affinis. They are presumed to be the native sources of HCoV-19. Bats are believed to be a possible animal pool for HCoV-19- and SARS-like [53] coronaviruses. Presently, non-comprehensive evidence is found to show the bats responsible for directly spreading HCoV-19-like coronaviruses to human beings. Recent research shows that the Malayan pangolin (Manisjavanica) has been considered a potential natural storehouse or transitional source of HCoV-19 [54–56]. In another study, community genomic sequencing of blood, intestine, and lung samples from Malayan pangolins was examined by Lam et al. [54, 57]. They detected virus sequences with a connection with a pair of subcategories of HCoV-19 like coronaviruses. Specifically, five analytical remnants of the pangolin virus, which play a significant role in human receptor binding, are similar in every detail to HCoV-19 [57]. Based on a re-evaluation conducted on a formerly announced virus metagenomics dataset of Malayan pangolins [58], it is recommended that there is a prospective pangolin origin of HCoV-19 [59]. The all-inclusive feature of HCoV-19 concerning Pangolin-CoV in pangolins has repeatedly suggested that Malayan pangolin could be a prospective transitional source for HCoV-19 [55]. It is believed that HCoV-19 could spring from a probable intermingling of the aforementioned

Bat-CoV-RaTG13-like virus [52] and Pangolin-CoV-like virus [55]. Malayan pangolins are reported to have been spotted in the natural habitat across Southeast Asia. However, it has never been considered to belong to China, where HCoV-19 was confirmed for the first time [3, 27, 45, 52] because it was significant as an origin of food and herbal treatment.

Irrespective of its whereabouts still not being identified, multiple cases of COVID-19 have been referred to those who have visited the Seafood Wholesale Market of Huanan, situated in the city of Wuhan, China. On February 11, 2020, the WHO came up with COVID-19, a shortened form for COVID 2019. The virus responsible for this flare-up is recognized as SARS-CoV-2; recently, it has been unearthed and is closely related to bat coronaviruses, SARS-Cov, and pangolin coronaviruses.

## 6. Spread of the virus

With highly changeable symptoms, COVID-19 ranges from none to fatal ailments. The virus of this illness is said to travel through the air from person to person nearby. Once an infected person coughs, breathes, or speaks, the virus is released and attacks the person next to him. It is also very likely to spread through surfaces already contaminated by virus-affected patients. The duration of this virus is at least 14 days, and it has the potential to spread asymptomatically as well (**Figure 3**).

## 7. Economic impact

The stock market collapse of 2020 was a serious and unprecedented global phenomenon that started on February 20, 2020 and lasted until April 7, 2020 (**Figure 4**).

A transitional bear was experienced in the market due to the COVID-19 disaster, but the bull returned by April 2020; it went on through December 2020

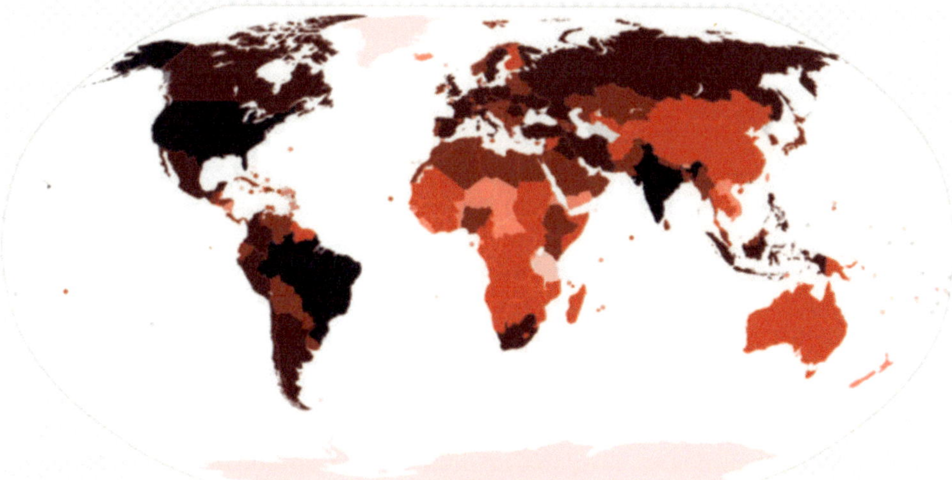

**Figure 3.**
*Total confirmed cases per country as of 10 May 2021. 10,000,000+ 1,000,000–9,999,999 100,000–999,999 10,000–99,999 1,000–9,999 100–999 1–99 0 [this file is licensed under the Creative Commons Attribution-Share Alike 4.0 International license. https://en.wikipedia.org/wiki/COVID-19_pandemic#/media/File:COVID 19_Outbreak_World_Map.Svg.*

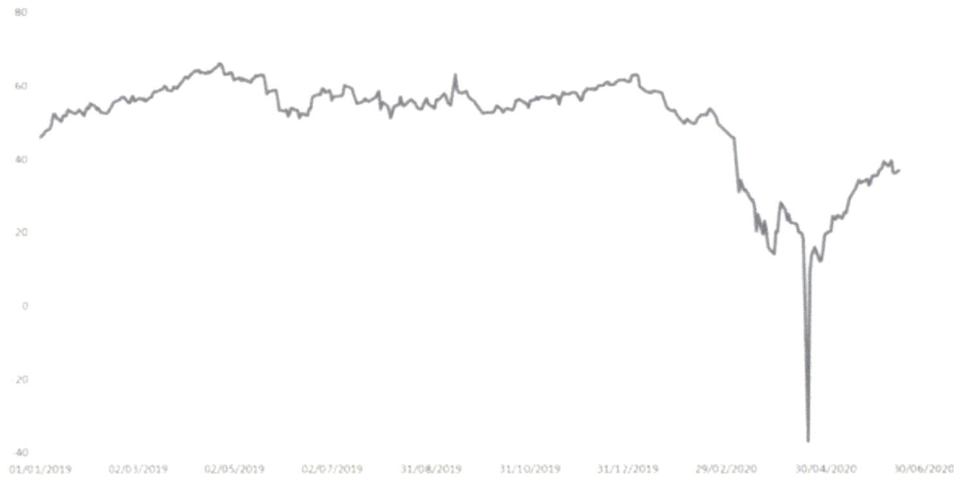


**Figure 4.**
*Movement of WTI (West Texas intermediate) price of crude oil from 2019. The collapse began on February 20, 2020. For the first time, on April 20, 2020, the prices went down to minus digits in petroleum history. Reference: Sheppard, David; McCormick, Myles; Brower, Derek; Lockett, Hudson (April 20, 2020). "US oil price below zero for first time in history." financial times. Retrieved April 20, 2020.*

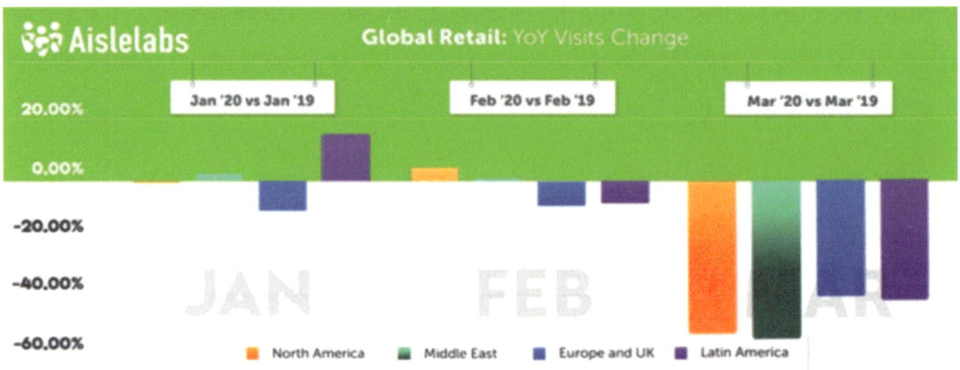


**Figure 5.**
*Retail experienced a 40–60% plummet in footfall in Mar 2020. Reference: Inc., Aislelabs (April 2, 2020), how retailers globally are responding to coronavirus by Aislelabs, retrieved June 2, 2020.*

despite the inability of the US markets to return to the levels of January 2020. This downturn remained until November 2020 because of a slowdown due to COVID-19 (**Figure 5**) [60–64].

The unexpected economic downturn due to COVID-19 trailed economic development and continued growth following the revival of a global monetary setback in 2009. Human history has given rise to unprecedented worldwide joblessness, an all-time low, while the quality of life has gradually settled to a better position worldwide. Over time, the 2020 COVID-19 outbreak—the most menacing upsurge since the Spanish flu of 1918—set out to eradicate the entire economy. The slowdown of the global economy occurred due to the pandemic and the panic caused by it; the equilibrium of demand and supply disrupted the market beyond measure. There is no denying that the International Monetary Fund (IMF) also spotted other diminishing variables before COVID-19, like a global synchronized slowdown in 2019, suggesting the already vulnerable condition of the market [65–70].

Although the collapse started on February 20, 2020, there was a considerable boost in sales in the first fortnight of March 2020. The collapse witnessed many serious daily falls in the stock market worldwide, the largest fall being on March 16; it was termed as 'Black Monday II' as there was a 12–13% fall in most of the business worldwide [71–73]. Two more important collapse dates became obvious: March 9, termed 'Black Monday I' [74–76], and March 12, termed 'Black Thursday' [77]. Banks and reserves worldwide lowered their cash flow and interest rates to manage the stock; furthermore, they offered the markets and investors extraordinary assistance to cope with the situation [78–80].

## 8. Recession during COVID-19

The slowdown due to COVID-19 is a serious worldwide economic catastrophe that has generated a downturn in many countries and depression in others. It has been considered the worst world economic disaster since the Great Depression [81]. The disaster began because of different government regulations against the production created to inhibit the ongoing outbreak. Significant slowdown symptoms in the collapse of stock markets appeared in late February 2020 and lasted until March 2020 [82–87]. However, the stock market devastation was transitory, and many market indices worldwide revived or established new records by the northern autumn of 2020. By September 2020, every developed economy experienced recession or depression, while all emerging economies were in recession [88–90]. According to the World Bank's anticipation, returning to normalcy would not be accomplished in many countries even by 2025 [91–94].

Due to the COVID-19 pandemic, half of the world population came to a halt to inhibit the spread of COVID-19 [95]. It has caused serious consequences on economies worldwide [96] just after the 2019 world economic slowdown that witnessed the inertia of higher magnitude in the stock markets and consumer activities globally [97, 98].

The slowdown due to the pandemic has caused massive unemployment, inability to sustain unemployment insurance, crashing computer systems, and struggling slow claims processing of the applications [99, 100]. More than 10 million unemployed people were registered in the US by October 2020 [101]. According to the UN forecast conducted in April 2020, the world would see more unemployed people, reducing working hours by nearly seven percent. It has been estimated that nearly 195 million full-time workers lost their jobs [102]. Unemployment, in some countries, was anticipated to reach ten percent; the countries seriously impacted by the COVID-19 outbreak had higher unemployment than before [103–105]. Regarding remittals, even developing countries were not unaffected [106], which exacerbated the global food crisis [107].

## Author details

Gaffar Sarwar Zaman* and Mesfer Al Shahrani
College of Applied Medical Sciences, King Khalid University, Abha, Kingdom of Saudi Arabia

*Address all correspondence to: gffrzaman@gmail.com

## References

[1] Huang C, Wang Y, Li X, Ren L, Zhao J, Hu Y, et al. Clinical features of patients infected with 2019 novel coronavirus in Wuhan, China. Lancet 2020; 395:497e506.

[2] N, Zhang D, Wang W, Li X, Yang B, Song J, et al. A novelcoronavirus from patients with pneumonia in China, 2019. NEngl J Med 2020;382:727e33.

[3] Wu F, Zhao S, Yu B, Chen YM, Wang W, Song ZG, et al. A newcoronavirus associated with human respiratory disease inChina. Nature 2020;579:265e9.

[4] Coronaviridae Study Group of the International Committee on Taxonomy of V. The species Severe acute respiratory syndrome-related coronavirus: classifying 2019-nCoV andnaming it SARS-CoV-2. Nat Microbiol 2020;5:536e44.

[5] Chan JF, Yuan S, Kok KH, To KK, Chu H, Yang J, et al. Afamilial cluster of pneumonia associated with the 2019 novelcoronavirus indicating person-to-person transmission: astudy of a family cluster. Lancet 2020;395:514e23.

[6] Johnson NP, Mueller J. Updating the accounts: globalmortality of the 1918-1920 "Spanish" influenza pandemic.Bull Hist Med 2002;76:105e15.

[7] Kain T, Fowler R. Preparing intensive care for the nextpandemic influenza. Crit Care 2019;23:337.

[8] Simonsen L, Clarke MJ, Schonberger LB, Arden NH, Cox NJ,Fukuda K. Pandemic versus epidemic influenza mortality: apattern of changing age distribution. J Infect Dis1998;178:53e60.

[9] Viboud C, Simonsen L, Fuentes R, Flores J, Miller MA,Chowell G. Global mortality impact of the 1957-1959influenza pandemic. J Infect Dis 2016;213:738e45.

[10] Weiss SR, Navas-Martin S. Coronavirus pathogenesis and the emerging pathogen severe acute respiratory syndrome coronavirus. Microbiol Mol Biol Rev. 2005; 69: 635-64.

[11] Su S, Wong G, Shi W, Liu J, Lai ACK, Zhou J, et al. Epidemiology, GeneticRecombination, and Pathogenesis of Coronaviruses. Trends Microbiol. 2016;24: 490-502.

[12] Lai MM, Cavanagh D. The molecular biology of coronaviruses. Adv Virus Res. 1997; 48: 1-100.

[13] Wong LY, Lui PY, Jin DY. A molecular arms race between host innate antiviral response and emerging human coronaviruses. Virol Sin. 2016; 31: 12-23.

[14] Schoeman D., Fielding B.C. Coronavirus envelope protein: current knowledge. *Virol J.* 2019;16:69. [PMC free article] [PubMed] [Google Scholar]

[15] Tai W., He L., Zhang X., Pu J., Voronin D., Jiang S. Characterization of the receptor-binding domain (RBD) of 2019 novel coronavirus: implication for development of RBD protein as a viral attachment inhibitor and vaccine. *Cell Mol Immunol.* 2020:1-8. [PMC free article] [PubMed] [Google Scholar]

[16] Xu H., Zhong L., Deng J., Peng J., Dan H., Zeng X. High expression of ACE2 receptor of 2019-nCoV on the epithelial cells of oral mucosa. *Int J Oral Sci.* 2020;12:1-5. [PMC free article] [PubMed] [Google Scholar]

[17] Rabi F.A., Al Zoubi M.S., Kasasbeh G.A., Salameh D.M., Al-Nasser A.D. SARS-CoV-2 and Coronavirus Disease 2019: what we

know so far. *Pathogens.* 2020;9:231. [PMC free article] [PubMed] [Google Scholar]

[18] Astuti I, Ysrafil. Severe Acute Respiratory Syndrome Coronavirus 2 (SARS-CoV-2): An overview of viral structure and host response. Diabetes Metab Syndr. 2020 Jul-Aug;14(4):407-412. doi: 10.1016/j.dsx.2020.04.020. Epub 2020 April 18. PMID: 32335367; PMCID: PMC7165108.

[19] Kan B, Wang M, Jing H, Xu H, Jiang X, Yan M, et al. Molecular evolution analysisand geographic investigation of severe acute respiratory syndromecoronavirus-like virus in palm civets at an animal market and on farms. JVirol 2005;79(18):11892-900.

[20] Zheng BJ, Guan Y, Wong KH, Zhou J, Wong KL, Young BWY, et al. SARS-relatedvirus predating SARS outbreak, Hong Kong. Emerg Infect Dis 2004;10(2):176.

[21] Shi Z, Hu Z. A review of studies on animal reservoirs of the SARS coronavirus.Virus Res 2008;133(1): 74-87.

[22] Memish ZA, Zumla AI, Al-Hakeem RF, Al-Rabeeah AA, Stephens GM. Familycluster of Middle East respiratory syndrome coronavirus infections. N Engl JMed 2013;368(26):2487-94.

[23] Paden C, Yusof M, Al Hammadi Z, Queen K, Tao Y, Eltahir Y, et al. Zoonotic origin and transmission of Middle East respiratory syndrome coronavirus in the UAE. Zoonoses Public Health 2018;65(3):322-33.

[24] Annan A, Baldwin HJ, Corman VM, Klose SM, Owusu M, Nkrumah EE, et al.Human betacoronavirus 2c EMC/2012–related viruses in bats, Ghana andEurope. Emerg Infect Dis 2013;19(3):456.

[25] Huynh J, Li S, Yount B, Smith A, Sturges L, Olsen JC, et al. Evidence supporting a zoonotic origin of human coronavirus strain NL63. J Virol 2012;86(23):12816-25.

[26] Lau SK, Li KS, Tsang AK, Lam CS, Ahmed S, Chen H, et al. Geneticcharacterization of Betacoronavirus lineage C viruses in bats reveals markedsequence divergence in the spike protein of pipistrellus bat coronavirus HKU5in Japanese pipistrelle: implications for the origin of the novel Middle Eastrespiratory syndrome coronavirus. J Virol 2013;87(15):8638-50.

[27] Lu R, Zhao X, Li J, Niu P, Yang B, Wu H, et al. Genomic characterisation andepidemiology of 2019 novel coronavirus: implications for virus origins andreceptor binding. The Lancet 2020.

[28] Chan JF-W, Yuan S, Kok K-H, To KK-W, Chu H, Yang J, et al. A familial cluster ofpneumonia associated with the 2019 novel coronavirus indicating person-topersontransmission: a study of a family cluster. Lancet 2020.

[29] Chan JF-W, Kok K-H, Zhu Z, Chu H, To KK-W, Yuan S, et al. Genomiccharacterization of the 2019 novel human-pathogenic coronavirus isolatedfrom a patient with atypical pneumonia after visiting. Wuhan. EmergingMicrobes & Infections 2020;9(1):221-36.

[30] Pan Y, Zhang D, Yang P, Poon LLM, Wang Q. Viral loadof SARS-CoV-2 in clinical samples. Lancet Infect Dis.2020;20:411-412. doi:10.1016/S1473-3099(20)30113-4

[31] Zhang W, Du RH, Li B, et al. Molecular and serological investigationof 2019-nCoV infected patients: implication of multipleshedding routes. Emerg

Microbes Infect. 2020;9:386-389.doi:10.1080/22221751.2020.1729071

[32] Zhang Y, Chen C, Zhu S, et al. Isolation of 2019-nCoV froma stool specimen of a laboratory-confirmed case of the coronavirusdisease 2019 (COVID-19) [in Chinese]. China CDCWeekly. 2020;2:123-124.

[33] Cai J, Xu J, Lin D, et al. A case series of children with 2019novel coronavirus infection: clinical and epidemiologicalfeatures [published online February 28, 2020]. Clin InfectDis. doi:10.1093/cid/ciaa198.

[34] Young BE, Ong SWX, Kalimuddin S, et al. Epidemiological features and clinical course of patients infected with SARSCoV-2 in Singapore. JAMA. 2020;323:1488-1494. doi:10.1001/jama.2020.3204

[35] Xie C, Jiang L, Huang G, et al. Comparison of different samples for 2019 novel coronavirus detection by nucleic acid amplification test. Int J Infect Dis. 2020;93:264-267. doi:10.1016/j.ijid.2020.02.050

[36] Hoehl S, Rabenau H, Berger A, et al. Evidence of SARS-CoV-2infection in returning travelers from Wuhan, China. N Engl JMed. 2020;382:1278-1280. doi:10.1056/NEJMc2001899

[37] Yu P, Zhu J, Zhang Z, Han Y. A familial cluster of infectionassociated with the 2019 novel coronavirus indicating potentialperson-to-person transmission during the incubation period[published online February 18, 2020]. J Infect Dis. doi:10.1093/infdis/jiaa077

[38] Zou L, Ruan F, Huang M, et al. SARS-CoV-2 viral load inupper respiratory specimens of infected patients. N Engl J Med. 2020;382:1177-1179. doi:10.1056/NEJMc2001737

[39] Bai Y, Yao L, Wei T, et al. Presumed asymptomatic carriertransmission of COVID-19. JAMA. 2020;323:1406-1407. doi:10.1001/jama.2020.2565

[40] Pan X, Chen D, Xia Y, et al. Asymptomatic cases in a familycluster with SARS-CoV-2 infection. Lancet Infect Dis.2020;20:410-411. doi:10.1016/S1473-3099(20)30114-6

[41] Kam KQ, Yung CF, Cui L, et al. A well infant with coronavirusdisease 2019 (COVID-19) with high viral load [published online February 28, 2020]. Clin Infect Dis. doi:10.1093/cid/ciaa201

[42] Imai N, Cori A, Dorigatti I, et al. Report 3: Transmissibilityof 2019-nCoV. Published January 25, 2020. Accessed May14, 2020. https://www.imperial.ac.uk/media/imperial-college/medicine/sph/ide/gida-fellowships/Imperial-College-COVID19-transmissibility-25-01-2020.pdf

[43] Wu JT, Leung K, Leung GM. Nowcasting and forecastingthe potential domestic and international spread of the2019-nCoV outbreak originating in Wuhan, China: a modellingstudy. Lancet. 2020;395:689-697. doi:10.1016/S01406736(20)30260-9

[44] Tuite AR, Fisman DN. Reporting, epidemic growth, and reproductivenumbers for the 2019 novel coronavirus (2019-nCoV)epidemic. Ann Intern Med. 2020;172:567-568. doi:10.7326/M20-0358

[45] Li Q, Guan X, Wu P, et al. Early transmission dynamicsin Wuhan, China, of novel coronavirus-infected pneumonia.N Engl J Med. 2020;382:1199-1207. doi:10.1056/NEJMoa2001316

[46] Cowling BJ, Leung GM. Epidemiological research prioritiesfor public health control of the ongoing global novel coronavirus(2019-nCoV)

outbreak. Euro Surveill. 2020;25(6). doi:10.2807/1560-7917. ES.2020.25.6.2000110

[47] Backer JA, Klinkenberg D, Wallinga J. Incubation period of2019 novel coronavirus (2019-nCoV) infections among travellersfrom Wuhan, China, 20-28 January 2020. Euro Surveill.2020;25(5). doi:10. 2807/1560-7917.ES.2020.25. 5.2000062

[48] Chen H, Guo J, Wang C, et al. Clinical characteristics and intrauterine vertical transmission potential of COVID-19 infection in nine pregnant women: a retrospective review of medical records. Lancet. 2020;395:809-815. doi:10.1016/ S0140-6736(20) 30360-3.

[49] Muhammad Adnan Shereen, Suliman Khan, Abeer Kazmi, Nadia Bashir, Rabeea Siddique. COVID-19 infection: Origin, transmission, and characteristics of human coronaviruses. Journal of Advanced Research 24 (2020) 91-98. DOI: 10.1016/j.jare.2020.03.005

[50] Andersen KG, Rambaut A, Lipkin WI, Holmes EC, Garry RF. 2020. The proximal origin of SARS-CoV-2. Nature Medicine, 26(4): 450–452.

[51] Liu SL, Saif LJ, Weiss SR, Su LS. 2020. No credible evidence supporting claims of the laboratory engineering of SARS-CoV-2. Emerging Microbes &Infections, 9(1): 505–507.

[52] Zhou H, Chen X, Hu T, Li J, Song H, Liu YR, Wang PH, Liu D, Yang J,Holmes EC, Hughes AC, Bi YH, Shi WF. 2020b. A novel bat coronavirusreveals natural insertions at the S1/S2 cleavage site of the Spike proteinand a possible recombinant origin of HCoV-19. bioRxiv, doi:10.1101/2020.03.02.974139.

[53] Shi JZ, Wen ZY, Zhong GX, Yang HL, Wang C, Huang BY, Liu RQ, He XJ,Shuai L, Sun ZR, Zhao YB, Liu PP, Liang LB, Cui PF, Wang JL, Zhang XF,Guan YT, Tan WJ, Wu GZ, Chen HL, Bu ZG. 2020. Susceptibility of ferrets,cats, dogs, and other domesticated animals to SARS-coronavirus 2.Science, doi: 10.1126/ science.abb7015.

[54] Lam TTY, Shum MHH, Zhu HC, Tong YG, Ni XB, Liao YS, Wei W, CheungWY, Li WJ, Li LF, Leung GM, Holmes EC, Hu YL, Guan Y. 2020. IdentifyingSARS-CoV-2 related coronaviruses in Malayan pangolins. Nature, doi:10.1038/s41586-020-2169-0. Lam et al., 2020;

[55] Xiao, K., Zhai, J., Feng, Y. et al. Isolation of SARS-CoV-2-related coronavirus from Malayan pangolins. Nature 583, 286-289 (2020). https://doi.org/10.1038/s41586-020-2313-x

[56] Zhang T, Wu QF, Zhang ZG. 2020a. Probable pangolin origin of SARSCoV-2 associated with the COVID-19 outbreak. Current Biology, 30(7):1346–1351.e2.

[57] Lam, T.TY., Jia, N., Zhang, YW. et al. Identifying SARS-CoV-2-related coronaviruses in Malayan pangolins. Nature 583, 282-285 (2020). https://doi.org/10.1038/s41586-020-2169-0. DOI: 10.1002/jmv.25965

[58] Liu J, Liu S. The management of coronavirus disease 2019 (COVID-19). J Med Virol. 2020;92:1484-1490. https://doi.org/10.1002/jmv.25965

[59] Zhang J et al. Changes in contact patterns shape the dynamics of the COVID-19 outbreak in China. Science 2020;368(6498):1481-1486. DOI: 10.1126/science.abb8001

[60] Smith, Elliot (February 28 2020). "Global stocks head for worst week since the financial crisis amid fears of a possible pandemic". CNBC. Archived from the original on February 28 2020.

[61] Huang, Eustance (February 28 2020). "Seven major Asia-Pacific markets have tumbled into correction territory". CNBC. Archived from the original on February 29 2020. Retrieved March 24 2020.

[62] GmbH, finanzen net. "Goldman Sachs now says US GDP will shrink 24% next quarter amid the coronavirus pandemic - which would be 2.5 times bigger than any decline in history | Markets Insider". markets. businessinsider.com. Archived from the original on March 26 2020. Retrieved March 24 2020.

[63] Rabouin, Dion. "Which asset classes performed best in the market frenzy of 2020". Axios. Retrieved January 6 2021.

[64] https://www.cnbc.com/2020/12/01/world-stocks-outperform-the-us-in-bumper-november.html

[65] "A Market Crash Was Coming, Coronavirus Was Just the Spark". Time. Archived from the original on March 2 2020. Retrieved March 24 2020.

[66] "Top three reasons behind the stock market crash 2020: is it coronavirus, oil price war or vanished liquidity?". capital. com. Retrieved March 24 2020.

[67] Partington, Richard; Wearden, Graeme (March 9 2020). "Global stock markets post biggest falls since 2008 financial crisis". The Guardian. ISSN 0261-3077. Archived from the original on March 14 2020. Retrieved March 15 2020.

[68] IMFBlog. "The World Economy: Synchronized Slowdown, Precarious Outlook". IMF Blog. Retrieved April 15 2020.

[69] Gurdus, Lizzy (October 10 2019). "'Yellow flag on recession risk': Top forecaster warns of cracks in consumer spending". CNBC. Retrieved April 15 2020.

[70] Lakshman Achuthan and Anirvan Banerji for CNN Business. "Opinion: Here's what is really causing the global economic slowdown". CNN. Retrieved April 15 2020.

[71] Huang, Eustance (March 16 2020). "Australia stocks drop nearly 10% as Asia markets tumble; Fed cuts rates to zero". CNBC. Archived from the original on March 16 2020. Retrieved March 16 2020.

[72] Smith, Elliot; Ellyatt, Holly (March 16 2020). "European stocks close down 5%, travel stocks tank 10% as EU proposes flight restrictions". CNBC. Archived from the original on March 16 2020. Retrieved March 16 2020.

[73] Hutchens, Gareth; Chalmers, Stephanie (March 16 2020). "ASX 200 posts biggest fall on record, Reserve Bank flags further measures amid coronavirus fears". ABC News. Archived from the original on March 16 2020. Retrieved March 16 2020

[74] "Global shares plunge in worst day since financial crisis". BBC. March 9 2020. Archived from the original on March 9 2020.

[75] Yun Li (March 8 2019). "Dow futures tumble as Saudi-Russia oil price war adds to coronavirus stress". NBC News. Archived from the original on March 9 2020.

[76] Stephanie Ruhle (9 March 2019). "Stocks plunge at market open, trading halts after Dow drops 1800 points". MSNBC.com.

[77] Imbert, Fred; Franck, Thomas (March 12 2020). "Dow drops more than 8%, heads for biggest one-day plunge since 1987 market crash". CNBC. Archived from the original on March 12 2020. Retrieved March 12 2020.

[78] Sanyal, Shreyashi (March 16 2020). "EMERGING MARKETS-Latam FX

caught in virus-driven rout; Chile central bank cuts rates". Reuters. Thomson Reuters. Archived from the original on March 16 2020. Retrieved March 17 2020.

[79] Komuves, Anita; Hovet, Jason (16 March 2020). "UPDATE 2-CEE MARKETS-Assets fall even as central banks act to fight virus impact". Reuters. Thomson Reuters. Retrieved March 31 2020.

[80] Menon, Praveen (March 15 2020). "New Zealand central bank slashes rates at emergency meeting as coronavirus worsens". Reuters. Thomson Reuters. Retrieved March 30 2020.

[81] Zumbrun, Josh (May 10 2020). "Coronavirus Slump Is Worst Since Great Depression. Will It Be as Painful?". *Wall Street Journal*. ISSN 0099-9660. Retrieved January 20 2021.

[82] Islam, Faisal (March 20 2020). "Coronavirus recession not yet a depression". BBC News. Retrieved April 16 2020.

[83] Hawkins, John. "How will the coronavirus recession compare with the worst in Australia's history?". The Conversation. Retrieved April 16 2020.

[84] Stewart, Emily (March 21 2020). "The coronavirus recession is already here". Vox. Retrieved April 16 2020.

[85] Islam, Faisal (March 20 2020). "Coronavirus recession not yet a depression". BBC News. Retrieved March 26 2020.

[86] "The coronavirus recession has arrived". The Canberra Times. March 25 2020. Retrieved March 26 2020.

[87] Elliott, Larry (April 14 2020). "'Great Lockdown' to rival Great Depression with 3% hit to global economy, says IMF". The Guardian. ISSN 0261-3077. Retrieved April 15 2020.

[88] "World Economic Outlook Update, June 2020: A Crisis Like No Other, An Uncertain Recovery". IMF. Retrieved September 11 2020.

[89] "The Great Lockdown: Worst Economic Downturn Since the Great Depression". IMF Blog. Retrieved April 16 2020.

[90] "COVID-19 to Plunge Global Economy into Worst Recession since World War II". World Bank. Retrieved September 11 2020.

[91] "The Great Recession Was Bad. The 'Great Lockdown' Is Worse". BloombergQuint. Retrieved April 15 2020.

[92] "IMF Says 'Great Lockdown' Worst Recession Since Depression, Far Worse Than Last Crisis". nysscpa.org. Retrieved April 15 2020.

[93] Winck, Ben (April 14 2020). "IMF economic outlook: 'Great Lockdown' will be worst recession in century". Business Insider. Retrieved April 27 2020.

[94] Larry Elliott Economics editor. "'Great Lockdown' to rival Great Depression with 3% hit to global economy, says IMF | Business". The Guardian. Retrieved April 27 2020.

[95] McFall-Johnsen, Juliana Kaplan, Lauren Frias, Morgan (March 14 2020). "A third of the global population is on coronavirus lockdown – here's our constantly updated list of countries and restrictions". Business Insider Australia. Retrieved April 15 2020.

[96] "World Economic Outlook, April 2020 : The Great Lockdown". IMF. Retrieved April 15 2020.

[97] Elliott, Larry (October 8 2019). "Nations must unite to halt global economic slowdown, says new IMF head". The Guardian. ISSN 0261-3077. Retrieved April 15 2020.

[98] Cox, Jeff (November 21 2019). "The worst of the global economic slowdown may be in the past, Goldman says". CNBC. Retrieved April 15 2020.

[99] Aratani, Lauren (April 15 2020). "'Designed for us to fail': Floridians upset as unemployment system melts down". The Guardian. ISSN 0261-3077. Retrieved April 15 2020.

[100] "The coronavirus has destroyed the job market. See which states have been hit the hardest". NBC News. Retrieved April 15 2020.

[101] "Unemployment cases jump in the United States".

[102] "ILO: COVID-19 causes devastating losses in working hours and employment". April 7 2020. Retrieved April 19 2020.

[103] Partington, Richard (April 14 2020). "UK economy could shrink by 35% with 2m job losses, warns OBR". The Guardian. ISSN 0261-3077. Retrieved April 15 2020.

[104] Sullivan, Kath (April 13 2020). "Unemployment forecast to soar to highest rate in almost 30 years". ABC News. Retrieved April 15 2020.

[105] Amaro, Silvia (April 15 2020). "Spain's jobless rate is set to surge much more than in countries like Italy". CNBC. Retrieved April 15 2020.

[106] "Covid stops many migrants sending money home". The Economist. ISSN 0013-0613. Retrieved April 23 2020.

[107] Picheta, Rob. "Coronavirus pandemic will cause global famines of 'biblical proportions,' UN warns". CNN. Retrieved July 13 2020.

Chapter 14

# Psychosocial Effects and Public Health Challenges of COVID-19 Pandemic in India

*Shankar Das and Julie Richards*


## Abstract

The COVID-19 pandemic is an ongoing global crisis that poses enormous and multifarious challenges to humanity since the end of 2019. The pandemic has severely devastated public health systems and universally affected socio-economic development. India is among the worst-hit nations owing to its massive population of 1.35 billion, and more significant socio-economic challenges than most other countries. Despite the current issues and challenges surrounding the COVID-19 pandemic, India has been making targeted efforts towards the fight against the spread of coronavirus, including medical, treatment, vaccination, community prevention and control strategies. The chapter examines the implications of the pandemic on Indian population which have certain unique challenges than other parts of the world. It delves on the gradual progression of the challenges among people especially the vulnerable and the disadvantaged in the existing public health systems. This chapter encompasses a wide array of human suffering and efforts for its mitigation. It highlights and brings to forefront the unique experiences of diverse populations who have faced a crisis within a crisis and its psychosocial ramifications, as well as the psychosocial adversities and public health challenges.


**Keywords:** Covid-19, Psychosocial effect, Public Health, India, Origin, Societal Impact, At-risk Population, Prevention and Control

## 1. Introduction

The COVID-19 pandemic is an ongoing global crisis that poses enormous multifarious challenges and threatening all of humanity since the end of 2019. The infectious disease COVID-19 (SARS-CoV-2) spread swiftly throughout the world and the outbreak placed most nations on a high public health alert. The pandemic has severely devastated public health systems and universally affected socio-economic development. India is among the worst-hit nations owing to its massive population of 1.35 billion, and more significant socio-economic challenges than most other countries.

By September 2020, the nation witnessed a considerable drop in new and active cases' and declining infection rates. However, during the second wave in April 2021, the virus started to spread faster than ever before. The country witnessed over 3 lakh new cases of COVID-19 daily while death rates surged to new peaks. Despite the current issues and challenges surrounding the COVID-19 pandemic, India has been making targeted efforts towards the fight against the spread of coronavirus, including community prevention and control strategies, COVID-19 RT-PCR tests, strengthening public health systems, immunization initiatives, nationwide lockdown, phased relaxation of restrictions, night curfews, doubled fines for not wearing masks and crowding, etc. However, the second wave of the pandemic in April 2021 had been enormous with very grim outcomes whereby oxygen, hospital beds and treatment facilities are in extremely short supply.

This chapter examines and discusses the range of societal challenges and public health burden that resulted from the COVID-19 pandemic in India. We examine the impact of the pandemic that has shaken the fundamental essence of social development and the response of public health systems. This chapter encompasses a wide array of human suffering and efforts for its mitigation. The findings are presented and several thematic psychosocial and public health areas which emerged are discussed, primarily the genesis and spread of the virus and its management, the physical impact of the disease and its psychosocial ramifications, as well as the psychosocial adversities and public health challenges.

More specifically, we describe the individualized experiences of varied high-risk groups in a densely populated country that posed unique challenges in the social and economic sphere. This rich learning may serve a significate value in the area of community prevention strategies. The authors further elucidate lessons learned about advancements and strategies of prevention, treatment and control of the pandemic in the country. The chapter concludes with a number of potentially fruitful research themes and directions.

## 2. Origin and progression of the pandemic

At the initial stage, on 31 December 2020, Chinese national authorities reported unspecified cases of pneumonia to the World Health Organization (WHO). Such cases of unknown etiology were identified in Wuhan city of Hubei province, China and within a mere 3 days, 44 patients were reported with such cases without any known causal agent [1]. Wang et al. [2] reported most common clinical symptoms among the hospitalized patients included fever (98.6 percent), fatigue (69.6 percentage) and dry cough (59.4 percent). Originally, the patients had a history of exposure to the Huanan Seafood Market - a live animal and seafood market in Jianghan District, Wuhan, Hubei, China [1]. On 30 January 2020, the World Health Organization [3] declared the pandemic a Public Health Emergency of International Concern and pandemic on 11 March 2020 [4]. At that point the agency also recommended that all countries should be ready with control strategies such as screening, early detection, containment, case management, contact tracing and prevention of further spread of COVID-19 infection and data sharing with WHO.

As per the available global data on 14 June 2021 there are total 91,451 confirmed COVID-19 cases in China with 86,344 recovered cases which indicates 94 percent recovery rate and 4,636 cases of deaths. Further, worldwide there have been 175,686,814 confirmed cases of COVID-19, including 3,803,592 deaths, reported to WHO [5]. To date, the pandemic rapidly spread across almost 222 countries and territories around the world. The top 10 most-affected countries include: United States of America, India, Brazil, France, Turkey, Russian Federation, the United Kingdom, Italy, Argentina and Spain. The infection levels, which continue to fight against the pandemic, are presented below (**Table 1**).

India reported a total 28,996,473 confirmed COVID-19 cases. The total number of patients who succumbed to the viral disease has reached 351,309 and thereby comprises 17 percent of the global share of case burden [4, 6].

| | Name | Cases – Cumulative Total | Cases – newly reported in last 24 hours | Death – Cumulative total | Death newly reported in last 24 hours | Transmission Classification |
|---|---|---|---|---|---|---|
| | Global | 173,331,478 | 308,911 | 3,735,571 | 7,801 | — |
| 1 | United States of America | 33,042,622 | 15,410 | 592,114 | 418 | Community transmission |
| 2 | India | 28,996,473 | 86,498 | 351,309 | 2,123 | Clusters of cases |
| 3 | Brazil | 16,947,062 | 39,637 | 473,404 | 873 | Community transmission |
| 4 | France | 5,611,217 | 946 | 109,209 | 88 | Community transmission |
| 5. | Turkey | 5,293,627 | 5,647 | 48,255 | 91 | Community transmission |
| 6. | Russian Federation | 5,145,843 | 9,977 | 124,496 | 379 | Clusters of cases |
| 7 | The United Kingdom | 4,522,480 | 5,584 | 127,841 | 1 | Community transmission |
| 8 | Italy | 4,233,698 | 1,270 | 126,588 | 65 | Clusters of cases |
| 9 | Argentina | 3,955,439 | 16,415 | 81,214 | 347 | Community transmission |
| 10 | Spain | 3,707,523 | 883 | 80,236 | 2 | Community transmission |

*Source: WHO [86], 09 June 2021 https://covid19.who.int/table1.*

**Table 1.**
*Top 10 countries with Most-affected by COVID-19 pandemic as on 9 June 2021.*

The first case of Coronavirus was reported on 30th January, 2020 and today the country has the second highest number of confirmed cases in the world after the USA. The first death due to COVID-19 was reported on 12 March 2020 from Kalburgi in Karnataka state in India [7].

During the first wave of the Coronavirus pandemic in September 2020, India witnessed the highest peak on 16th September 2021 with a total number of 97,894 infected persons. Again, after six months the country had a sharp upsurge from the first week of March indicating the second wave of the pandemic with the highest number of 4,14,188 infected cases on 6th May 2021. Fortunately, the national pandemic situation is steadily and rapidly improving with a decline in cases. Recent data recorded 100,636 new cases on 6th June 2021. Additionally, death rates and hospitalizations are also dropping [8].

## 3. Societal impact of COVID-19 in India

Amidst the unprecedented and devastating Coronavirus pandemic, particularly during the second wave, numerous issues related to crumbling public health infrastructures, increasing number of death tolls, psychosocial, economic, political, educational, agricultural effects and many more ramifications have created devastating impact on the lives of people across all states. For example, the social reality of human beings in the modern world revolves around unlimited social interaction.

This interaction came to a sudden halt with the advent of worldwide lockdowns and restrictions on social movement as a result of the coronavirus. Feelings of loneliness and boredom in the population ensued and had varied impacts on people's mental health (see ref. [9]). While this pandemic wreaked havoc in health systems across the world, the social aspects of the disease complicated the recovery process. The contagious character of the pandemic, along with its unpredictable nature of progression on various individuals, has resulted in catastrophic socioeconomic disruption caused by the coronavirus. It is estimated that there were nearly 690 million people globally undernourished in 2019, and by the end of 2021, an additional 132 million are expected to go hungry. Also in this short timeframe, it is anticipated that tens of millions of individuals will be further pushed into risk of extreme poverty [10].

India is not exempt from this prediction. The Covid-19 crisis has amplified the situation of poverty in the country, and left a large number of citizens grappling with inadequate access to clean water and nutritious food, insufficient access to livelihoods or employment, poor education and lack of infrastructure. There is strong underlying evidence between poverty and psychological health [11]. Additionally, studies also indicate that poverty leads to developmental and mental health problems that in turn prevent people from escaping the poverty trap; creating an intergenerational and causal nexus of poverty and ill-health [12]. A study conducted by Mukhtar [13] highlighted the psychological impact of COVID-19 making it a secondary health concern, which requires attention. "Globally implementing preventive and controlling measures, and cultivating coping and resilience are challenging factors; modified lifestyle (lockdown curfew, self-isolation, social distancing and quarantine); conspiracy theories, misinformation and disinformation about the origin, scale, signs, symptoms, transmission, prevention and treatment; global socioeconomic crisis; travel restrictions; workplace hazard control; postponement and cancellation of religious, sports, cultural and entertainment events; panic buying and hoarding; incidents of racism, xenophobia, discrimination, stigma, psychological pressure of productivity, marginalization and violence; overwhelmed medical centers and health organizations, and general impact on education, politics, socioeconomic, culture, environment and climate" ([13], p. 512) are the causative factors arousing challenge and concern.

These factors have diverse impact on people belonging to various strata of society. Demographics such as whether people reside in urban or rural communities and whether they are young or elderly contribute to their vulnerability. Further, hailing from different geographical locations with varying access to social networks, healthcare facilities and personal economic status also contribute to people's exposure to risk. Everyone struggled at his or her individual level with the double burden of the disease and its accompanying factors. In a cross-sectional study by Karmakar et al. [14], they reported that extensive sociodemographic risk factors such as socioeconomic position, family composition, environmental factors and racial/ethnic marginal status were all significantly linked with COVID-19 prevalence and mortality.

Regardless of the socioeconomic risk factors, the microorganism invaded every aspect of social life; individual, family, community and nation. The home environment changed into stressful office rooms and online schools. The personal space was compromised immediately and leaving no alternative. Children were confined to homes and their energy was bottled up causing frustration and loneliness. In some homes, other stressors (such as loss of jobs or ailing people) further dampened the spirit and caused anxiety about the future. While the sanitization rituals by individuals helped disease prevention, it is reported that rigorous hygiene routine to combat COVID-19 resulted in a rise in cases of obsessive–compulsive disorder [15]. There were countless stories of social isolation and its impact from around the nation and the world, each pointing towards the need to address this unsaid challenge.

## 4. Psychosocial aspects of COVID-19

Prolonged exposure to stress, regardless of age or race and ethnicity, adds another dimension to the pandemic's major public health threat. As a consequence, the COVID-19 infection and physical ailments produce pandemic-induced mental health issues that are critical challenges that must remain at the forefront of response. Studies reported heightened attention to evaluating social impact and community tension in order to facilitate psychosocial support to the population during this pandemic. The COVID-safe behavior such as social distancing, home isolation and security measures have grossly affected the social relationships among individuals and their perceptions of compassion towards fellow-beings. During the current unprecedented times in India, a large number of families are grieving their loss of near and dear ones. Prevailing mental health conditions triggered by a distressing or fearful event (either because of experiencing it first hand or by witnessing it) is commonly reported.

The current situation of COVID-19 is not only distressing for those grieving the loss of life, but it is also distressing individuals and families beyond, or irrespective of, their grief. People who are directly affected by the virus, or hit indirectly due to fear of infection, social isolation, and/or financial crisis, are struggling. More specifically, a large proportion of the Indian population have diverse and vulnerable life situations, such as people who are elderly and poor with chronic or acute ailments, migrant labourers, senior citizens, quarantined individuals in their homes or health facility, and families of those suffering or quarantined. Such large numbers of individuals are vulnerable and may show signs and symptoms of mental distress and emotional problems.

The pandemic has given rise to situations where these signs and symptoms of mental distress and emotional problems manifest in the risk of anxiety and depression, substance use, loneliness, and domestic violence; and with schools closed, there is a very real possibility of an epidemic of child abuse [16]. Several studies emphasized COVID-19's effect on mental well-being on vulnerable groups, including children, college students, and health care personnel, as they are more likely to develop post-traumatic stress disorder (PTSD), anxiety, depression, and other symptoms of distress [17]. While dealing with such public health emergencies, the past experiences have also testified that the generalized public fear and anxieties increase due to uncertainty, fatality, and lack of public health preparedness. Researchers must continue to investigate the strong link between mental and physical health [18, 19].

Across the world, anecdotal literature elucidates the large-scale reporting of mental health suffering of people. The literature calls for concentrated behavioral and mental health programmes to minimize and ameliorate psychosocial issues caused by the outbreak. In the current circumstances, crucial behavioral strategies such as physical distancing, hand hygiene and wearing masks, etc. are the only effective approaches to combat and survive the pandemic. Even so, there are a number of protective factors which may help alleviate these stressors and assist with maintaining good mental health among families and communities. Therefore, it is essential to systematically study the emerging psychosocial impacts and public health issues suffered by individuals in response to the lockdown or quarantining. Secondly, research needs to ascertain the psychosocial impact on specific vulnerable groups due to physical distancing, school closures, restricted health and social care provision, and loss of group activities. Thirdly, generating evidence for effective behavioral interventions, strategies and mechanisms to mitigate the psychosocial stressors and prevention of infections are equally important for developing policy and programmes for community mental wellbeing.

Similar to the recommendations above, comprehensive management and treatment of mental health issues at the institutional and community levels are just as significant as the various COVID-19 related protocols for physical health. Moreover, management and treatment of pre-existing mental disorders and new onsets are of an enormous concern. Lastly, it is imperative to understand the indirect effects of the pandemic and how these factors differ among population groups. The following discussions elucidate the psychosocial impact of Coronavirus disease on a few selected vulnerable populations. These notable lessons learned during the pandemic are highlighted here with a view to improving the effectiveness of policy planners, researchers and interventionist in the forthcoming months and improve future response.

## 5. COVID-19 and At-risk population

The country's coronavirus pandemic response with regard to the people living in poor urban and rural settlements, migrant workers and other vulnerable populations has been meager and slow. The current situation raises concerns about health inequity in terms of accessibility and availability of basic health care services to survive during the deadly pandemic.

Therefore, in order to best plan for preventative care and appropriate interventions to move public health policy and programming forward, it is essential to further understand the indirect effects of the pandemic, including the psychosocial impact of COVID-19 in India, which has been well documented [20–24]. While the pandemic has not discriminated among the Indian population, several population groups, and even their subgroups, have been particularly at-risk of psychosocial impact. In particular, special attention must be given to respond to the unique risk factors of women, children, health care professionals, migrant workers, and people with disabilities, who are among some of the populations that are disproportionately vulnerable to the impact of the pandemic in most facets of their lives.

Adverse effects, such as the risk of abuse, significantly rise during global emergencies [25–27]. Violence against women, including intimate partner violence (IPV), further presents a public health concern that is impacting already strained public health systems during the COVID-19 pandemic. Several factors contribute to the anticipated, and confirmed, rise of IPV during the pandemic. With restricted movement and stay-at-home orders, consistently close contact, additional stress, and potential income reduction or loss of livelihood, women who have previously been abused can experience increased violence in the home. Further, contact with supportive friends and family may also be reduced as a result of social/physical distancing. Concurrently, caregiving responsibilities for women increase while school closures also add to the care work of women. Since many women work in the informal wage-earning sector, the loss of their livelihoods leaves families further vulnerable to resource scarcity, ultimately resulting in placing women at "greater risk for experiencing economic abuse" [27–29]. A case vignette is provided below to exemplify the increased risk women face during this pandemic.

**COVID-19 and the Increased Risks for Women**
When a domestic worker and her husband have both lost their jobs, Mrs. T. takes the responsibility to make ends meet to manage the household and feed her children while her husband spends their savings on his alcohol use. Mrs. T. explains that prior to the pandemic, her husband beat her at night after he got home from work. However, since he lost his job (he was a rickshaw driver), he beats her unpredictably in the day [30].

Furthermore, for women experiencing IPV, access to essentials such as hand sanitizer and soap may be restricted, while information shared with them about COVID-19 may be misleading and stigmatize partners [27]. Access to services is also further limited due to the reduction in services resulting from organizations having to scale back services due to the pandemic.

Additionally, as options for essential travel are reduced, women may find themselves in a double bind. They may be both further exposed to risks of violence as well as infection. With metros shutting down, and any available transportation responsible for disinfection and limiting passengers to one at a time, the connection from home to destinations has significantly increased in cost while simultaneously reducing the cost saving opportunity to rideshare [27]. Several researchers note that women, comprise 81.6% of the informal work sector and are precluded from accessing social protections such as unemployment and cash transfers [31–33]. Moreover, women have reported being harassed both inside, and while waiting for, public transportation [34, 35]. An updated 2019 nationwide survey of women commuters found that only 9% of women felt very safe on public transportation [36]. Therefore, not only do women find themselves potentially further exposed to infection when commuting, but they also incur further expenses due to limited options and increased prices for intermediary public transportation. Finally, with women's reluctance to use public transportation for fear of being vulnerable to both sexual and other forms of violence, more effective urban planning to create a safer physical environment is essential. However, equally important are the coordinated efforts of civil society organizations, police, and transport authorities to ensure the protection of women travelers [37].

The violence against women often results in physical injuries, including affecting sexual and reproductive health, mental well-being, and perpetuating sexually transmitted diseases [38]. Risk factors that predispose vulnerability to violence, include economic stress, social isolation, poverty and associated factors (such as overcrowding and unemployment), poor neighborhood support and cohesion, unwillingness of neighbors to intervene when witnessing violence, and traditional gender norms and gender inequality [27–29]. Such risk factors are further exacerbated due to the pandemic. Although crimes against women are mostly unreported, or underreported at best, records suggest that this is a significant social and public health epidemic. Prior to the onset of the COVID-19 pandemic, of the 4.05 lakh registered crimes against women in 2019, over 30% of them were domestic violence occurrences [39]. Since the onset of the nationwide lockdown in response to the COVID-19 pandemic, the National Commission for Women has reported an increase of domestic violence being more than 2.5 times the previous rate of occurrence [40].

## 6. Children affected by COVID-19

The second wave of the Indian COVID-19 situation was certainly alarming compared to the first wave in 2020, as many more pediatric cases were reported across the country. Several children, including infants, are at greater risk of acquiring and spreading the infection. However, their condition remained under control and seldom turned fatal [41]. Notwithstanding, as per the Government of India [42] Protocol for Management of COVID-19 in the Pediatric Age Group indicates, a small percentage of children who are symptomatic may need hospitalization. Moreover, 1–3% of infected children may manifest severe symptoms necessitating intensive care treatment.

Nevertheless, a substantial number of families are undergoing a persistent sense of despair due to losses of livelihood, financial security, social support networks and threatened loss of loved ones. Such complexities tend to impact the quality of family cohesion and relationships among children and parents. The current pandemic-related uncertainties, fears, and worries certainly launched other crises among children which complicate and potentially hinder their developmental outcomes.

**School** - As the pandemic led to nationwide school closures beginning 16, March 2020, more than 290 million children were left to participate in education through virtual mode technology (e.g., smartphone, television, or computer). Although lessons pivoted to web links and TV, only 1 in 4 students have access to digital learning. Further, electricity and connectivity also present challenges for many students, highlighting the digital divide [43]. Across 23 states, 12% of school children do not have access to smartphones or basic phones [44], rendering education unattainable. Moreover, in Maharashtra, "only 50 percent of public-school students from classes I to VIII could access digital learning" [45]. Parents and teachers grappled with their own low levels of technology and digital literacy, further complicating education delivery. With such educational limitations, the incidence of school dropout risk increases significantly [46].

**Child Protection** - Issues of child protection have also seen a spike during the COVID-19 pandemic. In addition to families plunging further into poverty, violence against children (as with women) has also increased. CHILDLINE (a telephone helpline for children in distress) has received 4 million distressed calls from children requesting assistance; 92,000 calls reporting abuse and violence in just the early days of the 2020 lockdown [47]. As families come under duress responding to the pandemic, child labour, marriage and institutionalization are on the rise. With access to education compromised as described above, children are pressured to join the labour force and contribute to the family income [48]. Research demonstrates that during emergencies and crises, children are at higher risk for physical, verbal, and sexual abuse, as well as exploitation and trafficking [43, 49]. The case vignette below illustrates the desperation that can lead to child exploitation.

---

**COVID-19 and the Increase in Child Labour**

Despite it being a cognizable offense to employ a child as per the law, the last census indicated that "10 million of India's 260 million children "are child labourers [50]. The lockdown has caused parents to grapple with the decision to offer their child to human traffickers when they have gone for months with virtually no income. For example, Mr. L made the heart wrenching decision to offer his 13-year-old son to work in a bangle factory 1,000 km away from home after traffickers refused to bring Mr. L because they needed "nimble" fingers and an adult was "of no use." He told reporters that his children were going hungry and he felt he was left with no choice [50].

---

Considering children and adolescents' cognitive and emotional development, their inability to fully understand the pandemic and communicate their feelings fosters additional risk of mental health issues. Protective factors such as socialization and physical activity have all but come to a standstill. Social media, with its flood of information and misinformation further contributes to "anxiety, depression, sleep disturbance, and loss of appetite" [21, 51].

Children, particularly girls, have also seen a significant rise in their domestic workload responsibilities [52]. School-aged girls have become more vulnerable to child marriage in order to defray household expenditure. During the lockdown, 5,584 CHILDLINE interventions were related to child marriages (ToI, 27 June 2020). In addition, menstrual hygiene was also compromised during the pandemic. Menstrual hygiene products, such as sanitary napkins, were not initially designated as essential items and therefore inaccessible for menstruating girls, potentially leading to unhygienic practices that could have serious health consequences (such as toxic shock syndrome, infections, and vaginal diseases [45, 53].

Child malnutrition is also a concerning ramification of the pandemic [21, 54]. Not only with food insecurity on the rise in homes that have been economically hit by the pandemic, but children have also been hit with an additional blow as access to government food programmes have been disrupted in some states. And despite increased food insecurity, the risks of weight gain and other additional adverse physical effects of a sedentary lifestyle have increased. For example, children's average daily screen time has increased from 3.5 hours to 5.12 hours, leading to associated loss of physical fitness, increased psychosocial problems, ophthalmic issues, sleep disruption and decline in academic achievement [55–57].

In addition to these issues of malnutrition and childhood weight gain resulting from the shift to a more sedentary lifestyle living in a restricted mobility environment, it is also essential to consider the 486,000 children living in alternative care [21]. For these children, residential or institutional environments further increase their risk for poor outcomes during the pandemic. As Roy, S., [58] points out, non-residential care providers were unable to provide in-person services and therefore children have had to further rely on overworked residential staff for activities facilitation, schooling and therapeutic services. Overcrowded institutions are also challenged by finding adequate quarantine space for children infected with the virus. Issues of technology constraints (especially accessible learning materials for children with disabilities), understaffing, inadequate food, hygiene and medical supplies, and physical distancing with limited social connectivity are all prominent for children in childcare institutions and further exacerbate their anxiety and fear of the pandemic. For those children aging out of the system, limited options, concurrent with the inability to prepare for discharge during the pandemic, can hinder their ability to successfully transition into independent living and predispose them to exploitation, violence, and further adverse consequences [59].

On an encouraging note, however, immediately after the Ministry of Women and Child Development reported 577 children had been orphaned during the second wave, the Prime Minister (PM) announced support under the PM CARES for Children's scheme. Such support includes financial aid and free education for all COVID-19 orphans, the surviving parents, legal guardian or adoptive parents. In addition, the PM assured that the "GOI stands in solidarity with these families" [60].

## 7. Healthcare workers

Health care workers (HCW) are at high-risk for not only contracting the coronavirus, but also for the adverse psychosocial effects of the pandemic. However, the infection incident rate among healthcare workers is difficult to ascertain since there is no routine covid testing at health care facilities or accessible centralized repository for HCW prevalence data. Nevertheless, there are some recent studies that examine prevalence of infection among HCWs [61–63]. For example, Mahajan et al. [63] found 11% prevalence among the HCWs in their Mumbai study. Another study of healthcare workers in Kolkata suggests that routine COVID screening for HCWs is essential since they found 31% of their study participants who tested positive were asymptomatic; thereby increasing the risk of infection transmission unknowingly [63].

Dubey et al.'s [20] comprehensive literature review identified several factors that further compromise HCW well-being beyond the risk of infection exposure. Of particular relevance, they found that "burnout, anxiety, fear of transmitting infection, feeling of incompatibility, depression, increased substance-dependence, and PTSD" added to HCW's already concerns due to their high risk for contracting the virus. A cross sectional study of both HCWs and non-HCWs presented similar results with prevalent conditions such as depression, insomnia and anxiety as the significant psychological impacts of the pandemic [64]. Chew et al.'s [65] multinational study of HCWs reported that 79% of HCWs experienced moderate to very severe depression. Further, 2.2% reported feeling moderate to extremely severe stress, while 3.8% reported experiencing moderate to severe levels of psychological distress. These psychological impacts seemed to manifest in psychosomatic symptoms such as headaches, throat pain, anxiety, lethargy and insomnia.

The issue of stigmatization further adds to the stress and anxiety level of healthcare workers. Medical personnel, ward attenders and COVID-19 patient caregivers have all been targets of public outrage (including assaults) since they are perceived as high-risk infection transmitters [66, 67]. The following case vignette lucidly highlights the impact on a revered medical provider.

**COVID-19 Warriors**

An announcement was uploaded on Twitter as "It causes us immense pain to inform you that our dear Dr KK Aggarwal passed away at 11.30 pm on May 17, 2021, in New Delhi, after a lengthy battle with Covid-19...,". India's most prominent face of Medical Fraternity is no more. The 62-year cardiologist Dr. K K Agarwal, Padma Shri awardee and former national president of Indian Medical Association, was critical and he had been on ventilator support for the past few days but later succumbed to COVID-19 in All India Institute of Medical Sciences. His family put out a statement "KK Agarwal wanted his life to be celebrated not mourned." Ironically during the pandemic, Dr. Agarwal made relentless efforts to educate the common people and was able to reach out to 100 million people through several videos and education programmes and also saved innumerable lives. According to the report of the Indian Medical Association (IMA), 270 physicians have died in India's recent COVID-19 surge since early April and so far, more than 1,000 have died since the beginning of the pandemic. IMA also reported state-wise data on doctors' death, with the maximum figures in Bihar (78), Uttar Pradesh (37), and Delhi (28). The death toll is likely far higher since the association tracks only 350,000 registered members, but India has about 1.2 million doctors. A large number of them are survived by their families and children who need help for sustenance, education and rearing. The IMA very generously initiated the COVID Martyrs Fund by appealing for a minimum one-day income donation from members and citizenry [68].

## 8. Persons with disabilities (PWD) and the elderly

According to Census 2011, India is home to 26.8 million persons with disabilities; 2.21% of the total population [69]. This statistic may also underrepresent the total number of people coping with a disability since there is not yet an established universal definition of disability in either the international or national discussions. The Coronavirus pandemic, along with the subsequent lockdown, has brought diverse challenges for PWDs. For example, procuring essential supplies, accessing medical treatment, and adopting physical distancing practices have devolved into further obstacles. The following case of Mr. AK, illustrates his experience of additional challenges with activities of daily living during the pandemic.

**More Challenges for PWD During COVID-19**

Mr. AK, a 33-year-old with vision impairment, shared how he has organized his life for an independent existence. However, with the pandemic, Mr. AK is under tremendous stress as cleaning utensils, fixing broken gadgets, and the ability to differentiate and select particular food items at the market have become more complicated. No longer having domestic help available to assist with errands only further adds to his stress during the pandemic [70].

Further, the Secretary-General of the United Nations, has declared that COVID-19 has "disproportionately [impacted] PWDs both directly and indirectly" ([71], p. 2). PWDs may face barriers to several protective measures. Access to water, sanitation and hygiene facilities can be hindered, along with public health information access. Additionally, people with disabilities who are placed in institutional care can be further at risk of infection due to overcrowded and unhygienic conditions in many institutions. PWDs also often rely on physical contact for mobility and to complete activities of daily living, thereby diminishing physical distancing protective measures. Elders, too, often face these same barriers.

Moreover, skill training programs for PWDs have all but stopped dead in their tracks in response to the COVID-19 lockdown in March, 2020. In 2018–2019, 47,286 people with disabilities participated in skill training programs which dropped to merely 1,434 participants in 2019–2020. The Department for Empowerment of Persons with Disabilities has empaneled 75 programs to meet the more stringent expectations, compared with the previous 280 programs [72]. It is essential that rigorous safety protocols are followed as training programs reopen. As an additional option, online training program proposals for people who are differently-abled are currently being explored.

Of the persons with disabilities in India, nearly half of them have vision impairment. Senjam [73] points out that 13 million of those with vision impairment have functional low vision. However, appropriate and accessible information related to COVID-19 are inadequate, especially for people with visual disability in the areas of transmission, nature of the virus, and prevention and protective strategies. They also require personal assistance with activities of daily living and rely on tactile sensory for performing "routine activities or outdoor movement which may further increase the chance of getting the infection from the virus" ([73], p. 1368). Protective techniques such as handwashing and face mask wearing rely on visual functioning, while assistive devices require regular disinfection in order to prevent the transmission of infection. For people with visual impairment and other disabilities, the "sudden disruption of [their] support system, including personal assistance, and potential economic hardship ... will have serious consequences in health and wellbeing" ([73], p. 1368). The quality of life for people living with disabilities will be significantly impacted by the added risk factors and necessary precautions needed to interact with their surroundings during the pandemic [73–75].

The lack of priority given to establishing and distributing clear guidelines and recommendations for people with disabilities is further impacting persons with disabilities. If people with disabilities do not have disability certificates or ration card documentation, they can be denied food. Hospitals are closing their doors to non-COVID patients, leaving people with disabilities without the necessary and accessible healthcare infrastructure to support them [74, 76].

For elderly, as with people with disabilities, the physical risks of the pandemic and related issues are further exacerbated by the social isolation that they face [77, 78]. Elders have limited, if any, access and proficiency with technology to foster connections to information and alleviate social isolation. With such isolation and heightened anxiety, elders are also at an increased risk of suicide [79]. Further, with social isolation, particularly from their family systems, seniors are also predisposed to greater risks of "inactivity, smoking, alcohol abuse, unhealthy diet, depression, introversion, poor social skills, and post-traumatic stress disorder leading to greater risks of cardiovascular diseases, dementia, and premature mortality" ([78], p. 1).

## 9. Harder hit migrant workers

Throughout the Coronavirus pandemic, domestic migrant workers have been experiencing numerous adversities and destitution. With industries and factories closed down as a result of the nationwide lockdown, millions of migrant workers were left with loss of livelihood, food shortages, ambiguity about their future and unfortunate eventualities. The story of Mrs. SY, below, highlights the agony that some migrant workers and their families have faced during this time.

**Ordeal and Tragic Departure of a Migrant Family**

With excessive numbers of migrant workers without work and little hope once the lockdown began March 24, 2020, many began the journey back to their villages by foot, cycling, hitchhiking, etc. Mrs. SY and her family were living and working in Mumbai with their food cart. When their savings depleted in the first two months of the lockdown, they tried to book the special train tickets to return to their village some 1,500 km away. Their tickets never came so they left by Auto-rickshaw. Driving 11 hours/day and sleeping on the pavements, Mrs. SY, her husband and two children were eager for the safety of their village. However, on the fourth day of their journey home and just 200 km away, their Auto-rickshaw was struck by a truck and killed both Mrs. SY and one of her daughters [80].

Migrant workers comprise a significant sector of the population, and as such they have become particularly at-risk during the Coronavirus pandemic [77, 81, 82]. Presently, there is significant discrepancy among estimates of the migrant worker count in India. Estimates of the informal economic sector range from 70 to 400 million workers [83–85]. Further, the World Bank reports 471,689,092 workers in India's labour force [86]. The informal economy, therefore, comprises roughly anywhere between 14.8 and 76.2% of the workforce in India.

Regardless of the actual number of migrant labourers, the unique challenges and adverse psychosocial effects of the pandemic on the informal sector can be disproportionately significant and even fatal. With the initial lockdown, workers abruptly lost income and/or were subject to working conditions with suspended occupational safety precautions [81]. In addition to their susceptibility to communicable diseases due to migrant workers' factors relating to their socioeconomic status (e.g., malnutrition, substandard and crowded living and sanitation conditions, and pre-existing health issues related to their conditions), they also have had to contend with the absence of family support and economic constraints, as well as the burden of failing to provide financial support to their loved ones [81, 87].

Migrant workers' opportunities to meet their basic needs of food and shelter, coupled with the abrupt loss of income and concern with contracting the infection and developing anxiety, all converged in large-scale movements from the cities to return to home communities. However, such movements, supported by special train transportation, led to an increase in the spread of the infection, including migrant passengers losing their lives later to COVID-19 [87, 88]. The lack of available transportation during the lockdown has also led to "significant deaths of migrant workers in road accidents" ([77], p. 207). Further, even once migrant workers return home, they may further compromise their family's food and shelter access while employment opportunities back home are scarce. Moreover, social exclusion and the stigma of possibly transmitting the infection from the cities to their communities upon their return has also further alienated the worker and their family from their community. For those migrants who remained in their host cities, unsanitary, crowded living conditions and the inability to therefore adhere to social distancing guidelines only further jeopardized the remaining migrant workers' health [87]. Furthermore, accessing health care, particularly during the pandemic, has proven to be another obstacle for migrant workers. The dearth of trained health professionals to address communicable and noncommunicable diseases was already an issue for India's public health infrastructure prior to the onset of the pandemic.

## 10. Conclusion

The novel coronavirus impacted life in every facet, marking it as an epoch in human history. With the efforts of the scientific community, the mystery around the virus unfolded gradually as humanity grappled with the crisis each day over the last year and a half. To build a holistic picture, we touched upon multiple areas where the repercussions of the virus were felt. The chapter delineated the problem from multiple perspectives and endeavored to highlight the intervention strategies that were adopted at governmental, community and individual levels to fight the pandemic. There is a substantial amount of documentation to show the altruisms and resilience among the local communities of India during the time of the coronavirus pandemic. The citizens organized, offered and provided various types of assistance, such as setting up quarantine facilities, pooling resources for medical aids, oxygen, feeding millions of needy people and those stranded by lockdown, and assisting both the elderly and children affected directly or indirectly by COVID-19. Such fortitude of self-reliance and collective sense of purpose of Indian communities must be leveraged and empowered to fight the outbreak of the Corona pandemic and future challenges resulting from any health emergencies. As the second wave of the pandemic begins to decline, there is growing speculation and uncertainty yet again for a third wave. There is an urgent need to reflect and learn lessons for the future by undertaking evidence-based multi-disciplinary policy research that should pave the way to prepare for a public health challenge. In case of an anticipated third wave, the national and state health care systems and communities should be ready to invest in developing adequate public health infrastructure, effective prevention strategies and most importantly, enhancing societal participation in caring for vulnerable people.

## Author details

Shankar Das[1*] and Julie Richards[2]

1 Tata Institute of Social Sciences, Mumbai, India

2 Plattsburgh College, State University of New York, Plattsburgh, NY, USA

*Address all correspondence to: shankardass07@gmail.com

## References

[1] WHO (2020). Novel Coronavirus (2019-nCoV) Situation Report – 1, 21 January 2020 at https://www.who.int/docs/default-source/coronaviruse/situation-reports/20200121-sitrep-1-2019-ncov.pdf, Data as reported by: 20 January 2020

[2] Wang D, Hu B, Hu C, Zhu F, Liu X, Zhang J, et al., (2020). Clinical Characteristics of 138 hospitalized patients with 2019 novel coronavirus-infected pneumonia in Wuhan, China. JAMA, 323, 1061-1069.

[3] WHO (2020). COVID-19 Public Health Emergency of International Concern, (PHEIC) Global research and innovation forum; Towards a research; roadmap; 12 February 2020 at https://www.who.int/publications/m/item/covid-19-public-health-emergency-of-international-concern-(pheic)-global-research-and-innovation-forum

[4] WHO (2020). WHO characterizes COVID-19 as a pandemic. Rolling updates on coronavirus disease (COVID-19), 11 March 2020; at https://www.who.int/emergencies/diseases/novel-coronavirus-2019/events-as-they-happen

[5] World Health Organization (2021). WHO Coronavirus (COVID-19) Dashboard, Situation by Region, Country, Territory & Area. WHO Health Emergency Dashboard WHO (COVID-19) available at https://covid19.who.int/table (https://www.worldometers.info/coronavirus/country/china/)

[6] WHO (2020). Solidarity Therapeutics Trial produces conclusive evidence on the effectiveness of repurposed drugs for COVID-19 in record time 15 October 2020 News release, Geneva at https://www.who.int/news/item/15-10-2020-solidarity-therapeutics-trial-produces-conclusive-evidence-on-the-effectiveness-of-repurposed-drugs-for-covid-19-in-record-time

[7] Healthworld.com (2020). Karnataka Announces India's first Coronavirus death. From The Economic Times, AFP. March 13, 2020 available at https://health.economictimes.indiatimes.com/news/industry/state-minister-announces-indias-first-coronavirus-death/74604253#:~:text=Karnataka%20announces%20India's%20first%20coronavirus%20death%2C%20Health%20News%2C%20ET%20HealthWorld

[8] JHU CSSE COVID-19 Data (2021). JHU CSSE COVID-19 Data and Our World in Data. Statistics New cases and deaths. Available at https://github.com/CSSEGISandData/COVID-19, accessed on 8th June 2021.

[9] Banerjee, D. and Rai, M. (2020) Social isolation in Covid-19: The impact of loneliness. International Journal of Social Psychiatry, 66(6), 525-527

[10] WHO (2020). As more go hungry and malnutrition persists, achieving Zero Hunger by 2030 in doubt, UN report warns; 13 July 2020, News release, At https://www.who.int/news/item/13-07-2020-as-more-go-hungry-and-malnutrition-persists-achieving-zero-hunger-by-2030-in-doubt-un-report-warns

[11] Leventhal, T., Brooks-Gunn J. (2003). Moving to opportunity: an experimental study of neighborhood effects on mental health. American Journal of Public Health, 93, 1576-1582.

[12] McLoyd, V.C. (1998). Socioeconomic disadvantage and child development. American Psychology, 53, 185-204.

[13] Mukhtar, S. (2020). Psychological health during the coronavirus disease 2019 pandemic outbreak. International Journal of Social Psychiatry, 66(5) 512-516.

[14] Karmakar, M., Lantz, P.M. and Tipirneni, R. (2021) Association of Social and Demographic Factors With COVID-19 Incidence and Death Rates in the US. JAMA Netw Open. 2021;4(1): e2036462. doi:10.1001/ jamanetworkopen.2020.36462

[15] Fliess, C. (2020). Rigorous hygiene routine to beat COVID-19 increased OCD cases: Study. *Medindia*, Retrieved on December 20, 2020 from https:// www.medindia.net/news/rigorous-hygiene-routine-to-beat-covid-increased-ocd-cases-study-197991-1.htm

[16] Das, Shankar (2020): Mental Health and Psychosocial Aspects of COVID-19 in India: The Challenges and Responses, Journal of Health Management, Sage Publication, August 2020 https://doi.org /10.1177%2F0972063420935544

[17] Saladino,V., Algeri, D. & Auriemma, V. (2020) The Psychological and Social Impact of Covid-19: New Perspectives of Well-Being. Front. Psychol., 02 October 2020 | https://doi.org/10.3389/ fpsyg.2020.577684

[18] Nabi, H., Kivimaki M., R. De Vogli, M.G. Marmot, & A. Singh-Manoux (2008). Positive and negative affect and risk of coronary heart disease: Whitehall II prospective cohort study, BMJ, 337 (7660), 32-36.

[19] Surtees, P., N.W. Wainwright, R.N. Luben, N.J. Wareham, S.A. Bingham, K.T. Khaw (2008). Psychological distress, major depressive disorder, and risk of stroke, Neurology, 70(10), 788-794.

[20] Dubey, S., Biswas, P., Ghosh, R., Chatterjee, S., Dubey, M.J., Chatterjee, S., Lahiri, D., & Lavie, C. J. (2020). Psychosocial impact of COVID-19, Diabetes & Metabolic Syndrome: Clinical Research & Reviews, 14(5), 779-788, ISSN 1871-4021, https://doi. org/10.1016/j.dsx.2020.05.035.

[21] Ghosh, R., Dubey, MJ, Chatterjee, S. & Dubey, S. (2020). Impact of COVID-19 on children: Special focus on the psychosocial aspect. Minerva Pediatrica, 72(3), 226-235.

[22] Golechha, M. (2020). COVID-19, India, lockdown and psychosocial challenges: what's next? Indian Journal of Social Psychiatry, 66(8), 830-832.

[23] Joshi, A. (2021a). COVID-19 pandemic in India: through psycho-social lens. *Journal of Social and Economic Development*. https://doi. org/10.1007/s40847-020-00136-8

[24] Singh, K., Kondal, D., Mohan, S., Jaganathan, S., Deepa, M, Srinivasapura Venkateshmurthy N., Jarhyam, P., Mohan Anjana, R., Venkat Narayan, K.M., Mohan, V., Tandon, N., Ali, M., Prabhakaran, D., & Eggleston, K., (2021). Health, psychosocial, and economic impacts of the COVID-19 pandemic on people with chronic conditions in India: A mixed methods study, BMC Public Health, 21, 685-700.

[25] Das, M., Das, A., & Mandal, A. (2020). Examining the impact of lockdown (due to COVID-19) on Domestic Violence (DV): An evidence from India. Asian Journal of Psychiatry, *54*, 102335. https://doi.org/10.1016/j. ajp.2020.102335

[26] Ghoshal, R. (2020). Twin public health emergencies: COVID-19 and domestic violence, Indian *Journal of Medical Ethics*. Published online on May 7, 2020. DOI: 10.20529/ IJME.2020.056.

[27] WHO (2020). COVID-19 and violence against women: What the health sector/system can do? 7th April, 2020. Retrieved on May 17, 2021,

Retrieved on May 17, 2021, From https://apps.who.int/iris/bitstream/handle/10665/331699/WHO-SRH-20.04-eng.pdf?ua=1

[28] Joseph, S. J., Mishra, A., Bhandari, S. S., & Dutta, S. (2020). Intimate partner violence during the COVID-19 pandemic in India: From psychiatric and forensic vantage points. Asian Journal of Psychiatry, *54*, 102279. https://doi.org/10.1016/j.ajp.2020.102279

[29] Pal, A., Gondwal, R., Sayanti, P., Bohri, R., Pal Singh Aulakh, A., & Bhat, A. (2021). Effect of COVID-19-related lockdown on intimate partner violence in India: An online survey-based study, *Violence and Gender*. Retrieved on May 26,2021 from https://www.liebertpub.com/doi/abs/10.1089/vio.2020.0050

[30] Kotamraju, P. (2020). Local diaries: Untold stories of women in India's lockdown, *Oxfam*, Retrieved on May 25, 2021 from https://oxfamblogs.org/fp2p/local-diaries-untold-stories-of-women-in-indias-lockdown/.

[31] Joshi, S. (4, January 2021b). To sit or not to sit? Using intermediary public transport during COVID -19 pandemic. *Down to Earth,* Retrieved on 28 May, 2020, From https://www.downtoearth.org.in/blog/governance/to-sit-or-not-to-sit-using-intermediary-public-transport-during-covid-19-pandemic-74881

[32] Salcedo-La Vina, C., Singh, R., & Elwell, N. (September 21, 2020). Rural women must be at the heart of COVID-19 response and recovery, *World Resources Institute*. Retrieved on May 17, 2021, From https://www.wri.org/insights/rural-women-must-be-heart-covid-19-response-and-recovery

[33] Sinha, N. (July 27, 2020). The need for a gender responsive economy in the aftermath of COVID-19 in India. Retrieved on May 17, 2021, From https://blogs.lse.ac.uk/southasia/2020/07/27/the-need-for-a-gender-responsive-economy-in-the-aftermath-of-covid-19-in-india/.

[34] Jagori and UN Women (2011). Safe cities free of violence against women and Girl's initiative. http://www.jagori.org/wp-content/uploads/2011/03/Baseline-Survey_layout_for-Print_12_03_2011.pdf

[35] Valan, M. (2020). Victimology of sexual harassment on public transportation: evidence from India. Journal of Victimology and Victim Justice, 3(1), 24-37.

[36] OMI (March 2020). What do women and girls want from urban mobility systems? Ola Mobility Institute Retrieved 5/8/21 from https://olawebcdn.com/ola-institute/ola_women_and_mobility.pdf

[37] Paniker, L. (February 7, 2021). Make public transport safe for women, *The Hindustan Times*, Retrieved May 7, 2021, From https://www.hindustantimes.com/opinion/make-public-transport-safe-for-women-101612621008097.html

[38] Viveiros, N & Bonomi, A. (2020). Novel Coronavirus (COVID-19): Violence, reproductive rights and related health risks for women, opportunities for practice innovation, Journal of Family Violence, https://doi.org/10.1007/s10896-020-00169-x

[39] NCRB (2020). Crime in India 2019: Statistics Volume -1. National Crime Records Bureau, Retrieved on June 2, 2021 from https://ncrb.gov.in/sites/default/files/CII%202019%20Volume%201.pdf.

[40] Dhawan, H. (5, October 2020). *Not rape, domestic violence is top crime against women*. Times of India. Retrieved 2, June 2021, from https://timesofindia.indiatimes.com/india/not-rape-domestic-violence-is-top-crime-

against-women/articleshow/78494876.cms#:~:text=While%20cases%20of%20sexual%20assault,were%20that%20of%20domestic%20violence.

[41] UNICEF (2021). COVID-19 infection in children: Protecting and caring for children with COVID-19. AIIMS Delhi, WHO and UNICEF, India. Retrieved on June 3, 2021, From https://www.unicef.org/india/stories/covid-19-infection-children

[42] GoI (2021). Protocol for management of Covid - 19 in the pediatric age group, *Government of India Ministry of Health and Family Welfare*. Retrieved on June 3, 2021, From https://www.mohfw.gov.in/pdf/ProtocolforManagementofCovid19inthePaediatricAgeGroup.pdf

[43] UNICEF (17 November, 2020). *Impact of COVID-19 crisis on the lives of children in India*. https://www.unicef.org/india/media/4811/file/Impact%20of%20COVID-19%20crisis%20on%20the%20lives%20of%20children%20in%20India%20-%20Panel%20discussion%20with%20media%20for%20World%20Children's%20Day.pdf

[44] ToI (June 13, 2020). About 56% of children have no access to smartphones for e-learning: Study, The Times of India. Retrieved on June 3, 2021, From https://timesofindia.indiatimes.com/home/education/news/about56-of-children-have-no-access-to-smartphones-for-e-learning-study/articleshow/76355350.cms

[45] Bahl, D., Bassi, S., & Arora, M. (4 March 2021). The impact of COVID-19 on children and adolescents: Early evidence in India. *Issue Briefs and Special Reports*. Observer Research Foundation. Retrieved from https://www.orfonline.org/research/the-impact-of-covid-19-on-children-and-adolescents-early-evidence-in-india/

[46] Alvi, M. & Gupta, M. (2020). Learning in times of lockdown: How COVID-19 is affecting education and food security in India, Food Security, 12, 793-796. https://doi.org/10.1007/s12571-020-01065-4

[47] The Hindu, (April 8, 2020). Coronavirus lockdown: Government helpline receives 92,000 calls on child abuse and violence in 11 days, *The Hindu*. Retrieved on June 3, 2020 from https://www.thehindu.com/news/national/coronavirus-lockdown-govt-helpline-receives-92000-calls-on-child-abuse-and-violence-in-11-days/article31287468.ece#

[48] Tyagi, T. (July 5, 2020). Child labour cases rise in June, Hindustan Times, https://www.hindustantimes.com/cities/child-labour-cases-rise-in-june/story-7oDzLfO1x6U N0b3mMucNLI.html

[49] Dave, H. & Yagnik, P. (2020). Psycho-social impact of COVID-19 on children in India: The reality, Child Abuse & Neglect, 108. Doi:10.1016/j.chiabu.2020.104663.

[50] Arya, D. (2020). India's COVID crisis sees rise in child marriage and trafficking. (19, September 2020). *BBC*. Retrieved May 25, 2021 from https://www.bbc.com/news/world-asia-india-54186709

[51] Kumar, A., Nayar, K.R. and Bhat, L.D. (2020). Debate: COVID-19 and children in India. Child Adolescent Mental Health, 25, 165-166. https://doi.org/10.1111/camh.12398

[52] Ramaswamy, S. & Seshadri, S. (2020). Children on the brink: Risks for child protection, sexual abuse, and related mental health problems in the COVID-19 pandemic. Indian Journal of Psychiatry, 62(3), 404-413.

[53] Cousins, S. (2020). World report: COVID-19 has "devastating" effect on women and girls, The Lancet, 396, 301-302.

[54] Sandhu, K. (2020). COVID-19 - Affecting Malnutrition in India, International Journal of Organizational Business Excellence, 3(1), 35-40.

[55] Dutta, K., Mukherjee, R., Sen, D. & Sahay, S. (2020). Effect of COVID-19 lockdown on sleep behavior and screen exposure time: An observational study among Indian school children, Biological Rhythm Research, DOI: 10.1080/09291016.2020.1825284

[56] Roy, S., Tiwari, S., Kanchan, S., & Bajpai, P. (2020). Impact of COVID-19 pandemic led lockdown on the lifestyle of adolescents and young adults. *Indian Journal of Youth & Adolescent Health* doi: 10.24321/2349.2880.202008

[57] Stiglic N., & Viner, R.M. (2019). Effects of screen time on the health and well-being of children and adolescents: A systematic review of reviews, BMJ, Open 2019;9: e023191.

[58] Roy, S. (2021). Restructuring institutional care: Challenges and coping measures for children and caregivers in post-COVID-19 era, Institutionalised children Explorations and Beyond, 8(1), 65-78.

[59] Verma, R. & Verma, R. (2021). Child vulnerabilities and family-based childcare systems: COVID-19 challenges of foster care and adoption in India. Institutionalised Children Explorations and Beyond, 8(1), 79-89.

[60] ENS, (May 30 2021). PM announces aid, free education for Covid orphans; pension for employees' next of kin, *Express News Service*. Retrieved on June 2, 2021, From https://indianexpress.com/article/india/centre-to-help-children-left-orphaned-by-covid-with-education-loan-7335686/

[61] Banerjee, A., Mukherjee, K., Bhattacharjee, D., Garai, D., & Chakraborty, R. (2020). Status of health-care workers in relation to COVID-19 infection: A retrospective study in a level 4 COVID hospital in Eastern India, Journal of Association of Physicians India, 68(12), 55-57.

[62] Chatterjee, P., Anand, T., Singh, K.J., Rasaily, R., Singh, R., Das, S., Singh, H., Praharaj, I., Gangakhedkar, R.R., Bhargava, B., & Panda, S. (2020). Healthcare workers & SARS-CoV-2 infection in India: A case-control investigation in the time of COVID-19. Indian Journal of Medical Research, 151(5), 459-467.

[63] Mahajan, N. N., Mathe, A., Patokar, G.A., Bahirat, S., Lokhande, P.D., Rakh, V., Gajbhiye, R., Rathi, S., Tilve, A., Mahajan, K., & Mohite, S.C. (2020). Prevalence and Clinical Presentation of COVID-19 among Healthcare Workers at a Dedicated Hospital in India. Journal of Association of Physicians India. 68(12), 16-21.

[64] Raj R, Koyalada S, Kumar A, Kumari S, Pani P, Nishant, Singh KK. (2020). Psychological impact of the COVID-19 pandemic on healthcare workers in India: An observational study. Journal of Family Medicine Primary Care, 9, 5921-5926

[65] Chew, N., Lee, G., Tan, B., Jing, M., Goh, Y., Ngiam, N., Yeo, L., Ahmad, A., Khan, F., Shanmugam, G., Sharma, A., Komalkumar, R.N.., Meenakshi, P.V., Shah, K., Patel, B., Chan, B., Sunny, S., Chandra, B., Ong, J., Paliwal, P., Wong, L., Sagayanathan, R., Chen, J., Ng, A., Teoh, H., Tsivgoulis, G., Ho, C., Ho, R., & Sharma, V. (2020). A multinational, multicenter study on the psychological outcomes and associated physical symptoms amongst healthcare workers during COVID-19 outbreak, Brain, Behavior, and Immunity, 88, 559-565, ISSN 0889-1591, https://doi.org/10.1016/j.bbi.2020.04.049.

[66] Chaturvedi, S., & Sharma, M. (2020). Psychosocial aspects of Covid-19, the India way. World Social Psychiatry, 2(2), 129-131.

[67] Menon, V., Kumar Padhy, S., & Ispsita Pattnaik, J. (2020). Stigma and aggression against health care workers in India amidst COVID-19 times: Possible rivers and mitigation strategies, Indian Journal of Psychological Medicine, 42(4), 400-401.

[68] Indian Medical Association (2021). *IMA Headquarters, New Delhi*, Retrieved from https://www.ima-india.org/ima/

[69] SSD (2016). Social Statistics Division, Ministry of Statistics and Programme Implementation, Government of India. Disabled Persons in India" A statistical profile 2016. Retrieved on May 17, 2021, From http://mospi.nic.in/sites/default/files/publication_reports/Disabled_persons_in_India_2016.pdf.

[70] Narayanan, J. (September 22, 2020). Pandemic and a lockdown: Person with disabilities grapple with more challenges. *The Indian Express.* Retrieved May 28, 2021 from https://indianexpress.com/article/lifestyle/life-style/persons-with-disabilities-day-to-day-challenges-coronavirus-covid-19-lockdown-pandemic-handwashing-social-isolation-distancing-6383363/

[71] United Nations (May, 2020). Policy brief: A disability-inclusive response to COVID-19. Retrieved from https://www.un.org/sites/un2.un.org/files/sg_policy_brief_on_persons_with_disabilities_final.pdf

[72] Panit, A. (December 21, 2020). Skill programme for disabled hit by Covid, govt plans e-training. *Times of India*. Retrieved on June 3, 2021, From https://timesofindia.indiatimes.com/india/skill-programme-for-disabled-hit-by-covid-govt-plans-e-training/articleshow/79831291.cmsToI (June 27, 2020). Govt intervened to stop over 5,584 child marriages during Coronavirus-induced lockdown, *Times of India*, Retrieved on June 3, 2020 from https://timesofindia.indiatimes.com/india/govt-intervened-to-stop-over-5584-child-marriage-during-coronavirus-induced-lockdown/articleshow/76661071.cms

[73] Senjam, S. (2020). Impact of COVID-19 pandemic on people living with visual disability. Indian Journal of Ophthalmology, 68(7), 1367-1370.

[74] IDA, (2020). COVID 19 and disability in west Bengal, India: The story of two teachers, International Disability Alliance, May 15, 2020. Retrieved from https://www.internationaldisabilityalliance.org/west-bengal-covid19

[75] WHO (2020). Whose life matters? Challenges, barriers and impact of COVID-19 pandemic on persons with disabilities and their care givers. World Health Organization. Retrieved on May 25, 2021, From https://apps.who.int/iris/bitstream/handle/10665/336569/sea-disability-11-eng.pdf

[76] YUVA (2020). Living with multiple vulnerabilities: Impact of COVID-19 on the urban poor in the Mumbai metropolitan region. Final Report, Youth for Unity and Voluntary Action. Retrieved on May 25, 2021 from https://yuvaindia.org/wp-content/uploads/2017/03/COVID19_MMRImpact_UrbanPoor-1.pdf

[77] Bhandari, S., Shaktawat, A., Patel, B., Dube, A., Kakkar, S., Tak, A, Gupta, J. & Rankawat, G. (2020). The sequel to COVID-19: The antithesis to life. Journal of Ideas in Health, 3(1), 205-212.

[78] Gupta, R. & Dhamija, R. (2020). COVID-19: Social distancing or social isolation? BMJ, Retrieved May 28, 2021 from https://www.bmj.com/content/369/bmj.m2399

[79] Rana, U. (2020). Elderly suicides in India: An emerging concern during COVID-19 pandemic. International Psychogeriatrics, 32(10), 1251-1252.

[80] Pandey, V. (20, May 2020). Coronavirus lockdown: The Indian migrants dying to get home, *BBC*, Retrieved on June 3, 2021, From https://www.bbc.com/news/world-asia-india-52672764\

[81] Choudhari, R. (2020). COVID 19 pandemic: Mental health challenges of internal migrant workers of India, Asian Journal of Psychiatry, 54(38), 102-254.

[82] ILO, (2020). COVID-19 and the world of work, impact and policy responses, International Labour Organisation. Retrieved June 3 2021, from https://www.ilo.org/wcmsp5/groups/public/dgreports/dcomm/documents/briefingnote/wcms_738753.pdf

[83] Chaudhary, M., Sodani, P.R., & Das, S. (2020). effect of COVID-19 on economy in India: Some reflections for policy and programme. Journal of Health Management, 22(2), 169-180.

[84] Menon, A., Tare, K., & Srivastava, A. (January 4, 2021). COVID-19 fall-out: How the pandemic displaced millions of migrants, India Today. Retrieved May 20, 2021 from https://www.indiatoday.in/magazine/news-makers/story/20210111-displaced-distressed-1755084-2021-01-03

[85] Sharma, A. (September 16, 2020a). Migrant workers: The Indian government does not know their numbers, dead or alive. Retrieved on May 24, 2021, From https://en.gaonconnection.com/migrant-workers-the-indian-government-does-not-know-their-numbers-dead-or-alive/

[86] The World Bank. (2021). Labor Force, total - India. Retrieved on May 27, 2021, From https://data.worldbank.org/indicator/SL.TLF.TOTL.IN?locations=IN

[87] Suresh, R., James, J., & Balraju, R. (2020). Migrant workers at crossroads - The COVID-19 pandemic and the migrant experience in India. Social Work in Public Health, 35(7), 633-643.

[88] Azeez, A., Palzor Negi, D., Rani, A. & Sentil Kumar, A. P. (2021). The impact of COVID-19 on migrant women workers in India, Eurasian Geography and Economics, 62(1), 93-112.

Chapter 15

# Stress, Anxiety, Depression and Burnout in Frontline Healthcare Workers during COVID-19 Pandemic in Russia

*Ekaterina Mosolova, Dmitry Sosin and Sergey Mosolov*

## Abstract

During the COVID-19 pandemic, healthcare workers (HCWs) have been subject to increased workload while also exposed to many psychosocial stressors. Most studies reported high levels of depression and anxiety among HCWs worldwide. Our study is based on two online surveys of 2195 HCWs from different regions of Russia during spring and autumn epidemic outbreaks revealed the rates of anxiety, stress, depression, emotional exhaustion and depersonalization and perceived stress as 32.3%, 31.1%, 45.5%, 74.2%, 37.7%,67.8%, respectively. Moreover, 2.4% of HCWs reported suicidal thoughts. Revealed risk factors included: female gender, younger age, working for over 6 months, living outside of Moscow or Saint Petersburg, the fear of getting infected or infecting family and friends. These results demonstrate the need for urgent supportive programs for HCWs fighting COVID-19 that fall into higher risk factors groups.

**Keywords:** stress, anxiety, depression, suicide, burnout, healthcare workers, COVID-19

## 1. Introduction

A large group pf HCWs was involved in the treatment of patients with the novel SARS-COV-2 virus worldwide. Recently World Psychiatric Association states that HCWs, working long hours in life-threatening conditions, often without appropriate protective equipment, may develop anxiety, depression, post-traumatic stress disorder (PTSD), insomnia, and excessive irritability and anger. The paper also states that these HCWs feel it is important to engage psychiatrists to provide self-help techniques, offer group or individual support or treatments for distressed colleagues and their families [1].

The levels of depression, stress, anxiety and burnout are at disturbing levels in many parts of the world. Some studies report the level of moderate and severe depression and anxiety according to Patient Health Questionnaire-9 (PHQ-9) and General Anxiety Disorder-7 (GAD-7) scales as 44.71% [2], 32.8% [3], respectively. Moreover, many studies assessed and reported high levels of stress and burnout among HCWs worldwide [4–7].

Despite cultural and organizational differences, many risk factors are similar worldwide. Risk groups that previously displayed higher level of stress and affective symptoms include: frontline workers [8], women [9] nurses [6, 10], younger age [11] and HCWs with chronic illness [7], or mental disorders [12], respiratory therapists [13] intensive care unit workers [13]. Potentially controllable risk factors include: significant working demands [4], lack of personal protective equipment [15], insufficient training for protection [14], low income [2], lack of support [14], isolation from families [3], the fear of relatives getting infected [15].

However, due to the differences in assessment tools, cut-off scores, and percentage of frontline HCWs in different studies, it is difficult to compare results across countries, especially as it relates to stress and burnout. We did not find studies that reported rates of suicidal thoughts and/or behavior among HCWs. Moreover, today, there are only a few studies that compare HCW's mental health between the first and second waves of COVID-19 [16, 17], however there is evidence that longer duration of frontline work correlates with higher levels of stress [18]. Moreover, only a few studies assessed the state of mental health in HCWs in Russia [19, 20], where the HCWs mortality is among the highest in the world [21].

Therefore, we undertook a study to assess the range of psychopathological symptoms (anxiety, stress, depression, burnout) and risk factors in frontline HCWs during spring and autumn outbreaks of the new coronavirus infection in Russian Federation.

## 2. Materials and methods

We conducted two independent, cross-sectional hospital-based online surveys. Data were collected between May 19th and May 26th 2020 – sample 1, (S1) and between October 10th and October 17th 2020 - sample (S2). Participants answered online questionnaire spread through social networks. The surveys were anonymous, and confidentiality of information was assured. The study and the form of the survey were approved by the Local Ethical Committee of Moscow Research Institute of Psychiatry, waiving a written participation consent. Most participants worked in the hospitals treating patients with COVID-19 in Moscow.

Both questionnaires investigated stress and anxiety symptoms. These were assessed using the validated Russian version of Stress and Anxiety to Viral Epidemic Scale (SAVE-9) [22] and the Russian version of GAD-7 [23]. We also collected information on age, gender, occupation and the *duration* of *work with patients diagnosed with COVID-19*. The total score of anxiety using GAD-7 was interpreted as: normal (0–4), mild (5–9), moderate (10–14), and severe (15–21) anxiety [23]. The cut-off score for the Russian version of SAVE-9 was taken as 18 [24]. HCWs with SAVE-9 score $< 18$ was considered low stress and anxiety group (LSA), and with $\geq 18$ – high stress and anxiety group (HSA).

The second survey collected additional information about the place of residence, duration of work with COVID-19, health history of COVID-19, participation in the vaccine study for COVID-19. We also measured symptoms of depression using Patient Health Questionnaire (PHQ-9) [25]. The total score of depression was interpreted as: minimal (0–4), mild (5–9), moderate (10–14), moderately severe (15–19), severe (10–27) [25]. We used single items measures of emotional burnout and depersonalization derived from Maslach Burnout Inventory (MBI) scale to assess burnout [26]. We also used Perceived Stress Scale-10 (PSS-10) to access perceived stress [27]. The total score was interpreted as: low stress (0–13), moderate stress (14–26) and high stress (27–40).

Data analysis was performed using SPSS statistical software version 21.0 (IBM Corp., Armonk, NY). Given that all data were not normally distributed according to Kolmogorov–Smirnov test ($p < 0.05$), they were presented as medians with interquartile ranges (IQRs). Sample characteristics and median levels of symptoms were compared using $\chi 2$ test for categorial and Mann–Whitney U test for dependent variables. A multivariable logistic regression model was used in order to explore the association between the level of stress according to SAVE-9 score and age, gender and occupation for both pandemic waves and between the level of stress and age, gender, occupation, the duration of work with COVI D-19, place of residence, vaccination and positive test for COVID in the second survey. *Spearman rank correlation* was *used* to measure the degree of association scales total score. Associations between multiple variables were investigated using network analytic methods [28, 29]. These analyses were conducted in the R statistical environment. The chosen significance level for all tests was set as $\alpha = 0.05$.

## 3. Results

### 3.1 Demographics

S1 and S2 included 1090 and 1105 participants, respectively. LSA group included 1486 HCWs (67.7%), and HAS – 709 (32.2%). Demographic characteristics and differences in stress and anxiety symptoms between S1 and S2 as well as between LSA and HSA groups are outlined in **Table 1**. S1 and S2 samples did not differ by gender. However, S2 included significantly more physicians ($p < 0.001$) and HCWs in older age group ($p = 0.009$). The level of anxiety among the participants of the second study was higher relative to levels of participants in the first study according to GAD-7 score (<0.001), but both samples had equal severity of stress and anxiety symptoms according to SAVE-9 score. LSA group included significantly more men relative to HSA ($p < 0.001$). LSA group had significantly lower anxiety level according to GAD-7 scale ($p < 0.001$). The SAVE-9 total score significantly correlated with GAD-7 total score (rho = 0.565, $p < 0.001$).

Additional characteristics assessed in the second survey are presented in **Table 2**. Most participants (455 [41.2%]) worked with patients diagnosed with coronavirus disease for over 6 months. 316 [28.6%] have tested positive for COVID-19. Only 23 [2.1%] HCWs participated in the vaccine study for COVID-19. SAVE-9, GAD-7, PHQ-9 and PSS-10 scores did not differ significantly for HCWs who were involved in the 1st and 2nd wave (worked for over 6 months) and for those who worked less than 6 months as well for those who have been tested positively for COVID-19 and for those who have not.

According to the MBI, 416 [37.7] HCWs have become more callous toward people since they took this job (depersonalization), 827 [74.9%] feel burned out from their work (emotional exhaustion). We compared demographic characteristics between groups with high (4–6) and low (<4) emotional exhaustion. Those with high emotional exhaustion differed by gender, residence location, and duration of work with COVID-19: were women ($p < 0.001$), lived outside of Moscow or Saint Petersburg ($p < 0.001$), worked for less than 6 months ($p < 0.001$). HCWs with high emotional exhaustion also had significantly higher scores across all scales.

Moderate or severe depression was registered in 504 [45.5%] HCWs, according to PHQ-9. The PHQ-9 score significantly correlated with SAVE-9 score (rho = 0.476, $p < 0.001$). Moderate or high perceived stress was reported by 750 [67.8%] HCWs according to PPS-10 scale. PSS-10 score significantly correlated with SAVE-9 score (rho = 0.506, $p < 0.001$).

Vaccinated participants had significantly lower anxiety level ($p = 0.031$). HCWs from LSA group also had significantly lower MBI total and both items scores, as well as PHQ-9 and PSS-10 scores ($p < 0.001$).

| Parameter | S1 (n = 1 090) | S2 (n = 1 105) | p | LSA (n = 1486) | HSA (n = 709) | p | Total (n = 2 195) |
|---|---|---|---|---|---|---|---|
| Physicians | 548 [50.3%] | 941[85.1%] | <0.001* | 1012[68.1%] | 477[67.3%] | 0.699 | 1316 [60.0%] |
| Nurses | 542[49.7%] | 164 [14.9%] | | 474[31.9%] | 232[32.7%] | | 474 [21.6%] |
| Female | 740 [67.9%] | 742 [67.1%] | 0.711 | 516[34.7%] | 197[27.8%] | <0.001* | 1482 [67.5%] |
| Male | 350 [32.1%] | 363 [32.9%] | | 970[65.3%] | 512[72.2%] | | 713 [32.5%] |
| Age | Median (IQR) | Median (IQR) | p | Median (IQR) | Median (IQR) | p | Median (IQR) |
| | 33 (19) | 34 (17) | 0.009* | 34(18) | 33(17) | 0.177 | 34 (18) |
| Symptom assesement | | | | | | | |
| GAD-7 | Median (IQR) | Median (IQR) | p | Median (IQR) | Median (IQR) | p | Median (IQR) |
| | 5 (9) | 7 (9) | <0.001* | 4(7) | 10(9) | <0.001* | 6 (9) |
| normal | 503 [46.1%] | 361 [32.7%] | | 772[52.0%] | 92[13.0%] | | 864 [39.4%] |
| mild | 309 [28.4%] | 339 [30.7%] | | 438[29.5%] | 210 [29.6%] | | 648 [29.5%] |
| moderate | 144 [13.2%] | 220 [19.9%] | | 171[11.5%] | 193[27.3%] | | 364 [16.6%] |
| severe | 134[12.3%] | 185 [16.7%] | | 105[7.1%] | 214 [30.2%] | | 319 [14.5%] |
| SAVE-9 | Median (IQR) | Median (IQR) | p | Median (IQR) | Median (IQR) | p | Median (IQR) |
| | 14 (9) | 15 (10) | 0.051 | 11(7) | 21(5) | <0.001* | 15 (9) |

*Footnote: GAD-7 – general anxiety disorder-7 scale, HSA – high stress and anxiety group, IQR – interquartile range, LSA – low stress and anxiety group, SAVE-9- Stress and Anxiety to Viral Epidemic scale, S1 – Sample 1, S2 – sample 2. *P<0.05.*

**Table 1.**
*Comparison of demographics characteristics between S1 and S2 and between LSA and HAS groups.*

## 3.2 The frequency of symptoms

The frequency of participants' answers from S1 and S2 and from HSA and LSA groups on each SAVE-9 scale question are presented in **Table 3**. During the second wave HCWs worried more that the virus outbreak would continue indefinitely, felt more skeptical about their job after going through this experience, more frequently thought that they would avoid treating patients with viral illnesses, and more frequently thought that their colleagues would have more work to do due to their absence from a possible quarantine and might blame them. However, S2 participants worried less that others might avoid them even after the infection risk has been minimized. The frequency of all symptoms assessed with SAVE-9 were significantly higher in HSA group. 62.3% of HCWs have been often or always worrying that family or friends may become infected because of them, 34,7% have been more sensitive toward minor physical symptoms, 32.8% have been thinking that their colleagues might blame them, 29.6% have been worried about getting infection.

| Parameter | LSA (n = 727) | HSA (n = 378) | p | S2 total |
|---|---|---|---|---|
| The duration of work with COVID-19 | | | | |
| < 1 week | 22[3.0%] | 9[2.4%] | 0.787 | 31 [2.8%] |
| 1 week – 1 month | 59[8.1%] | 31[8.2%] | | 90 [8.1%] |
| 1 – 3 months | 116[16.0%] | 67[17.7%] | | 183 [16.6%] |
| 4 - 6 months | 235[32.3%] | 111[29.4%] | | 346 [31.3%] |
| >6 months | 295[40.6%] | 160[42.3%] | | 455 [41.2%] |
| Have you been tested positive for COVID-19? | | | | |
| Yes | 215[29.6%] | 101[32.0%] | 0.319 | 316 [28.6%] |
| No | 512[70.4%] | 277[73.3%] | | 789 [71.4%] |
| Have you been vaccinated against COVID-19? | | | | |
| Yes | 20[2.8%] | 3[0.8%] | 0.031* | 23 [2.1%] |
| No | 707[97.2%] | 375[99.2%] | | 1082 [97.9%] |
| MBI | Median (IQR) | Median (IQR) | p | Median (IQR) |
| | 7(4) | 9(3) | <0.001* | 7 (4) |
| Depersonalization | 3(3) | 4(3) | <0.001* | 3 (3) |
| Low (0-1) | 245[33.7%] | 70[18.6%] | | 315 [28.5%] |
| Moderate (2-3) | 256[35.2%] | 118[31.2%] | | 374 [33.8%] |
| High (4-6) | 226[31.1%] | 190[50.2%] | | 416 [37.7%] |
| Emotional exhaustion | 4(2) | 6(2) | <0.001* | 5 (3) |
| Low (0-1) | 58[8.0%] | 2[0.5%] | | 60 [5.4%] |
| Moderate (2-3) | 179[24.6%] | 39[10.4%] | | 218 [19.7%] |
| High (4-6) | 490[67.4] | 337[89.2%] | | 827 [74.9%] |
| PHQ-9 | Median (IQR) | Median (IQR) | p | Median (IQR) |
| | 7(9) | 12(9) | <0.001* | 9 (10) |
| Minimal (0-4) | 253[34.8%] | 35[6.6%] | | 278 [25.2%] |
| Mild (5-9) | 233[32.0%] | 90[23.8%] | | 323 [29.2%] |
| Moderate (10-14) | 132[18.2%] | 118[31.2%] | | 250 [22.6%] |
| Moderate Severe (15-19) | 76[10.5%] | 83[22.0%] | | 159 [14.4%] |
| Severe (20-27) | 33[4.5%] | 62[16.4%] | | 95 [8.6%] |
| PSS-10 | Median (IQR) | Median (IQR) | p | Median (IQR) |
| | 15(10) | 21(8) | <0.001* | 17 (11) |
| Low stress (0-13) | 312[42.9%] | 43[11.4%] | | 355 [32.2%] |
| Moderate stress (14-26) | 366[50.3%] | 262[69.3%] | | 628 [56.8%] |
| High stress (27-40) | 49[6.8%] | 73[19.3%] | | 122 [11.0%] |

*HSA – high stress and anxiety group, IQR – interquartile range, LSA – low stress and anxiety group, MBI -The Maslach Burnout Inventory, PHQ-9 - Patient Health Questionnaire, PSS-10 – perceived stress scale-10, S2 – sample 2.*
**P < 0.05.*

**Table 2.**
*Demographic characteristics of the participants from S2 with LSA and HSA.*

The frequency of participants' answers on each GAD-7 scale question are presented in **Table 4**. The frequency of all symptoms assessed with GAD-7 were significantly higher during the second wave and in HAS group. The most common

| **SAVE-9** | | | | | | |
|---|---|---|---|---|---|---|
| **Are you afraid the virus outbreak will continue indefinitely?** | | | | | | |
| | **Never** | **Rarely** | **Sometimes** | **Often** | **Always** | **p** |
| S1. No. (%) | 444 (40.7) | 232 (21.3) | 301(27.6) | 79(7.2) | 34(3.1) | <0.001* |
| S2. No. (%) | 315 (28.5) | 186 (16.8) | 378 (34.2) | 141(12.8) | 85(7.7) | |
| LSA | 703(47.3) | 322(21.7) | 371(25.0) | 68(4.6) | 22(1.5) | <0.001* |
| HSA | 56(7.9) | 96(13.5) | 308(43.4) | 152(21.4) | 97(13.5) | |
| Total. No. (%) | 759(34.6) | 418(19.0) | 679(30.9) | 220(10.0) | 119(5.4) | |
| Are you afraid your health will worsen because of the virus? | | | | | | |
| | Never | Rarely | Sometimes | Often | Always | p |
| S1. No. (%) | 180 (16.5) | 263 (24.1) | 412 (37.8) | 154(14.1) | 81(7.4) | 0.435 |
| S2. No. (%) | 192 (17.4) | 239 (21.6) | 405 (36.7) | 177(16.0) | 92 (8.3) | |
| LSA | 365(24.6) | 454(30.6) | 559(37.6) | 91(6.1) | 17(9.8) | <0.001* |
| HSA | 7(1.0) | 48(6.8) | 258(36.4) | 240(33.9) | 156(22.0) | |
| Total. No. (%) | 372(16.9) | 502(22.9) | 817(37.2) | 331(15.1) | 173(7.9) | |
| Are you worried that you might get infected? | | | | | | |
| | Never | Rarely | Sometimes | Often | Always | p |
| S1. No. (%) | 133(12.2) | 264(24.2) | 357(32.8) | 217(19.9) | 119(10.9) | 0.062 |
| S2. No. (%) | 174 (15.7) | 276 (25.0) | 341 (30.9) | 185 (16.7) | 129 (11.7) | |
| LSA | 300(20.2) | 484(32.6) | 531(35.7) | 146(9.8) | 25(1.7) | <0.001* |
| HSA | 7(2.3) | 56(7.9) | 167(23.6) | 256(36.1) | 223(31.5) | |
| Total. No. (%) | 307(14.0) | 540 (24.6) | 698(31.8) | 402(18.3) | 248(11.3) | |
| Are you more sensitive towards minor physical symptoms than usual? | | | | | | |
| | Never | Rarely | Sometimes | Often | Always | p |
| S1. No. (%) | 139(12.8) | 249(22.8) | 315(28.9) | 250(22.9) | 137(12.6) | 0.332 |
| S2. No. (%) | 159 (14.4) | 281 (25.4) | 292 (26.4) | 234(21.2) | 139(12.6) | |
| LSA | 287(19.3) | 476(32.0) | 456(30.7) | 201(13.5) | 66(4.4) | <0.001* |
| HSA | 11 (1.6) | 54(7.6) | 151(21.3) | 283(39.9) | 210(29.6) | |
| Total. No. (%) | 298(13.6) | 530(24.1) | 607(27.7) | 484(22.1) | 276(12.6) | |
| Are you worried that others might avoid you even after the infection risk has been minimized? | | | | | | |
| | Never | Rarely | Sometimes | Often | Always | p |
| S1. No. (%) | 414(38.0) | 198(18.2) | 243(22.3) | 158(14.5) | 77(7.1) | <0.001* |
| S2. No. (%) | 479 (43.3) | 235 (21.3) | 231 (20.9) | 102(9.2) | 58(5.2) | |
| LSA | 800(53.8) | 313(21.1) | 269(18.1) | 89(6.0) | 15(1.0) | <0.001* |
| HSA | 93 (13.1) | 120(16.9) | 205(28.9) | 171(24.1) | 120(16.9) | |
| Total. No. (%) | 893(40.7) | 433(19.7) | 474(21.6) | 260(11.8) | 135(6.2) | |
| Do you feel skeptical about your job after going through this experience? | | | | | | |
| | Never | Rarely | Sometimes | Often | Always | p |
| S1. No. (%) | 471(43.2) | 172(15.8) | 235(21.6) | 140(12.8) | 72(6.6) | <0.001* |
| S2. No. (%) | 365 (33.0) | 168(15.2) | 284(25.7) | 184(16.7) | 104(9.4) | |
| LSA | 728(49.0) | 254(17.1) | 297(20.0) | 142(4.4) | 65(4.4) | <0.001* |

| SAVE-9 | | | | | | |
|---|---|---|---|---|---|---|
| **Are you afraid the virus outbreak will continue indefinitely?** | | | | | | |
| | **Never** | **Rarely** | **Sometimes** | **Often** | **Always** | **p** |
| HSA | 108(15.2) | 86(12.1) | 222(31.3) | 182(25.7) | 111(15.7) | |
| Total. No. (%) | 836(38.1) | 340(15.5) | 519(23.6) | 324(14.8) | 176(8.0) | |
| After this experience. do you think you will avoid treating patients with viral illnesses? | | | | | | |
| | Never | Rarely | Sometimes | Often | Always | p |
| S1. No. (%) | 741(68.0) | 159(14.6) | 107(9.8) | 54(5.0) | 29(2.7) | 0.009* |
| S2. No. (%) | 669(60.5) | 195(17.6) | 140(12.7) | 67(6.1) | 34(3.1) | |
| LSA | 1134(76.3) | 202(13.6) | 103(6.9) | 30(2.0) | 17(1.1) | <0.001* |
| HSA | 276(38.9) | 152(21.4) | 144(20.3) | 91(12.8) | 46(6.5) | |
| Total. No. (%) | 1410(64.2) | 354(16.1) | 247(11.3) | 121(5.5) | 63(2.9) | |
| Do you worry your family or friends may become infected because of you? | | | | | | |
| | Never | Rarely | Sometimes | Often | Always | p |
| S1. No. (%) | 57(5.2) | 95(8.7) | 231(21.2) | 320(29.4) | 387(35.5) | 0.162 |
| S2. No. (%) | 69(6.2) | 114 (10.3) | 261(23.6) | 288(26.1) | 373(33.8) | |
| LSA | 125 (8.4) | 194(13.1) | 437(29.4) | 429(28.9) | 301(20.3) | <0.001* |
| HSA | 1(0.1) | 15(2.1) | 55(7.8) | 179(25.2) | 459(64.7) | |
| Total. No. (%) | 126(5.7) | 209(9.5) | 492(22.4) | 608(27.7) | 760(34.6) | |
| Do you think that your colleagues would have more work to do due to your absence from a possible quarantine and might blame you? | | | | | | |
| | Never | Rarely | Sometimes | Often | Always | p |
| S1. No. (%) | 337(30.9) | 185(17.0) | 249(22.8) | 174(16.0) | 145(13.3) | <0.001* |
| S2. No. (%) | 334(31.1) | 124(11.2) | 236(21.4) | 228(20.6) | 172(15.7) | |
| LSA | 599(40.3) | 248(16.7) | 329(22.1) | 205(13.8) | 105(7.1) | <0.001* |
| HSA | 82(11.6) | 61(8.6) | 156(22.0) | 197(27.8) | 213(30.0) | |
| Total. No. (%) | 681(31.0) | 309(14.1) | 485 (22.1) | 402(18.3) | 318(14.5) | |

*HSA – high stress and anxiety group, LSA – low stress and anxiety group, SAVE-9- Stress and Anxiety to Viral Epidemic scale, S1 – Sample 1, S2 – sample 2.*
**P < 0.05.*

**Table 3.**
*The frequency of S1 and S2 participants' answers on each SAVE-9 scale question.*

symptoms included: have been feeling nervous, anxious, or on edge (40.8% more than half the days or nearly every day), have had trouble relaxing (36.5%) have been easily annoyed or irritable (31.4%).

The level of emotional burnout and depersonalization according to two single-item MBI question scale differed significantly between LSA and HSA groups (**Table 5**). 32.5% every day felt burned out from their work, and 9.7% became more callous toward people.

All the symptoms assessed with PHQ-9 and PSS-10 differed significantly between groups with low and high stress according to SAVE-9 during the second COVID-19 wave (**Tables 6** and **7**). Most participants felt tired or had little energy (31.0%), had little interest or pleasure in doing things (22.0%), had trouble falling or staying asleep, or sleeping too much (21.4%). 2.4% of participants had suicidal thoughts that they would be better off dead, or of hurting themselves.

| **GAD-7** | | | | | |
|---|---|---|---|---|---|
| **How often have you been bothered by feeling nervous, anxious, or on edge over the past 2 weeks?** | | | | | |
| | **Not at all** | **Several days** | **More than half the days** | **Nearly every day** | **p** |
| S1. No. (%) | 335(30.7) | 408(37.4) | 131(12.1) | 216(19.8) | <0.001* |
| S2. No. (%) | 176 (15.9) | 381 (34.5) | 216 (19.5) | 332 (30.0) | |
| LSA | 469(31.6) | 586(39.4) | 195(13.1) | 236(15.9) | <0.001* |
| HSA | 42(5.9) | 203(789) | 152(21.4) | 312(56.9) | |
| Total. No. (%) | 511 (23.3) | 789(35.9) | 347(15.8) | 548(25.0) | |
| How often have you been bothered by not being able to stop or control worrying over the past 2 weeks? | | | | | |
| | Not at all | Several days | More than half the days | Nearly every day | |
| S1. No. (%) | 608(55.8) | 312(28.6) | 83(7.6) | 87(8) | <0.001* |
| S2. No. (%) | 448(40.5) | 412(37.3) | 124(11.2) | 121(11.0) | |
| LSA | 896(60.3) | 436(29.3) | 84(5.7) | 70(4.7) | <0.001* |
| HSA | 160(22.6) | 288(39.8) | 123(17.3) | 138(19.5) | |
| Total. No. (%) | 1056(48.1) | 724 (33.0) | 207(9.4) | 208 (9.5) | |
| How often have you been bothered by worrying too much about different things over the past 2 weeks? | | | | | |
| | Not at all | Several days | More than half the days | Nearly every day | |
| S1. No. (%) | 407(37.3) | 422(38.7) | 130(11.9) | 131(12.1) | <0.001* |
| S2. No. (%) | 289(26.2) | 465(42.1) | 165(14.9) | 186(16.8) | |
| LSA | 620(41.7) | 608(40.9) | 138(9.3) | 120(8.1) | <0.001* |
| HSA | 76(10.7) | 279(39.4) | 157(22.1) | 709(32.3) | |
| Total. No. (%) | 696(31.7) | 887 (40.4) | 295(13.4) | 317(14.4) | |
| How often have you been bothered by trouble relaxing over the past 2 weeks? | | | | | |
| | Not at all | Several days | More than half the days | Nearly every day | |
| S1. No. (%) | 405(37.2) | 341(31.3) | 154(14.1) | 190(17.4) | <0.001* |
| S2. No. (%) | 271(24.5) | 375(33.9) | 185(16.7) | 274(24.8) | |
| LSA | 589(39.6) | 503(33.8) | 194(13.1) | 200(13.5) | <0.001* |
| HSA | 87(12.3) | 213(30.0) | 145(20.5) | 264(37.2) | |
| Total. No. (%) | 676(30.8) | 716 (32.6) | 339(15.4) | 464 (21.1) | |
| How often have you been bothered by being so restless that it's hard to sit still over the past 2 weeks? | | | | | |
| | Not at all | Several days | More than half the days | Nearly every day | |
| S1. No. (%) | 657(60.3) | 288(26.4) | 82(7.5) | 63(5.8) | <0.001* |
| S2. No. (%) | 556 (50.3) | 329(29.8) | 126(11.4) | 94(8.5) | |
| LSA | 1006(67.7) | 350(23.6) | 87(5.9) | 43(2.9) | <0.001* |
| HSA | 207(29.2) | 267(37.7) | 121(17.1) | 114(16.1) | |
| Total. No. (%) | 1213 (55.3) | 617 (28.1) | 208 (9.5) | 157 (7.2) | |
| How often have you been bothered by becoming easily annoyed or irritable over the past 2 weeks? | | | | | |
| | Not at all | Several days | More than half the days | Nearly every day | |
| S1. No. (%) | 398(36.5) | 418(38.4) | 128(11.7) | 146(13.4) | <0.001* |
| S2. No. (%) | 249(22.5) | 441(39.9) | 209(18.9) | 206(18.6) | |

| GAD-7 | | | | | |
|---|---|---|---|---|---|
| **How often have you been bothered by feeling nervous, anxious, or on edge over the past 2 weeks?** | | | | | |
| | **Not at all** | **Several days** | **More than half the days** | **Nearly every day** | **p** |
| LSA | 575(38.7) | 595(40.0) | 173(11.6) | 143(9.6) | <0.001* |
| HSA | 72(10.2) | 264(37.2) | 164(23.1) | 209(29.5) | |
| Total. No. (%) | 647(29.5) | 859(39.1) | 337(15.4) | 352(16.0) | |
| How often have you been bothered by feeling afraid as if something awful might happen over the past 2 weeks? | | | | | |
| | Not at all | Several days | More than half the days | Nearly every day | |
| S1. No. (%) | 579(53.1) | 351(32.2) | 66(6.1) | 94(8.6) | <0.001* |
| S2. No. (%) | 526(47.6) | 357(32.3) | 121(11.0) | 101(9.1) | |
| LSA | 959(64.5) | 407(27.4) | 66(4.4) | 54(3.6) | <0.001* |
| HSA | 146(20.6) | 301(42.5) | 121(17.1) | 141(19.9) | |
| Total. No. (%) | 1105(50.3) | 708(32.3) | 187(8.5) | 195(8.9) | |

*GAD-7- general anxiety disorder-7 scale, HSA – high stress and anxiety group, LSA – low stress and anxiety group, S1 – Sample 1, S2 – sample 2.*
**P < 0.05.*

**Table 4.**
*The frequency of S1 and S2 participants' answers on each GAD-7 scale question.*

| MBI | | | | | | | | |
|---|---|---|---|---|---|---|---|---|
| **I feel burned out from my work** | | | | | | | | |
| | **Never** | **A few times a year** | **Once a month or less** | **A few times a month** | **Once a week** | **A few times a week** | **Every day** | **p** |
| LSA | 12(1.7) | 46(6.3) | 54(7.4) | 125(17.2) | 184(25.3) | 140(19.3) | 166 (22.8) | <0.001* |
| HSA | 0(0.0) | 2(0.5) | 4(1.1) | 35(9.3) | 58(15.3) | 86(22.8) | 193(51.1) | |
| Total. No. (%) | 12(1.1) | 48(4.3) | 58(5.2) | 160 (14.5) | 242 (21.9) | 226 (20.5) | 359(32.5) | |
| I have become more callous toward people since I took this job | | | | | | | | |
| | Never | A few times a year | Once a month or less | A few times a month | Once a week | A few times a week | Every day | p |
| LSA | 151(20.8) | 94(12.9) | 101(13.9) | 155(21.3) | 114(15.7) | 64(8.8) | 48(6.6) | <0.001* |
| HSA | 34(9.0) | 36(9.5) | 40(10.6) | 78(20.6) | 75(19.8) | 56(14.8) | 59(15.6) | |
| Total. No. (%) | 185(16.7) | 130(11.8) | 141(12.8) | 233(21.1) | 189(17.1) | 120(10.9) | 107(9.7) | |

*HSA – high stress and anxiety group, LSA – low stress and anxiety group, MBI -The Maslach Burnout Inventory.*
**P < 0.05.*

**Table 5.**
*The frequency of S2 participants' answers on each MBI single-item.*

| **PHQ-9** | | | | | |
|---|---|---|---|---|---|
| **Little interest or pleasure in doing things** | | | | | |
| | **Never** | **Rarely** | **Sometimes** | **Often** | **p** |
| LSA | 220(30.3) | 264(36.3) | 118(16.2) | 125(17.2) | <0.001* |
| HSA | 31(8.2) | 123(32.5) | 106(28.0) | 118(31.2) | |
| Total. No. (%) | 251 (22.7) | 387 (35.0) | 224 (20.3) | 243 (22.0) | |
| Feeling down. depressed. or hopeless | | | | | |
| | Never | Rarely | Sometimes | Often | p |
| LSA | 243(33.4) | 307(42.2) | 105(14.4) | 72(9.9) | <0.001* |
| HSA | 35(9.3) | 141(37.3) | 118(31.2) | 84(22.2) | |
| Total. No. (%) | 278 (25.2) | 448 (40.5) | 223 (20.2) | 156 (14.1) | |
| Trouble falling or staying asleep. or sleeping too much | | | | | |
| | Never | Rarely | Sometimes | Often | p |
| LSA | 242(33.3) | 240(33.0) | 122(16.8) | 123(16.9) | <0.001* |
| HSA | 45(11.9) | 110(29.1) | 109(28.8) | 114(30.2) | |
| Total. No. (%) | 287 (26.0) | 350 (31.7) | 231 (20.9) | 237 (21.4) | |
| Feeling tired or having little energy | | | | | |
| | Never | Rarely | Sometimes | Often | p |
| LSA | 74(10.2) | 314(43.2) | 155(21.3) | 184(25.3) | <0.001* |
| HSA | 9(2.4) | 91(24.1) | 120(31.7) | 158(41.8) | |
| Total. No. (%) | 83 (7.5) | 405 (36.7) | 275 (24.9) | 342(31.0) | |
| Poor appetite or overeating | | | | | |
| | Never | Rarely | Sometimes | Often | p |
| LSA | 329(45.3) | 212(29.2) | 89(12.2) | 97(13.3) | <0.001* |
| HSA | 73(19.3) | 110(29.1) | 92(24.3) | 103(27.2) | |
| Total. No. (%) | 402(36.4) | 322 (29.1) | 181 (16.4) | 200(18.1) | |
| Feeling bad about yourself or that you are a failure or have let yourself or your family down | | | | | |
| | Never | Rarely | Sometimes | Often | p |
| LSA | 482(66.3) | 148(20.4) | 47(6.5) | 50(6.9) | <0.001* |
| HSA | 135(35.7) | 111(29.4) | 72(19.0) | 60(15.9) | |
| Total. No. (%) | 617 (55.8) | 259 (23.4) | 119 (10.8) | 110(10.0) | |
| Trouble concentrating on things. such as reading the newspaper or watching television | | | | | |
| | Never | Rarely | Sometimes | Often | p |
| LSA | 387(53.2) | 188(25.9) | 70(9.6) | 82(11.3) | <0.001* |
| HSA | 84(22.2) | 134(35.4) | 73(19.3) | 87(23.0) | |
| Total. No. (%) | 471 (42.6) | 322(29.1) | 143(12.9) | 169(15.3) | |
| Moving or speaking so slowly that other people could have noticed. Or the opposite being so figety or restless that you have been moving around a lot more than usual | | | | | |
| | Never | Rarely | Sometimes | Often | p |
| LSA | 490(67.5) | 162(22.3) | 43(5.9) | 31(4.3) | <0.001* |
| HSA | 160(42.3) | 117(31.0) | 62(16.4) | 39 (3.4) | |
| Total. No. (%) | 650(58.8) | 279(25.2) | 105(9.5) | 70(6.3) | |

| **PHQ-9** | | | | | |
|---|---|---|---|---|---|
| **Little interest or pleasure in doing things** | | | | | |
| | **Never** | **Rarely** | **Sometimes** | **Often** | **p** |
| Thoughts that you would be better off dead. or of hurting yourself | | | | | |
| | Never | Rarely | Sometimes | Often | p |
| LSA | 647(89.0) | 54(7.4) | 12(1.7) | 14(1.9) | <0.001* |
| HSA | 299(79.1) | 48(12.7) | 18(4.8) | 13(3.4) | |
| Total. No. (%) | 946(85.6) | 102(9.2) | 30(2.7) | 27(2.4) | |

*HSA – high stress and anxiety group, LSA – low stress and anxiety group, PHQ-9-Patient Health Questionnaure-9, S1 – Sample 1, S2 – sample 2.*
**P < 0.05.*

**Table 6.**
*The frequency of S2 participants' answers on each item of PHQ-9 scale.*

| **PSS-10** | | | | | | |
|---|---|---|---|---|---|---|
| **In the last month. how often have you been upset because of something that happened unexpectedly?** | | | | | | |
| | **Never** | **Almost never** | **Sometimes** | **Fairly often** | **Very often** | **p** |
| LSA | 169(23.2) | 191(26.3) | 244(33.6) | 92(12.7) | 31(4.3) | <0.001* |
| HSA | 8(2.1) | 50(13.2) | 156(41.3) | 116(30.7) | 48(12.7) | |
| Total. No. (%) | 177 (16.0) | 241 (21.8) | 400 (36.2) | 208 (18.8) | 79(7.1) | |
| In the last month. how often have you felt that you were unable to control the important things in your life? | | | | | | |
| | Never | Almost never | Sometimes | Fairly often | Very often | |
| LSA | 237(32.6) | 195(26.8) | 180(24.8) | 83(11.4) | 32(4.4) | <0.001* |
| HSA | 23(6.1) | 73(19.3) | 145(38.4) | 90(23.8) | 47(12.4) | |
| Total. No. (%) | 260 (23.5) | 268 (24.3) | 325 (29.4) | 173 (15.7) | 79(7.1) | |
| In the last month. how often have you felt nervous and "stressed"? | | | | | | |
| | Never | Almost never | Sometimes | Fairly often | Very often | |
| LSA | 71(9.8) | 116(16.0) | 250(34.4) | 174(23.9) | 116(49.8) | <0.001* |
| HSA | 3(0.8) | 13(3.4) | 92(24.3) | 153(40.5) | 117(31.1) | |
| Total. No. (%) | 74 (6.7) | 129 (11.7) | 342 (31.0) | 327 (29.6) | 233(21.1) | |
| In the last month. how often have you felt confident about your ability to handle your personal problems? | | | | | | |
| | Never | Almost never | Sometimes | Fairly often | Very often | |
| LSA | 36(5.0) | 45(6.2) | 168(23.1) | 294(40.4) | 184(25.3) | <0.001* |
| HSA | 9(2.4) | 37(9.8) | 175(46.3) | 116 (30.7) | 41(10.8) | |
| Total. No. (%) | 45(4.1) | 82 (7.4) | 343(31.0) | 410 (37.1) | 225 (20.4) | |
| In the last month. how often have you felt that things were going your way? | | | | | | |
| | Never | Almost never | Sometimes | Fairly often | Very often | |
| LSA | 42(5.8) | 100(13.8) | 254(34.9) | 236(32.5) | 95(13.1) | <0.001* |
| HSA | 29(7.7) | 98(25.9) | 153(40.5) | 77 (20.4) | 21(5.6) | |
| Total. No. (%) | 71 (6.4) | 198 (17.9) | 407 (36.8) | 313(28.3) | 116(10.5) | |

| **PSS-10** | | | | | | |
|---|---|---|---|---|---|---|
| **In the last month. how often have you been upset because of something that happened unexpectedly?** | | | | | | |
| | **Never** | **Almost never** | **Sometimes** | **Fairly often** | **Very often** | **p** |
| In the last month. how often have you found that you could not cope with all the things that you had to do? | | | | | | |
| | Never | Almost never | Sometimes | Fairly often | Very often | |
| LSA | 141(19.4) | 203(27.9) | 248(34.1) | 93(12.8) | 42(5.8) | <0.001* |
| HSA | 11(2.9) | 62(16.4) | 168(44.4) | 100(26.5) | 37(9.8) | |
| Total. No. (%) | 152 (13.8) | 265 (24.0) | 416 (37.6) | 193(17.5) | 79(7.1) | |
| In the last month. how often have you been able to control irritations in your life? | | | | | | |
| | Never | Almost never | Sometimes | Fairly often | Very often | |
| LSA | 39 (5.4) | 67(9.2) | 194(26.7) | 273(37) | 154(21.2) | <0.001* |
| HSA | 10(2.6) | 40(10.6) | 161(42.6) | 121(32.0) | 46(12.2) | |
| Total. No. (%) | 49 (4.4) | 107(9.7) | 355(32.1) | 394(35.7) | 200(18.1) | |
| In the last month. how often have you felt that you were on top of things? | | | | | | |
| | Never | Almost never | Sometimes | Fairly often | Very often | |
| LSA | 12(1.7) | 34(4.7) | 193(26.5) | 333(45.8) | 155(21.3) | <0.001* |
| HSA | 10(2.6) | 50(13.2) | 166(43.9) | 120(31.7) | 32(8.5) | |
| Total. No. (%) | 22(2.0) | 84(7.6) | 359(32.5) | 453(41.0) | 187(16.9) | |
| In the last month. how often have you been angered because of things that were outside of your control? | | | | | | |
| | Never | Almost never | Sometimes | Fairly often | Very often | |
| LSA | 100(13.8) | 185(25.4) | 276(38.0) | 128 (17.6) | 38(5.2) | <0.001* |
| HSA | 14(3.7) | 41(10.8) | 159(42.1) | 118(31.2) | 46(12.2) | |
| Total. No. (%) | 114(10.3) | 226(20.5) | 435(39.4) | 246(22.3) | 84(7.6) | |
| In the last month. how often have you felt difficulties were piling up so high that you could not overcome them? | | | | | | |
| | Never | Almost never | Sometimes | Fairly often | Very often | |
| LSA | 247(34.0) | 191(26.3) | 184(25.3) | 74(10.2) | 31(4.3) | <0.001* |
| HSA | 31(8.2) | 73(19.3) | 136(36.0) | 85(22.5) | 53(14.0) | |
| Total. No. (%) | 278 (25.2) | 264 (23.9) | 320 (29.0) | 159 (14.4) | 84 (7.6) | |

*HSA – high stress and anxiety group, LSA – low stress and anxiety group, PSS-10 -Perceived Stress Scale-10, S1 – Sample 1, S2 – sample 2.*
**P < 0.05.*

**Table 7.**
*The frequency of S2 participants' answers on each PSS-10 scale.*

The most common symptoms according to PSS-10 scale included: fairy or very often felt nervous and "stressed" (50.9%), fairy or very often have been angered because of things that were outside of their control (29.9%), fairy or very often have been upset because of something that happened unexpectedly (25.9%).

| Categories | p | OR | Lower limit | Upper limit |
|---|---|---|---|---|
| Male | 0.001* | 0.710 | 0.581 | 0.866 |
| Female | 0 | 0 | 0 | 0 |
| Age | 0.077 | 0.992 | 0.984 | 1.001 |
| Physicians | 0.727 | 1.035 | 0.852 | 1.259 |
| Nurses | 0 | 0 | 0 | 0 |

**Table 8.**
*Influence of gender, age, position in participants from HAS group (total sample – S1+S2).*

### 3.3 Logistic regression and network analysis

The regression model for total sample (N = 2195) was reliable (−2Log likelihood ratio = 571.5; $p = 0.05$). The group with LSA (SAVE-9 score < 18) was used as the reference category. Male sex (Odds Ratio (OR) 0,710 [95%CI 0.581–0.866, p = 0.001]) was associated with lower anxiety level among the participants from HAS group (see **Table 8**).

The regression model for second wave sample (N = 1105) was reliable (−2Log likelihood ratio = 1067.1; $p = 0.05$). The LSA group (SAVE-9 score < 18) was used as the reference category. Male sex (OR 0.686 [95%CI 0.512–0.908, p = 0.008]) and working in Moscow (OR 0,544 [95%CI 0.402–0.736, p = 0.001]) or Saint Petersburg (OR 0,357 [95%CI 0.181–0.704, p = 0.003]) were associated with lower anxiety level among the participants from HAS group (see **Table 9**).

| Categories | p | OR | Lower limit | Upper limit |
|---|---|---|---|---|
| Male | 0.008* | 0.686 | 0.512 | 0.908 |
| Female | 0 | 0 | 0 | 0 |
| Age | 0.904 | 0.999 | 0.987 | 1.012 |
| Physicians | 0.727 | 1.035 | 0.852 | 1.259 |
| Nurses | 0 | 0 | 0 | 0 |
| Place of residence: Moscow | 0.001* | 0.544 | 0.402 | 0.736 |
| Place of residence: St. Petersburg | 0.003* | 0.357 | 0.181 | 0.704 |
| Place of residence: Other | 0 | 0 | 0 | 0 |
| Duration of work with COVID-19: < 1 week | 0.465 | 0.739 | 0.328 | 1.664 |
| Duration of work with COVID-19: 1 week – 1 month | 0.607 | 0.880 | 0.541 | 1.431 |
| Duration of work with COVID-19: 1 – 3 months | 0.952 | 0.880 | 0.541 | 1.431 |
| Duration of work with COVID-19: 4 - 6 months | 0.174 | 0.810 | 0.598 | 1.097 |
| Duration of work with COVID-19: >6 months | 0 | 0 | 0 | 0 |
| Have been tested positive for COVID-19 | 0.590 | 0.924 | 0.694 | 1.230 |
| Haven't been tested positive for COVID-19 | 0 | 0 | 0 | 0 |
| Have been vaccinated against COVID-19 | 0.057 | 0.301 | 0.87 | 1.034 |
| Haven't been vaccinated against COVID-19 | 0 | 0 | 0 | 0 |

**Table 9.**
*Influence of gender, age, position, place of residence, the duration of work with COVID-19, the history of COVID-19 and vaccination in participants from HAS group (S2 sample).*

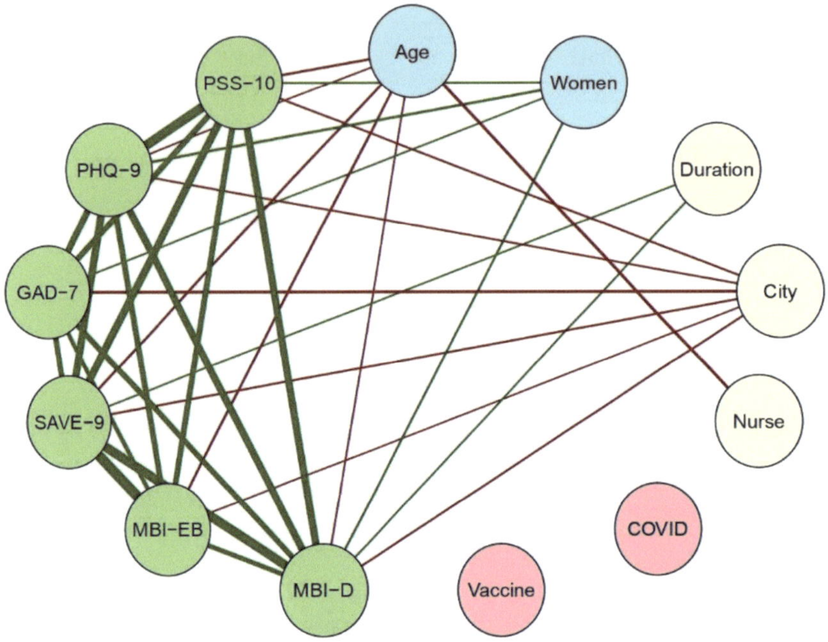


**Figure 1.**
*Relationships between multiple variables for 2195 HCWs during first and second waves of COVID-19 in Russia (network analysis). Nodes represent variables. The coloring of the nodes indicates different groups of variables (green = mental health, blue = demographics, light yellow = work-related factors, pink = COVID-19-related factors); edges represent associations between the nodes (continuous /green = positive, dashed/red = negative, thickness = magnitude of the relationship); age = years of age, women = gender (levels: men = 1, women = 2); duration = the duration of work with patients with COVID-19 (levels: less than 6 months = 1, 6 months and over = 2); city = hospital location (levels: Moscow/ Saint Petersburg = 1,other location = 0); nurse = working position (levels: physician = 1, nurse = 2); COVID = the history of COVID-19 (positive test) (levels: No = 0, Yes = 1), Vaccine = the history of vaccination against COVID-19 (levels: No = 0, Yes = 1); MBI-D = depersonalization according to MBI, MBI-EB = emotional burnout according to MBI; SAVE-9 = total SAVE-9 score, GAD-7 = total GAD-7 score, PHQ-9 = total PHQ-9 score, PSS-10 = total PSS-10 score.*

The results of the network analyses are presented in **Figure 1**.

Scores across all scales significantly correlated with each other. Age negatively correlated with perceived stress according to PSS-10, emotional exhaustion, total score of SAVE-9 and being a nurse. Being a woman positively correlated with perceived stress according to PSS-10, anxiety, depression, emotional exhaustion. Living in Moscow or Saint Petersburg negatively correlated with all symptoms. Working for over 6 months positively correlated with level of stress and anxiety according to SAVE-9 and emotional burnout.

## 4. Discussion

This study revealed that a substantial proportion of HCWs working during the COVID-19 pandemic in Russia have mental health problems that have exacerbated since the first wave in the spring. High level of stress by SAVE-9 and moderate or severe anxiety by GAD-7 were registered in 32,3% and 31,1% HCWs, respectively. The level of anxiety in Russia was higher when compared with other countries [10, 12–14]. This at least partially can be explained by higher contamination and mortality rates among HCWs in Russia [21]. Another possible reason is that all participants were directly involved in treating patients with COVID-19 and worked as frontline personnel. However, mean total score of SAVE-9 in our sample was lower than in some other studies [30, 31].

All studies consistently reported the main symptom of the fear that family or a friend may become infected because of the HCWs [31]. Therefore, providing HCWs with appropriate PPE and training them how to use it to stay safe is essential. Another potential solution could be providing an opportunity for HCWs to live separately from family and friends to protect them from infecting others. It is important to note, however, that previous studies reported that living alone was associated with higher levels of stress and anxiety [11].

The level of anxiety among the participants of the second study was higher when compared to the level of anxiety of participants from the first study according to GAD-7 mean score. Some studies confirm that duration of work with COVID-19 was associated with higher stress levels [18]. Other studies reported lower levels of anxiety in May compared to those in April in Switzerland [16] as well as in China in March compared to January [17]. The results of our study may be different given that our survey dates correspond to the peak of two outbreaks of COVID-19 in Russia, while dates of other mentioned studies correspond to the first outbreak and the subsequent decline in incidence of COVID-19 cases and deaths after the initial peak.

Network analysis also revealed that working for over 6 months positively correlated with level of stress and anxiety according to SAVE-9 and emotional burnout. On the other hand, HCWs who worked for less than 6 months reported higher emotional exhaustion. Similarly, some previous studies reported higher levels of anxiety and stress in those who have less working experience [32]. Therefore, the effect of the duration of work with COVID-19 on mental health of HCWs needs further investigation.

During the second wave HCWs worried more that the virus outbreak would continue indefinitely, felt more skeptical about their job after going through this experience, more frequently thought that they would avoid treating patients with viral illnesses, and more frequently thought that their colleagues would have more work to do due to their absence from a possible quarantine and might blame them. Indirectly these data could be the evidence of depressive ideas of guilt. However, during the second wave participants worried less that others might avoid them even after the contamination risk has been minimized that can be associated with lower stigmatization of HCWs. The main finding of the second survey was that 74,2% of participants felt burned out from their work. Almost half of the respondents (45,5%) had moderate or severe depression according to PHQ-9. Most participants had asthenic complaints (feeling tired or having little energy), anhedonia (little interest or pleasure in doing things), and insomnia (trouble falling or staying asleep). The level of moderate or severe depression in our sample was higher relative to other studies [2, 5, 9, 10, 12]. Moreover 2,4% of participants had thoughts that they would be better off dead, or of hurting themselves, which reflects a higher potential risk of suicide. Our study shows the importance of assessing the risk of suicide in HCWs perhaps with using more specific and valid scales like C-SSRS [33] or SAD PERSONS [34]. Two thirds of participants (67,8%) had moderate or high perceived stress according to PPS-10 scale that was also higher relative to other studies [11]. The most common symptoms included: feeling nervous and "stressed", have been angered because of things outside of their control, have been upset because of something that happened unexpectedly.

In discussing possible risk factors of psychological problems in frontline HCWs we should note that women had higher levels of stress and anxiety according to both surveys. This result corresponds to other studies [6, 8, 11, 12], and female gender seems to be the main risk factor. According to the network analysis being a woman also positively correlated with perceived stress according to PSS-10, anxiety, depression, emotional exhaustion. Age was also associated with higher perceived stress and emotional exhaustion according to the network analysis similar to other studies [11, 14]. Working in Moscow or Saint Petersburg (two major cities of Russian Federation) were associated with lower anxiety level as well as other symptoms among HCWs. This result can be explained by having better working conditions, including sufficient PPE, higher salaries and full personnel strength in big cities compared to others. Mortality rates of HCWs in Russia were higher in cities other than Moscow [21]. Vaccinated participants in our study had significantly lower stress and anxiety levels. This finding once again indicates that the main factor contributing to the anxiety level is the fear of getting infected or infecting family and friends.

Therefore, risk groups of HCWs should be defined at early stages of work and provided with additional social and psychological support. Unfortunately, nowadays, many barriers limit the immediate formation of such support programs due to the quarantine policy; however, self-help interventions [35], spread of online materials on stress and anxiety reduction, access to psychological assistance hotlines, and involvement in leisure activities among HCWs may be helpful [36].

This study has several limitations. The bias related to anonymous online survey could not be excluded; we had to follow this design due to the pandemic, although face-to-face interviews would have been more accurate in assessing the levels of depression, anxiety, stress and burnout. The levels of depression and burnout have not been specifically assessed during the first wave; therefore, it was difficult to compare their rates.

## 5. Conclusions

Our study has shown high rates of stress, anxiety, depression and burnout especially among frontline HCWs in Russia. Female gender, living outside of Moscow or Saint Petersburg and not being vaccinated for COVID-19 were factors associated with higher level of stress and anxiety in HCWs. It is known that high level of depression may lead to increased suicide rate. Therefore, these results demonstrate the urgent need for supportive programs to the frontline HCWs at risk fighting COVID-19.

## Acknowledgements

This study was not financially supported. We are thankful to all the HCWs in Russian COVID-19 medical centers who voluntarily participated in our online survey.

## Conflict of interest

The authors declare no conflict of interest.

## Nomenclature

| | |
|---|---|
| GAD -7 | General Anxiety Disorder-7 scale |
| HCWs | healthcare workers |
| IQR | interquartile range |
| MBI | Maslach Burnout Inventory scale |
| LSA | low stress and anxiety group |
| PHQ-9 | Patient Health Questionnaire −9 scale |

| | |
|---|---|
| PSS-10 | Perceived Stress Scale-10 |
| PTSD | post-traumatic stress disorder |
| SAVE-9 | Stress and Anxiety to Viral Epidemic scale-9 |
| S1 | sample 1 (May 19th and May 26th 2020) |
| S2 | sample 2 (between October 10th and October 17th) |

## Author details

Ekaterina Mosolova[1], Dmitry Sosin[2] and Sergey Mosolov[2,3]*

1 Faculty of Basic Medicine, Lomonosov Moscow State University, Moscow, Russia

2 Department of Psychiatry, Russian Medical Academy of Continuous Professional Education Ministry of Public Health of Russian Federation, Moscow, Russia

3 Moscow Research Institute of Psychiatry, Moscow, Russia

*Address all correspondence to: profmosolov@mail.ru

## References

[1] Stewart DE, Appelbaum PS. COVID-19 and psychiatrists' responsibilities: a WPA position paper. *World Psychiatry.* 2020;19(3):406-407. DOI:10.1002/wps.20803

[2] Naser AY, Dahmash EZ, Al-Rousan R, Alwafi H, Alrawashdeh HM, Ghoul I et al. Mental health status of the general population, healthcare professionals, and university students during 2019 coronavirus disease outbreak in Jordan: A cross-sectional study. *Brain Behav.* 2020 Aug;10(8): e01730. DOI: 10.1002/brb3.1730

[3] Luceno-Moreno L, Talavera-Velasco B, Garcia-Albuerne Y, Martin-Garcia J. Symptoms of Posttraumatic Stress, Anxiety, Depression, Levels of Resilience and Burnout in Spanish Health Personnel during the COVID-19 Pandemic. *Int J Environ Res Public Health.* 2020;17(15): 5514. DOI: 10.3390/ijerph17155514

[4] Song X, Fu W, Liu X, Luo Z, Wang R, Zhou N, et al. Mental health status of medical staff in emergency departments during the Coronavirus disease 2019 epidemic in China. Brain *Behav Immun.* 2020;88:60-65. DOI: 10.1016/j.bbi.2020.06.002

[5] Zhan YX, Zhao SY, Yuan J, Liu H, Liu YF, Gui LL, et al. Prevalence and Influencing Factors on Fatigue of First-line Nurses Combating with COVID-19 in China: A Descriptive Cross-Sectional Study. *Curr Med Sci.* 2020;40(4):625-635. DOI: 10.1007/s11596-020-2226-9

[6] Barello S, Palamenghi L, Graffigna G. Burnout and somatic symptoms among frontline healthcare professionals at the peak of the Italian COVID-19 pandemic. *Psychiatry Res.* 2020;290:113129. DOI: 10.1016/j.psychres.2020.113129

[7] Duarte I, Teixeira A, Castro L, Marina S, Ribeiro C, Jacome C, et al. Burnout among Portuguese healthcare workers during the COVID-19 pandemic. *BMC Public Health.* 2020 (20):1885. DOI: https://doi.org/10.1186/s12889-020-09980-z

[8] Alshekaili M, Hassan W, Al Said N, Al Sulaimani F, Jayapal SK, Al-Mawali A, et al. Factors associated with mental health outcomes across healthcare settings in Oman during COVID-19: frontline versus non-frontline healthcare workers. *BMJ Open.* 2020;10(10): e042030. DOI: 10.1136/bmjopen-2020-042030

[9] Azoulay E, Cariou A, Bruneel F, Demoule A, Kouatchet A, Reuter D, et al. Symptoms of Anxiety, Depression, and Peritraumatic Dissociation in Critical Care Clinicians Managing Patients with COVID-19. A Cross-Sectional Study. *Am J Respir Crit Care Med.* 2020;202(10):1388-1398. DOI: 10.1164/rccm.202006-2568OC

[10] Lai J, Ma S, Wang Y, Cai Z, Hu J, Wei N, et al. Factors Associated with Mental Health Outcomes Among Health Care Workers Exposed to Coronavirus Disease 2019. *JAMA Netw Open.* 2020;3 (3):e203976. DOI: 10.1001/jamanetworkopen.2020.3976

[11] Liu Y, Chen H, Zhang N, Wang X, Fan Q, Zhang Y, et al. Anxiety and depression symptoms of medical staff under COVID-19 epidemic in China. *J Affect Disord.* 2021; 278:144-148. DOI: 10.1016/j.jad.2020.09.004

[12] Zhu Z, Xu S, Wang H, Liu Z, Wu J, Li G, et al. COVID-19 in Wuhan: Sociodemographic characteristics and hospital support measures associated with the immediate psychological impact on healthcare workers. *EClinicalMedicine.* 2020;24:100443. DOI: 10.1016/j.eclinm.2020.100443

[13] Lu W, Wang H, Lin Y, Li L. Psychological status of medical workforce during the COVID-19

pandemic: A cross-sectional study. *Psychiatry Res.* 2020; 288:112936. DOI: 10.1016/j.psychres.2020.112936

[14] Wanigasooriya K, Palimar P, Naumann D, Ismail K, Fellows J, Logan P, et al. Mental health symptoms in a cohort of hospital healthcare workers following the first peak of the Covid-19 pandemic in the United Kingdom. medRxiv [Preprint] 2020. DOI: https://doi.org/10.1101/2020.10.02.20205674

[15] Dai Y, Hu G, Xiong H, Qui H, Yuan X. Psychological impact of the coronavirus disease 2019 (COVID-19) outbreak on healthcare workers in China. medRxiv [Preprint] 2020. DOI: h ttps://doi.org/10.1101/2020.03.03.20030874

[16] Spiller TR, Mean M, Ernst J, Sazpinar O, Gehrke S, Paolercio F, et al. Development of health care workers' mental health during the SARS-CoV-2 pandemic in Switzerland: two cross-sectional studies. *Psychol Med*. 2020:1-4. DOI: 10.1017/S0033291720003128

[17] Liu Z, Wu J, Shi X, Ma Y, Ma X, Teng Z et al. Mental Health Status of Healthcare Workers in China for COVID-19 Epidemic. *Ann Glob Health.* 2020;86(1):128. DOI: 10.5334/aogh.3005

[18] Wang H, Liu Y, Hu K, Zhang M, Du M, Huang H, et al. Healthcare workers' stress when caring for COVID-19 patients: An altruistic perspective. *Nurs Ethics.* 2020;27(7):1490-1500. DOI: 10.1177/0969733020934146

[19] Petrikov SS, Kholmogorova AB, Suroegina AY, Mikita OY, Roy AP, Rakhmanina AA. Professional Burnout, Symptoms of Emotional Disorders and Distress among Healthcare Professionals during the COVID-19 Epidemic. *Counseling Psychology and Psychotherapy.* 2020; 28 (2):8—45. DOI: https:// doi.org/10.17759/cpp.2020280202

[20] Bachilo E, Barylnik J, Shuldyakov A, Efremov A, Novikov D. Mental Health of Medical Workers During the COVID-19 Pandemic in Russia: Results of a Cross-Sectional Study. medRxiv [Preprint] 2020. DOI: https://doi.org/10.1101/2020.07.27.20162610

[21] Lifshits M, Neklyudova N. COVID-19 mortality rate in Russia: forecasts and reality evaluation. medRxiv [Preprint] 2020. DOI: https://doi.org/10.1101/2020.09.25.20201376

[22] Chung S, Kim HJ, Ahn MA, Yeo S, Lee J, Kim K, et al. Development of the Stress and Anxiety to Viral Epidemics-9 (SAVE-9) scale for assessing work-related stress and anxiety in healthcare workers in response to viral epidemics. PsyArXiv [Preprint] 2020. DOI: 10.31234/osf.io/a52b4

[23] Spitzer RL, Kroenke K, Williams JBW, Löwe B. A Brief Measure for Assessing Generalized Anxiety Disorder: The GAD-7. *Arch Intern Med*. 2006;166(10):1092–1097. DOI:10.1001/archinte.166.10.1092

[24] Mosolova E, Chung S, Sosin D, Mosolov S. P 663 Stress and anxiety among healthcare workers during the coronavirus disease 2019 pandemic in Russia. *Eur Neuropsychopharmacol.* 2020;40:S375. DOI: 10.1016/j.euroneuro.2020.09.486

[25] Kroenke K, Spitzer RL, Williams JB. The PHQ-9: validity of a brief depression severity measure. *J Gen Intern Med.* 2001;16(9):606-13. DOI: 10.1046/j.1525 1497.2001.016009606.x

[26] West CP, Dyrbye LN, Sloan JA, Shanafelt TD. Single item measures of emotional exhaustion and depersonalization are useful for assessing burnout in medical professionals. *J Gen Intern Med.* 2009;24 (12):1318-21. DOI: 10.1007/s11606-009-1129-z

[27] Cohen S, Williamson G. Perceived stress in a probability sample of the United States. In: Spacapam S and Oskamp S (eds) The Social Psychology of Health. Newbury Park, CA: Sage. 1998:31–67.

[28] Jones PJ, Mair P, McNally RJ. Visualizing Psychological Networks: A Tutorial in R. *Front Psychol.* 2018; 9:1742. DOI:10.3389/fpsyg.2018.01742

[29] Epskamp S, Borsboom D, Fried EI. Estimating psychological networks and their accuracy: A tutorial paper. *Behavior Research Methods.* 2018;50(1): 195–212. DOI:10.3758/s13428-017-0862-1

[30] Lee J, Lee H, Hong Y, Shin Y, Chung S, Park J. The Hazardous Workplace, Work-related Stress, and Unhealthy Behaviors among Healthcare Workers: The Relationships with Depressive and Insomnia symptoms during COVID-19. medRxiv [Preprint] 2020. DOI: 10.31234/osf.io/ph3ny

[31] Tavormina G, Tavormina MGM, Franza F, Aldi G, Amici P, Amorosi M, et al. A New Rating Scale (SAVE-9) to Demonstrate the Stress and Anxiety in the Healthcare Workers During the COVID-19 Viral Epidemic. *Psychiatr Danub.* 2020;32:5-9.

[32] Wang H, Huang D, Huang H, Zhang J, Guo L, Liu Y, et al. The psychological impact of COVID-19 pandemic on medical staff in Guangdong, China: a cross-sectional study. Psychol Med. 2020:1-9. DOI: 10.1017/S0033291720002561

[33] Posner K, Oquendo MA, Gould M, Stanley B, Davies M. Columbia Classification Algorithm of Suicide Assessment (C-CASA): classification of suicidal events in the FDA's pediatric suicidal risk analysis of antidepressants. *Am J Psychiatry.* 2007; 164(7):1035-43. DOI: 10.1176/ajp.2007.164.7.1035

[34] Juhnke GE. SAD PERSONS scale review. Measurement and Evaluation in Counseling & Development. 1994;27: 325–328.

[35] Yang L, Yin J, Wang D, Rahman A, Li X. Urgent need to develop evidence-based self-help interventions for mental health of healthcare workers in COVID-19 pandemic. *Psychological Medicine.* 2020: 1-2. DOI: 10.1017/S0033291720001385

[36] Chen Q, Liang M, Li Y, Guo J, Fei D, Wang L, et al. Mental health care for medical staff in China during the COVID-19 outbreak. *Lancet Psychiatry.* 2020;7(4):e15-e16. DOI: 10.1016/S2215-0366(20)30078-X

Section 6

# Impact of Architecture and Urbanism on Epidemics/Pandemics

Chapter 16

# The Role of Architecture and Urbanism in Preventing Pandemics

*Bogdan Andrei Fezi*

## Abstract

This chapter aims to assess the historical role of architecture and urbanism in the prevention and mitigation of pandemics and the place it may occupy in future international strategies. During COVID-19, the contemporary healthcare system response to pandemics showed its limits. There must be investigated a more interdisciplinary answer in which the role of the built environment in the One Health should be clarified. Since the 19th century, the built environment traditionally occupied a decisive role in mitigating pandemics. The war against tuberculosis led to the Hygiene movement which set the principles of the Modernist architectural and urban movement. With the discovery of antibiotics, the medicine emancipated from architecture. In the absence of health implications, the social and environmental counterreactions to the Modernist movement led to the Green Architecture, New Urbanism or Urban Village movements. After the last decades warnings about future pandemics, some of the present COVID-19 scientific findings have notable impact on the built environment design: pollution, green areas, urban population density or air quality control. Finally, the chapter analyses architectural and urban measures for preventing and mitigating future pandemics: air control, residential approaches, public spaces, green areas design, working, transportation and mixed neighborhoods.

**Keywords:** architecture, urbanism, green buildings, built environment, pandemics, health, environment, ecology, COVID-19, SARS-CoV-2

## 1. Introduction

This chapter aims to reveal the role of architecture and urbanism in the prevention and mitigation of pandemics. Although since the 19th century the built environment traditionally had a decisive role in mitigating pandemics, such as tuberculosis, the emancipation of medicine, after the discovery of antibiotics, gradually excluded architecture and urbanism from the strategies against pandemics. In the context of COVID-19, there are relevant reasons for an interdisciplinary scientific approach of pandemics including the built environment and for a reevaluation of the future international strategies.

 

## 2. The limits of the contemporary healthcare system response to pandemics

In the second half of the 20th century, a complex set of measures was set in place that successfully fought against pandemics. Pharmaceutical interventions brought substances such as antibiotic drugs against tuberculosis or such as vaccine products against influenzas. In 1997, International Coordination Group (ICG) was established by the World Health Organization (WHO) "to manage and coordinate the provision of emergency vaccine supplies and antibiotics to countries [1]". Unfortunately, although existing influenza vaccines are among the most effective protections and strategic stockpiles for several influenza types are gathered, they are ineffective against new strains. Developing and distributing a new vaccine takes several months, delaying the pharmaceutical response. As for antibiotics, WHO started, since the 1990s, to strengthen the surveillance of the drug resistance for the tuberculosis.

Lack of pharmaceutical means, non-pharmaceutical interventions "should be put in place, at the early stage of a pandemic [1]". The foreseen interventions included hygiene, social distancing, using facemasks and schools' closures. The non-pharmaceutical interventions were established as part of the international response interventions: anticipation, early detection, containment, control and mitigation as well as elimination or eradication. These measures were regulated, since 1969, by the International Health Regulations that aimed to "prevent, protect against, control and respond to the international spread of disease". Events that might have international consequences were supposed to be promptly reported by the states to WHO for assessment.

The COVID-19 pandemic showed the limits of the existing healthcare system strategies. By the end of 2020, lack of adequate response, the pandemic led to a dramatic health impact, with more than 1.5 million deaths by December 2020 [1], to a huge social disruption and an economic result that brought to the biggest global recession since the 1930s Great Depression.

**Without an effective treatment for COVID-19, governments adopted the 19th century traditional measures concerning people and the built environment**. The 2020 approach was contrary to the WHO politics of 2018, which stated that "many traditional containment measures are no longer efficient" and that "measures such as quarantine, for example, once regarded as a matter of fact, would be unacceptable to many populations today [1]". People oriented measures in 2020 addressed individuals, like hygiene or wearing face masks, or were related to contacts with people, like the social distancing (or physical distancing), curfew, isolation, quarantine and confinement (lockdown). Building oriented measures were also adopted by interior air control through ventilation.

The COVID-19 pandemic brought into attention other **non-pharmaceutical methods** that may prevent or mitigate the effects of pandemics. One of the directions concerns the environmental approaches. As for the role of the built environment in fighting against pandemics, scientific studies undergone during 2020 concerning pollution, urban heat islands, land use, green areas, urban density and interior air quality suggest that the buildings and the built environment may play a decisive role in the international strategies against future pandemics.

## 3. The One Health system response to pandemics and the role of the built environment

In the 1980s, after increased outbreaks of zoonoses, human healthcare system became aware of the benefits in approaching human and animal diseases together with the unifying concept of One Medicine [2]. In the 1990s, due to the alteration of the ecosystems which led to new ways of diseases spread, the role of the environment in human health became relevant [3]. During the decade of the 2000s, the unification was extended to the humans, animals and environment resulting the One Health system in the 2000's [4, 5]. A broader spectrum of professions was brought together, gathering **veterinarians, ecologists, economists, sociologists or wildlife managers**.

The 2010 decade brought an increased awareness of the urbanization risks for pandemics. The approaches were quantitative and focused on the **overlapping of habitats, the heat that provide high-risk habitats for animals and the high density of people**. As for the building health, there is also consistent literature about its role in supporting physical, social or psychological health. One of the key aspects is the indoor environmental quality, focused on the **air quality**.

Despite these advances in understanding the role of the built environment in human health, by the end of 2020 the was still not international strategy that included buildings and the built environment in the fighting against pandemics.

## 4. The historical role of the built environment in pandemics before the advent of antibiotics

Until the arrival of antibiotics in the middle of the 20th century, the main historical methods against bacterial pandemics were limiting the contacts between individuals through **isolation, quarantine and confinement** (**lockdown**) and, from the 19th century, the architectural and urban measures concerning air quality and sunlight.

In the case of leprosy, containment led to the appearance of the first dedicated architectural program, the leprosarium. The measure was common in Medieval Europe [6], although "less uniform and prescriptive [7]".

Plagues were the deadliest pandemics. The 1346–1353 Black Death supposedly killed up to half of Europe's population [8]. They pushed to a diversification of measures aiming the limitation of contacts between individuals, such as isolation, quarantine, confinement, the use of plague mask and the introduction of the medical passport. They also led to dedicated constructions, such as the 27 km long, six feet tall, Plague Wall in the French Vaucluse mountains traced in 1721 [9, 10]. Since the 19th century, plagues impact diminished.

The tuberculosis, "the white plague", took the relay, with a peak mortality rate in Western Europe in 1800 [11]. Tuberculosis deaths counts for 45% between 1790 and 1796 in Bristol, 33.2% of deaths between 1751 and 1778 in Marseille [12] and for 25% of death between 1810 and 1815 in New York City [13]. In 1900, it remained the third cause of mortality after cardiovascular diseases and influenza–pneumonia in the US [14].

In France, the backbone of the fight against tuberculosis was the **Hygiene movement** in which public health was supposed to scientifically guide political decisions, architecture and urbanism. The movement started in the 1820s, continued with the creation of the Hygiene Commissions (1848) and of the Commission for Unhealthy Housing (1950) [15] and reached its peak in the urban renewal during the Haussmann period as Seine (Paris) prefect (1853–1870). The French capital applied the hygiene reform at the largest scale ever seen: **sewage, wastewater treatment, waste removal, air circulation inside and between buildings, sunlight**.

**Hygiene movement derived principles definitively marked architecture and urbanism.** The sunlight that kills bacteria imposed the sanatoriums as general architectural models, with vast windows stretching from one side to the other of the room and terraces for sun baths. Sunlight and ventilation at the 45th parallel north are the reason for imposing distances in between buildings greater than the building height.

At the turn of the 20th century emerged the British **Garden City movement**, started with the Ebenezer Howard's 1898 book, republished in 1902 as *Garden Cities of To-morrow*. In Germany and Switzerland appeared the *Lebensreform* (Life Reform) movement.

The turn of the 20th century brought the first *International Congresses on Tuberculosis*: Berlin (1899), London (1901), Paris (1905). The *First International Congress for Sanitation and Housing Health Safety* was held in Paris (1904). The congress report correlates population density and health. The European research of the French dr. Samuel Bernheim concludes that "The tuberculosis mortality is proportional to the housing density; the danger of infection is all the greater when the residents are more cramped in their housings [15]".

The hygiene measures led to a decline of tuberculosis and, at the turn of the 20th century, mortality was reduced at half in Paris between 1872–1900 and 1901–1925 periods [12].

The 19th century Hygiene movement marked the Interwar modernist architecture. Architect's **Le Corbusier** *Five Points of a New Architecture* are derived from Hygiene movement theories. The **house on *pilotis***, reinforced concrete columns raising the house from the ground, allows aeration. The **roof garden** is inspired by the sanatorium sunbath terraces. The **free plan** allows the liberation from being the "slave of the load-bearing walls". The **horizontal window**, "essential goal of the house", which "runs from one end to the other of the façade" is directly taken from the 19th century recommendations. The **free façade** in front of the columns is a "lightweight membrane made of isolating walls or windows". Modernist urbanism is synthesized by the Le Corbusier architect book *Athens Charter* (1933) and the Josep Lluís Sert architect *Can our cities survive?* (1942). Hygiene movement principles were employed, emphasizing lighting and sunlight, light-oriented buildings and air circulation inside and between buildings.

One year later, in 1943, the discovery of the streptomycin antibiotic brought the first effective treatment for tuberculosis. The health strategies against bacterial pandemics no longer needed the support of architecture and urbanism.

## 5. Architecture and urbanism after the emancipation of medicine

As human health ceased to be an architectural and urban issue, Modernist movement, that promoted air, sun and light, was judged by social and environmental concerns determined by the functional segregation and the automobile-based traffic. In 1972 was symbolically declared the death of the modernist movement with the demolishment of a 1955 modernist US housing planned according to the principles of Le Corbusier [16].

The environmental counterreaction appeared in the late 1960s with the **green architecture**, as a reaction to the suburban sprawl and to the energy crisis. Different approaches are green city, sustainable city, eco city, zero & low carbon cities, zero energy city, livable city, compact city, smart city or resilient city. They concern pollution, carbon emission, energy, water, waste management and recycling, green-space ratios, forests and agricultural land loss.

The counterreaction to the social environment led in the US to the **New Urbanism** movement, in the 1980s. It emphasized mixed-use neighborhood and encouraged walking and bicycle transportation [17]. At the same time emerged in Europe the **Urban Village** movement that also promotes mixed use zoning aiming for partial self-containment by combining working, leisure and living, leads to medium-density housing, encourages walking and bicycling as well as public space encounters.

## 6. Health engaged architecture and urbanism certifications

At the end of the 20th century were introduced building certification systems. At the architectural level, green building certifications of the 1990s concerned health issues, such as the 1990 Building Research Establishment's Environmental Assessment Method (BREEAM) and the 1993 Leadership in Energy and Environmental Design (LEED). They relate to **indoor air quality, ventilation, interior lighting and daylight, thermal comfort, acoustic performance and the quality of views**.

More health-oriented certifications started in the 2010s with the 2012 Fitwel, a joint initiative led by the US Centers for Disease Control and Prevention (CDC) and General Services Administration (GSA), or WELL Building Standard from the International WELL Building Institute, launched in 2014.

At the urban scale, healthy cities topics are only generally addressed by initiatives such as the WHO European Healthy Cities Network or the Urban Low Emissions Development Strategy (Urban LEDS). As for the LEED for Neighborhood Development, it repeatedly addressed health as a main issue: preferred location within existing cities to **avoid the health consequences of sprawl**, reduced motor vehicle use to reduce pollution, **promote bicycling, walkable streets** "to improve public health", **compact development, access to public space** and **connected community** "to improve public health", access to recreation facilities to "improve public health by providing **recreational facilities close to work and home**", **neighborhood schools** "to improve students' health by encouraging walking and bicycling to school [18]".

## 7. The last decades warnings about future pandemics

According to a 2008 *Nature* paper, emerging infectious diseases, dominated by zoonoses, "are increasing significantly over time", with "the emergence of 335 infectious diseases between 1940 and 2004" and "reflecting a large number of drug-resistant microbes [19]". The most commonly cited reasons for this increase are the environmental issues, such as overlapping of habitats due to the agricultural intrusion in the ecosystems [20–22] or the global warming [23, 24] and urban heat islands [25, 26].

During the last decades, there was such concern about the zoonotic diseases impact that the COVID-19 pandemic seems the precise illustration: "**Virtually every expert on influenza believes another pandemic is nearly inevitable, that it will kill millions of people, and that it could kill tens of millions**—and a virus like 1918, or H5N1, might kill a hundred million or more—and that it could cause economic and social disruption on a massive scale. This disruption itself could kill as well. Given those facts, every laboratory investigator and every public health official involved with the disease has two tasks: first, to do his or her work, and second, to make political leaders aware of the risk. The preparedness effort needs resources. Only the political process can allocate them [27]."
In the 2016 United Nations *Environment Programme* report about the "Emerging Issues of Environmental Concern", zoonosis arrived second out of the six issues [28]. In 2018, WHO estimated that "another influenza pandemic is inevitable but unpredictable [1]".

## 8. COVID-19 scientific findings with impact on the built environment design

The inevitable came with the COVID-19 pandemic. It led to an important allocation of resources in scientifically addressing the pandemic. Although the most notorious studies concern vaccines and antivirals, other research directions regard non-pharmaceutical measures aimed to prevent or mitigate pandemics. As in the 19th century, the implementation of some of these findings needs a **dedicated built environment approach**.

### 8.1 Pollution

Air pollution was already subject to studies that proved the effects on human health, such as respiratory diseases or lung cancer [29]. The correlation between road traffic, pollution and health has been associated with heart disease mortality [30].

**Studies undergone in 2020 almost unanimously found that the relationship between air pollution and the COVID-19** led to a "large increase [31]" in the US, clear increases in the Netherlands [32], to a "significant relationship [33]" in China, "aggravating [34]" in a study on nine cities form India, China, Pakistan, and Indonesia and "increase vulnerability [35]" or positively associated with higher fatality rates [36] in Italy.

### 8.2 Green areas

Pre-pandemic studies already concluded not only that "the percentage of green space in people's living environment has a positive association with the perceived general health [37]" but also "consistent negative association between urban green space exposure and mortality, heart rate, and violence, and positive association with attention, mood, and physical activity [38]".

**In the context of the COVID-19 pandemic, studies interpreted the distribution of green areas as part of the environment role on the infection's risks** [39]. Green spaces are also interpreted as a barometer for health inequity [39]. The green spaces help regulate the heat islands [40], generally considered as a zoonotic pandemic aggravating factor. There are studies that show how suburban forest fragmentation led to increased human disease risk.

### 8.3 Urban population density

Studies carried over time aimed to determine the correlation between population density and pandemics. For the 1918 Spanish flu, in England and Wales, research found "30–40% higher rates in cities and towns compared with rural areas" but "no association between transmissibility, death rates and indicators of population density and residential crowding [41]". A research on India stretches that districts with a lower density experienced lower rates of population loss [42]. A US research revealed "the positive correlation between population density and influenza mortalities [43]" although another paper finds no significant correlation between population density and transmissibility measured by the reproductive number (R) [44]. As for Japan, a paper concluded that "lower morbidity in the towns and cities is likely explained by effective preventive measures in urban areas [45]."

Other researchers investigated the correlation between population density and epidemics of tuberculosis or avian flu [46–49]. Paper also discussed on the impact of urban form and land use on the transmission of vector-borne viruses [50].

**During the COVID-19 pandemic, most of the researches consider increased population density as a health risk.** Papers in Japan concluded that "the correlations between the morbidity and mortality rates and population density were statistically significant [51]" or "the population density was shown to be a major factor [52]". In India, there was a "moderate association between Covid-19 spread and population density [53]". In Algeria, "there is a strong correlation [54]". In Turkey, "population density mediated the effect of wind speed (9%) on the number of COVID-19 cases [55]". US studies show contradictory results which must be further analyzed through different criteria. A paper concludes that "counties with greater population density have greater rates of transmission [56]". Some concluded that denser locations more likely to have an early outbreak but did not found evidence that linked the population density to the COVID-19 cases and deaths [57]. Another study pointed that "county density leads to significantly lower infection rates and lower death rates [...] possibly due to superior health care systems [58]".

Those conclusions must be correlated with studies that include income, education or health care systems [36, 59]. A study involving more variables was realized in Italy, showing that population density was not statistically significant but, instead, car and firm density were positively associated with higher fatality rates [36].

These researches are limited though by the ability of collecting geolocation data. In the US and in the EU, gathering spatial data about people movements was neither intended by the governments nor embraced by citizens' free participation [60].

### 8.4 Air control

Respiratory route transmitted diseases can spread either by droplets or by aerosols (suspensions in air of finer particles). By 2020, "virtually all infectious disease dynamics models on influenza have thus far ignored aerosol-transmission [61]".

Research conducted during the COVID-19 pandemic showed that aerosols could be one of the most dangerous way of transmission in the interior spaces. A paper concluded that "virus could be detected in aerosols up to 3 hours post aerosolization [61]". The badly ventilated rooms present the highest risk as an article on a Wuhan Hospital shows that the highest virus concentration was found in the toilets [62].

A 2020 research shows that **3 air changes per hour**, which is common in most countries legislation, "generated reductions in expected outbreak sizes that would normally only be possible with a substantial **vaccination coverage of 50–60%,** which is within the range of observed vaccination rates in school settings [63]".

Studies show also that recirculating the air without proper filtration presents a potential risk. According to the study of a closed restaurant in Guangzhou, published on 2 April 2020, "droplet transmission was prompted by air-conditioned ventilation" and therefore the virus might have traveled through the central HVAC system [64]. The finding was confirmed by the April 2020 statement of the American Society of Heating, Refrigerating and Air-Conditioning Engineers (ASHARE) that "infectious aerosols can be disseminated through buildings by pathways that include air distribution systems and interzone airflows [65]".

## 9. Architectural and urban measures in mitigating pandemics

During the COVID-19 pandemic, the established principles were opposed to contrary solutions:

- the need for creating public spaces for encounters was replaced by social distancing
- the dense city paradigm, as opposed to the urban sprawl, posed virus transmission problems
- encouraging public transport was replaced by the individual transportation.

Based on the scientific findings during the COVID-19 pandemic and based on previous experiences, architecture and urbanism can provide solution with the design of the buildings and of the built environment:

- interior spaces: air quality
- residential: middle density and the intermediate housing
- public spaces: the key for the social interaction
- green areas: a perennial goal
- working: downsizing and dispersion
- shopping: proximity and downscaling
- transportation: walking, bicycling, shared mobility and robo-taxies
- city scale: mixed use neighborhoods

### 9.1 Interior spaces: air quality

In the interior spaces, the virus transmission can be reduced by air control through ventilation, humidifying and filtering.

A 2020 research shows that 3 air changes per hour, which is common in most countries legislation, "generated reductions in expected outbreak sizes that would normally only be possible with a substantial vaccination coverage of 50–60%, which is within the range of observed vaccination rates in school settings [63]".

As for filtering, pre-pandemic experiments have been conducted since 1968 on the efficiency of HEPA filters that "showed an average reduction of 99.996% [66]" or in which "aerosol transmission of PRRSV occurred in 0 of the 10 HEPA-filtration replicates [67]". During COVID-19 pandemic, HEPA filters were recommended in hospitals for air filtering in operating rooms or in the breathing circuit [68, 69]. Some papers recommend HEPA for filtering the recirculating air in closed rooms or vehicles [70, 71], although certain studies are reserved concerning the HEPA filters capacity of filtering submicron size particles [70].

Humidifying could play an important role as long as a 2013 research concluded that "maintaining indoor relative humidity >40% will significantly reduce the infectivity of aerosolized virus [72]".

As in the 19th century, air control becomes a key measure in mitigating pandemics in 2020.

### 9.2 Residential: middle density and the intermediate housing

There seems to be a conflict between epidemiologic studies that suggest a lower people density and the environmental approach that recommends the increasing of the built density. The urban sprawl is considered to increase pollution, to cause the loss of a sense of community [73], global warming [74], higher transportation costs and create health effects due to the dependence on automobiles [75]. It is addressed by professional organizations such as Architects' Council of Europe, the American Institute of Architects and the American Planning Association, by agencies such as European Environment Agency or by national legislation, such as the French law for Solidarity and Urban Renewal.

On the other hand, lowering the people density is not only implied by studies carried over time that correlate population density and pandemics but also the public preference. Pre-pandemic surveys showed that 76% of French [76] and 80% of US Americans [77] would choose to live in single-family houses. The COVID-19 pandemic increased this desire. Teleworking and the reduced access to shops, "led to a reduced demand for housing in neighborhoods with high population density", trend which strengthen after the market recovery in June 2020 [78].

**The solution to reconcile the dense city environmental paradigm with the low density of population suggested by epidemiologic studies can only find the answer in architecture and urbanism.** For most epidemiological approaches, people density is a figure in a quantitative approach while for architecture and urbanism there is also a shape-related morphological and typological building approach. Urban approach also considers different densities, such as population density (related to inhabitants' number), residential density (related to number of housings) or built density (related to gross floor area). Moreover, the same people density can be achieved with different urban typologies, such as parallel buildings, courtyard or scattered. Architectural approach also takes into account building morphology. The same people density can be achieved under different morphologies, such as detached houses, row houses or blocks. Therefore, addressing population density as a figure is not enough for analyzing the complexity of the built environment.

A more detailed approach should also be based on studies carried over the virus transmission in the interior spaces. Small, confined and poorly ventilated spaces, such as stairs or elevators, must be carefully planned as they are the most susceptible for aerosol contamination [79].

Medium density environments are the mostly supposed to reach this goal. Both New Urbanism and Urban village movements promote medium density housing. There are urban and architectural approaches that stay in between the single family detached house and the block paradigm. The French Intermediate Housing concept addresses buildings with more than one superposed apartments and with private access to each apartments. The definition appears in a French 1973 decree: the social intermediate housing (*habitat social intermédiaire*) is supposed to have a private access, a private exterior space of one quarter of the apartment surface and a height of no more than three floors. The organization led to densities of 80 to 100 dwellings per hectare for intermediate housing compared to the 10–50 dwellings per hectare for dense single-family houses [80].

### 9.3 Public spaces: the key for the social interaction

One of the problems the COVID-19 pandemic created was the social disruption. The public space was put under scrutiny [81]. In this matter, exterior public spaces could play a key role. The COVID-19 droplets transmission occurs up to 6 feet (2 meters). According to Edward T. Hall's proxemics theories, the social distance far phase is in between 7 and 12 ft. (2.1–3.7 m) and the public distance is in between 12 and 25 ft. (3.7–7.6 m) for the close phase and more than 25 ft. (7.6 m) for the far phase. Therefore, far social and public contacts could be achieved in exterior spaces without transmission risks.

According to Jan Gehl's theories, social contacts in public spaces are among the most important. They have the characteristic of being spontaneous because people interact as a result of necessary or optional activities. The space in between the buildings is ideal for conversation, greetings, children playing: "life between buildings as dimension of architecture, urban design and city planning to be carefully treated [82]".

### 9.4 Green areas: a perennial goal

As recent scientific studies show, green areas can improve the response to pandemics. They were already present in the 1900s urban theories and they maintain their permanent importance.

### 9.5 Working: downsizing and dispersion

Architectural measures can be taken in the case of office buildings. Some approaches concern general building measures, such as air control by ventilation filtration and humidification. Other methods should lean on morphologic changes that consider access separation and office space distribution.

There is also question of the offices size and their urban distribution. During the COVID-19 pandemic, an Italian multicriterial research concluded that firm density, based on an over 250 employees firm index for each region, was positively associated with higher fatality rates [36].

The COVID-19 pandemic also accelerated the use of telecommuting (teleworking or working from home). In 2019, 5.5% of workers in the US already worked from home [83] and, in April 2020, already 20% of Americans were able to work from home and doing so [84]. Estimations from 2020 are that "37 percent of U.S. jobs that can plausibly be performed at home account for 46 percent of all wages [85]". Telecommuting has an indirect environment impact by reducing the greenhouse emissions, fuel and energy usage and network congestion [86, 87].

### 9.6 Shopping: proximity and downscaling

Apart air quality methods, different measures can be taken for shops. Reducing the size cold lead to a better ventilation and less potential contacts. Proximity shopping is also an environmental desideratum as it allows for less automobile transportation, lead to pedestrian cities, reduced pollution, less energy consumption and less environmental impacts. Recent study shows that "to achieve a balance between energy consumption, GHG [Greenhouse Gas] emissions and energy generation potential, a neighborhood should contain an optimal ratio of commercial to residential buildings of about 0.25 [88]."

The proximity and downscaling decision have long term social and environment motivations more than short term economic reasons. An example are hypermarkets, huge stores combing supermarkets to department stores. It is symptomatic how France, the country that first implemented hypermarkets with Carrefour, in 1963, prevented their implantation in cities ten years later, by the Royer law which regulated the creation of shops over 1500 $m^2$ inside towns.

### 9.7 Transportation: walking, bicycling, shared mobility and robo-taxis

Before the pandemic there was already very strong evidence of aerosol transmission over long distances [89]. Studies during 2020 showed substantial transmission in closed vehicles and suggest "future efforts at prevention and control must consider the potential for airborne spread of SARS-CoV-2, which is a highly transmissible pathogen in closed environments with air recirculation [90]". At the beginning of 2020, studies drew a warning about public transportation showing that, for New York City, the subway system was the major disseminator of COVID-19 [91].

To keep the present transportation system there could be applied methods that reduce the viral transmission. Airborne virus spread in public transport can be reduced by installing HEPA filters and surface disinfection can be done by UV disinfection.

There is also question of changing the current transportation paradigm. Changes that may reduce the virus transmission in the transportation system already begun before the COVID-19 pandemic. Cities designed at the scale of walking or bicycle distances were proposed by the 1900s Garden City movement, the 1970s Intermediate Housing or 1980s New Urbanism and Urban Village movements.

Mobility sharing with bicycles can increase the efficiency of an urban public transport network [92] and has health benefits [93]. Starting with the white bicycle and white path proposed by the Provo movement in Amsterdam, in 1965, the Vélib' in Paris, launched in 2007 and reached the Chinese bike sharing system where the two largest operators, Ofo, launched in 2014, and Mobilke 2015, totalize over 50 million orders per day [94]. Electric car sharing, on which UV disinfection could be applied, could be a pandemic and environmental solution too. It has a positive environmental approach by "reducing 29% of CO2 emissions and increasing 36% electric vehicle adoption, when compared to the business-as-usual scenario [95]". Along with UV disinfection, robo-taxis (robo-cabs, self-driving taxis or driverless taxis) could be used. Experiment in Beijing with electric robo-taxis showed a good impact in lower energy consumption, zero tailpipe emissions, traffic decongestion and reduced health risks [96] while simulation in Milan "propose that introducing a robo-taxi fleet of 9500 vehicles, centered around mid-size 6 seaters, can solve traffic congestion and emission problems in Milan [97]".

From the larger urban point of view, transportation is influenced not only by the means of transport but also by the overall cities' organization.

### 9.8 City scale: mixed use neighborhoods

Reducing transportation while maintaining social contacts and the access to urban facilities is a key aspect in preventing and mitigating pandemics. Research done during the 2020 pandemic suggest that "connectivity matters more than density in the spread of the COVID-19 pandemic [98]". The risks are represented by commuting, tourists and businesspeople. Studies emerged during pandemic concern health inequities derived from the urban development [99].

This desideratum can be reached by designing mixed use neighborhoods that could concentrate transportation on walking and bicycling. These neighborhoods are likely to lead to a medium density environments [100]. They should combine living with working, leisure, education and public space encounters.

The concept is not new, as it is already present in Ebenezer Howard's Garden City with self-contained mixed-use new towns and socially mixed population. It is also relevant for the US 1980s New Urbanism or for the European Urban Village.

## 10. Opportunities

There is a consistent scientific literature about the opportunities highlighted by COVID-19 pandemic in different domains. There is also an expressed confidence that "architecture and urbanism after the COVID-19 epidemic will never be the same [101]". Some built environment related trends may be accelerated by the pandemic:

- the recognition of the role of environmental impacts on zoonosis, such as deforestation and destroying natural habitats
- an increased awareness of the public space importance
- the architectural research on new medium density typologies
- the acceleration of promoting mixed-use neighborhood and encouraging walking and bicycle transportation
- accelerate advancements in transportation such as shared mobility and robo-taxis.

## 11. Conclusion

Healthcare shape our cities and vice versa.

Although fighting against pandemics was traditionally associated with the built environment, the 20th century pharmaceutical progress allowed medicine to emancipate from architecture and urbanism. As WHO stated in 2018, "Will history repeat itself? The answer must be: Yes, it will [1]." Last decades evolutions which culminated with the COVID-19 pandemic stretched the role of a new interdisciplinary strategy in both combating and mitigating future outbursts.

There is an important COVID-19 scientific literature concerning pollution, green areas role, urban population density or air control that can be addressed mainly through built environment measures. These measures include air control, residential measures, public spaces, green areas design, working, transportation and mixed neighborhoods.

The COVID-19 pandemic dramatic implications can be also perceived as an opportunity for setting up a more stable health and built environment systems. Scientific evidence is not enough and it should be doubled by public awareness and by political implication. Otherwise, it may end like *The Great Illusion*, the 1910 book of the Nobel Prize winner Sir Norman Angell, which, although scientifically proved that economic interconnection among nations made future wars illogical and counterproductive, was followed by two World Wars.

## Author details

Bogdan Andrei Fezi
"Ion Mincu" University of Architecture and Urbanism, Bucharest, Romania

*Address all correspondence to: bogdan.fezi@arcvision.ro

## References


[1] World Health Organization. WHO Coronavirus Disease (COVID-19) Dashboard, retrieved from https://covid19.who.int/table, accessed on December 11, 2020

[2] Schwabe CW. Veterinary medicine and human health. Baltimore: Williams & Wilkins, 1984

[3] Rapport, D., Böhm, G., Buckingham, D., Cairns, J., Jr., Costanza, R., Karr, J., De Kruijf, H., Levins, R., McMichael, A., Nielsen, N. and Whitford, W. (1999), Ecosystem Health: The Concept, the ISEH, and the Important Tasks Ahead. Ecosystem Health, 5: 82-90. https://doi.org/10.1046/j.1526-0992.1999.09913.x

[4] Osofsky SA, Cleaveland S, Karesh WB, et al. Conservation and development interventions at the wildlife/livestock interface: implications for wildlife, livestock and human health. IUCNed. Gland, Switzerland and Cambridge, UK: the World Conservation Union IUCN, 2005

[5] Wildlife Conservation Society, One World, One Health symposium. September 29, 2004. Retrieved from www.oneworldonehealth.org, accessed on December 1, 2020

[6] Touati, François-Olivier. Maladie et société au Moyen âge: la lèpre, les lépreux et les léproseries dans la province ecclésiastique de Sens jusqu'au milieu du xive siècle, Paris; Bruxelles: De Boeck université, 1998

[7] Carole Rawcliffe. Leprosy in Medieval England. Woodbridge, U.K.: Boydell Press, 2006, p. 7

[8] Hatcher J, The Black Death: an intimate history. London: Weidenfeld & Nicolson, 2010

[9] Lassure C, Larcena D et al., La Muraille de la Peste, Les Alpes de Lumière, No 114, September 1993. First published in L'Architecture vernaculaire, tome 17, 1993. Retrieved from http://www.pierreseche.com/recension_4.html on December, 11, 2020.

[10] Duranty. La peste de 1720 à Marseille et en France: d'après des documents inédits... /Paul Gaffarel et Mis de Duranty. Paris, 1911

[11] Murray J. A Century of Tuberculosis, Am J Respir Crit Care Med Vol 169. pp 1181-1186, 2004, DOI: 10.1164/rccm.200402-140OE

[12] Bello S. La mortalité par tuberculose en France du XVI e au XX e siècle: approche paléoépidé-miologique, Médecine Maladies Infectieuses 2000; 30: 27.5-2783

[13] Holmberg SD. The rise of tuberculosis in America before 1820. American Review of Respiratory Disease, 1990, Volume 142, Issue 5. https://doi.org/10.1164/ajrccm/142.5.1228

[14] U.S. Bureau of the Census. Historical statistics of the United States: colonial times to 1970. Bicentennial edition, Parts 1 and 2. Washington, DC: U.S. Government Printing Office, 1975, p. 6.

[15] Marié-Davy F. (1905). Premier Congrès international d'assainissement et de salubrité de l'habitation [de 1904] : Compte rendu, p. 19-20

[16] Jenks C. The Language of Post Modern Architecture, New York: Rizzoli, 1977

[17] Congress for the New Urbanism, Charter of the New Urbanism, https://www.cnu.org/resources/what-new-urbanism, retrieved on 05.20.2020.

[18] LEED (2018), LEED v4 for NEIGHBORHOOD DEVELOPMENT, July 2, 2018

[19] Jones, K., Patel, N., Levy, M. et al. (2008) Global trends in emerging infectious diseases. Nature 451, 990-993 (2008). https://doi.org/10.1038/nature06536

[20] Jones, B.A., Grace, D., Kock, R., Alonso, S., Rushton, J., Said, M.Y., McKeever, D., Mutua, F., Young, J., McDermott, J. and Pfeiffer, D.U. (2013). Zoonosis emergence linked to agricultural intensification and environmental change. Proceedings of the National Academy of Science, 110(21), 8399-8404. http://www.pnas.org/content/110/21/8399.full.pdf

[21] Allen, T., Murray, K.A., Zambrana-Torrelio, C. et al. (2017) Global hotspots and correlates of emerging zoonotic diseases. Nat Commun 8, 1124 (2017). https://doi.org/10.1038/s41467-017-00923-8.

[22] IPBES (2020) Workshop Report on Biodiversity and Pandemics of the Intergovernmental Platform on Biodiversity and Ecosystem Services. Daszak, P., das Neves, C., Amuasi, J., Hayman, D., Kuiken, T., Roche, B., Zambrana-Torrelio, C., Buss, P., Dundarova, H., Feferholtz, Y., Foldvari, G., Igbinosa, E., Junglen, S., Liu, Q., Suzan, G., Uhart, M., Wannous, C., Woolaston, K., Mosig Reidl, P., O'Brien, K., Pascual, U., Stoett, P., Li, H., Ngo, H. T., IPBES secretariat, Bonn, Germany, DOI:10.5281/zenodo.4147317

[23] Naicker PR, The impact of climate change and other factors on zoonotic diseases, Archives of Clinical Microbiology, 2011, Vol. 2 No. 2:4, doi: 10:3823/226

[24] Grace D, Bett B, Lindahl J, Robinson T. (2015). Climate and livestock disease: assessing the vulnerability of agricultural systems to livestock pests under climate change scenarios. CCAFS Working Paper no. 116. Copenhagen, Denmark. CGIAR Research Program on Climate Change, Agriculture and Food Security (CCAFS). Available online at: www.ccafs.cgiar.org

[25] Akhtar R., Gupta P.T., Srivastava A.K. (2016) Urbanization, Urban Heat Island Effects and Dengue Outbreak in Delhi. In: Akhtar R. (eds) Climate Change and Human Health Scenario in South and Southeast Asia. Advances in Asian Human-Environmental Research. Springer, Cham. http://doi-org-443.webvpn.fjmu.edu.cn/10.1007/978-3-319-23684-1_7

[26] Ooi, Eng. (2015). The re-emergence of dengue in China. BMC medicine. 13. 99. 10.1186/s12916-015-0345-0.

[27] Barry J. (2005), 1918 Revisited: Lessons and Suggestions for Further Inquiry, in Institute of Medicine (US) Forum on Microbial Threats; Knobler SL, Mack A, Mahmoud A, et al., editors. The Threat of Pandemic Influenza: Are We Ready? Workshop Summary. Washington (DC): National Academies Press (US); 2005. 1, The Story of Influenza. Available from: https://www.ncbi.nlm.nih.gov/books/NBK22148/

[28] UNEP (2016). UNEP Frontiers 2016 Report: Emerging Issues of Environmental Concern. United Nations Environment Programme, Nairobi

[29] Kampa M, Castanas E. Human health effects of air pollution, Environmental Pollution, Volume 151, Issue 2, 2008, Pages 362-367, https://doi.org/10.1016/j.envpol.2007.06.012.

[30] Wen Qi Gan, Hugh W. Davies, Mieke Koehoorn, Michael Brauer, Association of Long-term Exposure to Community Noise and Traffic-related Air Pollution With Coronary Heart Disease Mortality, American Journal of Epidemiology, Volume 175, Issue 9, 1 May 2012, Pages 898-906, https://doi.org/10.1093/aje/kwr424

[31] Wu, X., Nethery, R.C., Sabath, M.B., Braun, D. and Dominici, F., 2020. Air pollution and COVID-19 mortality in the United States: strengths and limitations of an ecological regression analysis. Science Advances 04 Nov 2020: Vol. 6, no. 45, eabd4049, DOI: 10.1126/sciadv.abd4049

[32] Cole, Matthew A. and Ozgen, Ceren and Strobl, Eric, Air Pollution Exposure and COVID-19. IZA Discussion Paper No. 13367, Available at SSRN: https://ssrn.com/abstract=3628242

[33] Yongjian Zhu, Jingui Xie, Fengming Huang, Liqing Cao, Association between short-term exposure to air pollution and COVID-19 infection: Evidence from China, Science of The Total Environment, Volume 727, 2020, 138704, ISSN 0048-9697, https://doi.org/10.1016/j.scitotenv.2020.138704.

[34] Gupta, A., Bherwani, H., Gautam, S. et al. Air pollution aggravating COVID-19 lethality? Exploration in Asian cities using statistical models. Environ Dev Sustain (2020). https://doi.org/10.1007/s10668-020-00878-9

[35] Contini, Daniele. Costabile, Francesca. Does Air Pollution Influence COVID-19 Outbreaks? Atmosphere 2020, 11(4), 377; https://doi.org/10.3390/atmos11040377

[36] Gaetano Perone, The determinants of COVID-19 case fatality rate (CFR) in the Italian regions and provinces: An analysis of environmental, demographic, and healthcare factors, Science of The Total Environment, Volume 755, Part 1, 2021, 142523, ISSN 0048-9697, https://doi.org/10.1016/j.scitotenv.2020.142523.

[37] Maas J, Verheij RA, Groenewegen PP, et al Green space, urbanity, and health: how strong is the relation? Journal of Epidemiology & Community Health 2006;60:587-592.

[38] Kondo, M.C.; Fluehr, J.M.; McKeon, T.; Branas, C.C. Urban Green Space and Its Impact on Human Health. Int. J. Environ. Res. Public Health 2018, 15, 445.

[39] Helen V. S. Cole, Isabelle Anguelovski, Francesc Baró, Melissa García-Lamarca, Panagiota Kotsila, Carmen Pérez del Pulgar, Galia Shokry & Margarita Triguero-Mas (2020) The COVID-19 pandemic: power and privilege, gentrification, and urban environmental justice in the global north, Cities & Health, DOI: 10.1080/23748834.2020.1785176

[40] Wood E, Harsant A, Dallimer M, Cronin de Chavez A, McEachan RRC and Hassall C (2018) Not All Green Space Is Created Equal: Biodiversity Predicts Psychological Restorative Benefits From Urban Green Space. Front. Psychol. 9:2320. doi: 10.3389/fpsyg.2018.02320

[41] Chowell Gerardo, Bettencourt Luís M.A, Johnson Niall, Alonso Wladimir J and Viboud Cécile 2008The 1918-1919 influenza pandemic in England and Wales: spatial patterns in transmissibility and mortality impact Proc. R. Soc. B.275501-509. http://doi.org/10.1098/rspb.2007.1477

[42] Chandra, S., Kassens-Noor, E., Kuljanin, G. et al. A geographic analysis of population density thresholds in the influenza pandemic of 1918-19. Int J Health Geogr 12, 9 (2013). https://doi.org/10.1186/1476-072X-12-9

[43] Garrett, Thomas. (2007). Economic Effects of the 1918 Influenza Pandemic Implications for a Modern-day Pandemic. Working paper CA0721.

[44] Mills, C., Robins, J. & Lipsitch, M. Transmissibility of 1918 pandemic influenza. Nature 432, 904-906 (2004). https://doi.org/10.1038/nature03063

[45] H. Nishiura, G. Chowell. Rurality and pandemic influenza: geographic

heterogeneity in the risks of infection and death in Kanagawa Prefecture, Japan, from 1918-1919. The New Zealand Medical Journal 121(1284):18-27 (2008).

[46] Wallace, D. (1994), The resurgence of tuberculosis in New York City: a mixed hierarchical and spatially diffused epidemic. American Journal of Public Health, June 1994, Vol. 84, No. 6, p. 1000-1002.

[47] Wallace, D., & Wallace, R. (2008). Urban Systems during Disasters: Factors for Resilience. Ecology and Society, 13(1). www.jstor.org/stable/26267922, retrieved on 04.26.2020

[48] Diez-Roux A. V. (1998). Bringing context back into epidemiology: variables and fallacies in multilevel analysis. American journal of public health, 88(2), 216-222. https://doi.org/10.2105/ajph.88.2.216

[49] Fan, Y., & Song, Y. (2009). Is sprawl associated with a widening urban-suburban mortality gap?. Journal of urban health : bulletin of the New York Academy of Medicine, 86(5), 708-728. https://doi.org/10.1007/s11524-009-9382-3

[50] Ruiz, M.O., Walker, E.D., Foster, E.S. et al. Association of West Nile virus illness and urban landscapes in Chicago and Detroit. Int J Health Geogr 6, 10 (2007). https://doi.org/10.1186/1476-072X-6-10.

[51] Kodera, S.; Rashed, E.A.; Hirata, A. Correlation between COVID-19 Morbidity and Mortality Rates in Japan and Local Population Density, Temperature, and Absolute Humidity. Int. J. Environ. Res. Public Health 2020, 17, 5477.

[52] Rashed E, Kodera S, Gomez-Tames J, Hirata A. Influence of Absolute Humidity, Temperature and Population Density on COVID-19 Spread and Decay Durations: Multi-Prefecture Study in Japan. Int. J. Environ. Res. Public Health 2020, 17(15), 5354; https://doi.org/10.3390/ijerph17155354

[53] Bhadra, A., Mukherjee, A. & Sarkar, K. Impact of population density on Covid-19 infected and mortality rate in India. Model. Earth Syst. Environ. (2020). https://doi.org/10.1007/s40808-020-00984-7

[54] Kadi, N., Khelfaoui, M. Population density, a factor in the spread of COVID-19 in Algeria: statistic study. Bull Natl Res Cent 44, 138 (2020). https://doi.org/10.1186/s42269-020-00393-x

[55] Hamit Coşkun, Nazmiye Yıldırım, Samettin Gündüz, The spread of COVID-19 virus through population density and wind in Turkey cities, Science of The Total Environment, Volume 751, 2021, 141663, https://doi.org/10.1016/j.scitotenv.2020.141663

[56] Therese KL, Sy, White LF, Nichols BE. Population density and basic reproductive number of COVID-19 across United States counties, medRxiv 2020.06.12.20130021; doi: https://doi.org/10.1101/2020.06.12.20130021

[57] Carozzi, Felipe, Urban Density and Covid-19. IZA Discussion Paper No. 13440, Available at SSRN: https://ssrn.com/abstract=3643204

[58] Shima Hamidi, Reid Ewing, Sadegh Sabouri, Longitudinal analyses of the relationship between development density and the COVID-19 morbidity and mortality rates: Early evidence from 1,165 metropolitan counties in the United States, Health & Place, Volume 64, 2020, 102378, https://doi.org/10.1016/j.healthplace.2020.102378

[59] Jack Cordes, Marcia C. Castro, Spatial analysis of COVID-19 clusters

and contextual factors in New York City, Spatial and Spatio-temporal Epidemiology, Volume 34, 2020, 100355, https://doi.org/10.1016/j.sste.2020.100355.

[60] Rosenkrantz, Leah & Schuurman, Nadine & Bell, Nathaniel & Amram, Ofer. (2020). The need for GIScience in mapping COVID-19. Health & Place. 102389. 10.1016/j.healthplace.2020.102389

[61] Doremalen, N. van et at. (2020) Aerosol and surface stability of HCoV-19 (SARS-CoV-2) compared to SARS-CoV-1, In The New England Journal of Medicine doi: 10.1056/NEJMc2004973.

[62] Liu Y. et al. (2020), Aerodynamic Characteristics and RNA Concentration of SARS-CoV-2 Aerosol in Wuhan Hospitals during COVID-19 Outbreak, bioRxiv 2020.03.08.982637; doi: https://doi.org/10.1101/2020.03.08.982637, retrieved on 26.04.2020

[63] Smieszek, T., Lazzari, G. & Salathé, M. Assessing the Dynamics and Control of Droplet- and Aerosol-Transmitted Influenza Using an Indoor Positioning System. Sci Rep 9, 2185 (2019). https://doi.org/10.1038/s41598-019-38825-y, retrieved on 05.20.2020.

[64] Lu J. et al. (2020) COVID-19 outbreak associated with air conditioning in restaurant, Guangzhou, China, 2020. Emerg Infect Dis. 2020 Jul. https://doi.org/10.3201/eid2607.200764, retrieved on 04.26.2020.

[65] ASHARE (2020), ASHRAE Position Document on Infectious Aerosols, April 14, 2020.

[66] Roelants P., Boon B., Lhoest W. (1968), Evaluation of a Commercial Air Filter for Removal of Virus from the Air, Applied Microbiology, Oct 1968, 16 (10) 1465-1467.

[67] Dee SA, Deen J, Cano JP, Batista L, Pijoan C. (2006), Further evaluation of alternative air-filtration systems for reducing the transmission of Porcine reproductive and respiratory syndrome virus by aerosol. Can J Vet Res. 2006;70(3):168-175.

[68] Ti, L. K., Ang, L. S., Foong, T. W., & Ng, B. (2020). What we do when a COVID-19 patient needs an operation: operating room preparation and guidance. Canadian journal of anaesthesia = Journal canadien d'anesthesie, 67(6), 756-758. https://doi.org/10.1007/s12630-020-01617-4.

[69] Wong, J., Goh, Q.Y., Tan, Z. et al. (2020) Preparing for a COVID-19 pandemic: a review of operating room outbreak response measures in a large tertiary hospital in Singapore. Can J Anesth/J Can Anesth 67, 732-745 (2020). https://doi.org/10.1007/s12630-020-01620-9

[70] Blake Elias and Yaneer Bar-Yam (2020), Could air filtration reduce COVID-19 severity and spread?, New England Complex Systems Institute (March 9, 2020).

[71] Rodrigues-Pinto, R., Sousa, R., & Oliveira, A. (2020). Preparing to Perform Trauma and Orthopaedic Surgery on Patients with COVID-19. The Journal of bone and joint surgery. American volume, e20.00454. Advance online publication. https://doi.org/10.2106/JBJS.20.00454.

[72] Noti JD, Blachere FM, McMillen CM, Lindsley WG, Kashon ML, et al. (2013) High Humidity Leads to Loss of Infectious Influenza Virus from Simulated Coughs. PLoS ONE 8(2): e57485. February 27, 2013. doi:10.1371/journal.pone.0057485

[73] Nechyba, Thomas, J., and Randall P. Walsh. 2004. "Urban Sprawl." Journal of Economic Perspectives, 18 (4): 177-200. DOI: 10.1257/0895330042632681

[74] George A Gonzalez (2005) Urban Sprawl, Global Warming and the Limits

of Ecological Modernisation, Environmental Politics, 14:3, 344-362, DOI: 10.1080/0964410500087558

[75] Frumkin H. Urban Sprawl and Public Health, Public Health Reports, Volume: 117 issue: 3, May 1, 2002, page(s): 201-217, https://doi.org/10.1093/phr/117.3.201

[76] Damon J. (2017), Les Français et l'habitat individuel : préférences révélées et déclarées, *SociologieS* [online], Dossiers, Où en est le pavillonnaire ?, published 02.21.2017, http://journals.openedition.org/sociologies/5886, retrieved on 05.20.2020.

[77] National Association of Realtors (2011). The 2011 Community Preference Survey What Americans are looking for when deciding where to live Analysis of a survey of 2,071 American adults nationally, Belden Russonello & Stewart.

[78] Liu, Sitian and Su, Yichen, The Impact of the COVID-19 Pandemic on the Demand for Density: Evidence from the U.S. Housing Market (October 17, 2020). Available at SSRN: https://ssrn.com/abstract=3661052 or http://dx.doi.org/10.2139/ssrn.3661052

[79] Liu J, Huang J, Xiang D. Large SARS-CoV-2 Outbreak Caused by Asymptomatic Traveler, China. Emerging Infectious Diseases. 2020;26(9):2260-2263. doi:10.3201/eid2609.201798.

[80] Allen B., Bonetti M., Werlen J. (2010) Entre individuel et collectif : l'habitat intermédiaire. Plan Urbanisme Construction Architecture et Union sociale de l'Habitat, p. 10.

[81] Honey-Roses, J., Anguelovski, I., Bohigas, J., Chireh, V. K., Mr., Daher, C., Konijnendijk, C., ... Nieuwenhuijsen, M. (2020, April 21). The Impact of COVID-19 on Public Space: A Review of the Emerging Questions. https://doi.org/10.31219/osf.io/rf7xa

[82] Gehl J (2011), Life Between Buildings, Island Press, p. 7.

[83] US Census, apud. Kopf D. (2019), Slowly but surely, working at home is becoming more common, Quartz, https://qz.com/work/1392302/more-than-5-of-americans-now-work-from-home-new-statistics-show/, retrieved on 22.05.2020

[84] Statista (2020), Work situation of adults in the United States during the COVID-19 outbreak as of April 2020. May 6, 2020, https://www.statista.com/statistics/1110076/share-adults-work-situation-covid-19-us/, retrieved on 05.22.2020.

[85] Dingel J., and Neiman B. (2020) How Many Jobs Can be Done at Home? University of Chicago, Booth School of Business, NBER, and CEPR April 16, 2020.

[86] Shabanpour, R. et al. (2018). Analysis of telecommuting behavior and impacts on travel demand and the environment. Transportation Research Part D Transport and Environment. 62. 10.1016/j.trd.2018.04.003

[87] Shamshiripour A, Rahimi E, Shabanpour R, Mohammadian A. How is COVID-19 reshaping activity-travel behavior? Evidence from a comprehensive survey in Chicago, Transportation Research Interdisciplinary Perspectives, Volume 7, 2020, 100216, ISSN 2590-1982, https://doi.org/10.1016/j.trip.2020.100216.

[88] Hachem-Vermette C, Grewal KS. Investigation of the impact of residential mixture on energy and environmental performance of mixed use neighborhoods, Applied Energy, Volume 241, 2019, Pages 362-379, https://doi.org/10.1016/j.apenergy.2019.03.030.

[89] Jones, Rachael M. PhD; Brosseau, Lisa M. ScD Aerosol Transmission of Infectious Disease, Journal of Occupational and Environmental Medicine: May 2015 - Volume 57 - Issue 5 - p 501-508 doi: 10.1097/JOM.0000000000000448

[90] Shen Y, Li C, Dong H, et al. Community Outbreak Investigation of SARS-CoV-2 Transmission Among Bus Riders in Eastern China. JAMA Intern Med. 2020;180(12):1665-1671. doi:10.1001/jamainternmed.2020.5225

[91] Harris J. (2020), The Subways Seeded the Massive Coronavirus Epidemic in New York City, Department of Economics, Massachusetts Institute of Technology, Cambridge MA 02139 USA, updated April 24, 2020, http://web.mit.edu/jeffrey/harris/HarrisJE_WP2_COVID19_NYC_24-Apr-2020.pdf retrieved on 05.04.2020.

[92] Yang X-H et al. (2018), The impact of a public bicycle-sharing system on urban public transport networks, Transportation Research Part A: Policy and Practice, Volume 107, January 2018, pages 246-256.

[93] Woodcock J. et al. (2014). Health effects of the London bicycle sharing system: health impact modelling study BMJ 2014; 348 :g425.

[94] Zheyan Chen Z., van Lierop D., & Ettema D. (2020) Dockless bike-sharing systems: what are the implications?, Transport Reviews, 40:3, 333-353, DOI: 10.1080/01441647.2019.1710306.

[95] Luna T.F. et al. (2020), The influence of e-carsharing schemes on electric vehicle adoption and carbon emissions: An emerging economy study, *Transportation Research Part D: Transport and Environment*, Volume 79, February 2020, 102226, https://doi.org/10.1016/j.trd.2020.102226.

[96] Taiebat M. and Ming X (2017), Environmental Benefits of Robotaxi Fleet. Proceedings of 2017 AEESP Research and Education Conference. June 20-22, 2017, Ann Arbor, MI. (Paper #237).

[97] Alazzawi S. (2018), Simulating the Impact of Shared, Autonomous Vehicles on Urban Mobility – a Case Study of Milan, EPiC Series in Engineering Volume 2, 2018, Pages 94-110. SUMO 2018- Simulating Autonomous and Intermodal Transport Systems.

[98] Shima Hamidi, Sadegh Sabouri & Reid Ewing (2020) Does Density Aggravate the COVID-19 Pandemic?, Journal of the American Planning Association, 86:4, 495-509, DOI: 10.1080/01944363.2020.1777891

[99] Helen V. S. Cole, Isabelle Anguelovski, Francesc Baró, Melissa GarcíaLamarca, Panagiota Kotsila, Carmen Pérez del Pulgar, Galia Shokry & Margarita Triguero-Mas (2020): The COVID-19 pandemic: power and privilege, gentrification, and urban environmental justice in the global north, Cities & Health, DOI: 10.1080/23748834.2020.1785176

[100] Moudon AV, Hess PM, Snyder MC, Stanilov K. Effects of Site Design on Pedestrian Travel in Mixed-Use, Medium-Density Environments. Transportation Research Record. 1997;1578(1):48-55. doi:10.3141/1578-07

[101] Megahed, N. A., & Ghoneim, E. M. (2020). Antivirus-built environment: Lessons learned from Covid-19 pandemic. Sustainable cities and society, 61, 102350. https://doi.org/10.1016/j.scs.2020.102350

Section 7

# Bioethical Approach to Prevent Zoonotic Disease Pandemics

Chapter 17

# Why a Bioethical Approach is Needed in Addressing Health Risks Stemming from Pandemics Due to Zoonoses Linked to Human Impact on Biodiversity?

*Tullia Penna*

## Abstract

This chapter aims to demonstrate why a precautionary and bioethical approach is needed to avert forthcoming pandemics due to zoonosis. Precautionary principle should be intended as a conceptual tool for assessing whether human action, and its arising environmental alterations, exceed the absorption capacity of Nature. Likewise, original meaning of *bioethics*, namely the questioning of unsustainable progress and human survival, should be resumed to reflect on human footprint on biodiversity. This reflection seems to be even more pressing if we consider how national policies are struggling to face the pandemic's socio-economic consequences. Focusing on how to prevent zoonosis' events, by pondering on the concept of 'biological wisdom' coined by Van Rensselaer Potter, might be more effective than suggesting complex reforms of healthcare systems. Furthermore, a bioethical approach, by its very definition, consists of a multidisciplinary approach, increasingly worthwhile in present-day societies characterized by strong complexity. Indeed, the SARS-CoV-2 pandemic has demonstrated how dense is the network of nature, human beings and socio-economic structures. It seems appropriate to think origins of SARS-CoV-2 pandemic as a warning for the future, by questioning methods and extension of human impact on biodiversity.

**Keywords:** SARS-CoV-2 Origin, COVID-19, Bioethics, Wildlife Preservation, Precautionary Principle, Anthropocene, Public Health

## 1. Introduction

On February 11, 2020, World Health Organization (WHO) named COVID-19 a new severe acute respiratory syndrome, provoked by a new coronavirus isolated a month earlier. WHO declared this disease an international health emergency and the virus, SARS-CoV-2, has entered to take part of our daily lives. Life as we know it has changed rapidly, and the evolving pandemic scenario has made us realize how deep globalization is. Every country around the world willing to curb the spread of COVID-19 has placed precautionary principle at the core of public health policies. At EU level, precautionary principle is defined as principle enabling "decision-makers to adopt precautionary measures when scientific evidence about an environmental or human health hazard is uncertain and stakes are high" [1]. In the case of SARS-CoV-2, reflecting on human health means reflecting on environmental conditions as well, given the strong interconnection between human beings and their surrounding environment. Indeed, even if the whole causal sequence between ecological changes and emerging zoonosis is not thoroughly clear, there is strong evidence of their bonding. Especially, when we consider that the epoch we are living in could be termed 'Anthropocene', since the devastating impact of human activity on our planet. This much is clear: addressing pandemic tightly as a national healthcare issue would prove to be unsuccessful, likewise conceiving it as a merely human health matter. Indeed, multidimensional connection between human health and environment is nowadays very clear and we have a pressing need to choose an ethical and legal approach that takes due account of this link.

## 2. Zoonosis as an environmental and human health crisis

SARS-CoV-2 belongs to the family of coronaviruses, whose preferred hosts in nature are various animal species [2], and which were identified in human beings for the first time in 1966 [3, 4]. In the event of transmission of disease or infection from vertebrate animals to humans, we refer to "zoonosis". Nowadays we know over 200 types of zoonoses, whose conspicuous portion consists of existing diseases in humans (rabies, AIDS, etc.) [5]. The possibility of infection and disease transmission from other vertebrates to human being testifies to the belonging of humans to the animal kingdom, as a memorandum of the interdependence amongst animal species.

When it comes to zoonosis, infectious disease is due to a pathogen (such as a bacterium, virus, parasite or prion) affecting a reservoir animal, which actually can remain undamaged by this infective agent. Pathogens hosted by reservoir animals may need an intermediate to gain access to humans, and this intermediate serves as an amplifier of the infectious strength [6]. That is, sometimes the last victim in a zoonotic infection chain requires higher dose of pathogens or prolonged contact to get infected [7]. A differentiated infection threshold ensures significant protection to humans against viruses, but more considerable degree of protection is ensured by high biodiversity and an unhindered ecosystem. In such a context, possibility of contact and transmission decrease sharply. Pathogens are definitely unconscious, therefore their transfer responds to an evolutionary mechanism: they move from one host to another since this solution, randomly found, turned out to be successful from both reproductive and survival standpoint. Amongst pathogens, viruses are undoubtedly the most troubling due to their evolutionary rapidity, flexibility, and resulting mortality rate. Moreover, "viruses have no locomotion yet many of them have traveled around the world" [8].

Describing zoonotic mechanism requires also to stress the difference between spillover and emerging infectious diseases. Spillover indicates the point at which a pathogen moves from one animal species to another; while an emerging infectious disease is the one which has been increasing after introduced in a specific population. These notions are clearly linked, especially if we consider that, under ordinary conditions, infectious diseases are natural events, which bond individuals and species in their ecosystems. Cross-species transmission is not rare, but rarely it is the result of chance. In fact, last decades have been heavily characterized by an increasing disruptive human activity perpetrated on the environment: Transforming natural habitats, altering ecosystems, reducing biodiversity and damaging patterns of interactions between different species [9–12]. Climate change, deforestation, overfishing, natural resources extraction, intensive farming, wildlife poaching and trade are all key drivers of increased rates of zoonotic emerging diseases. Human communities find themselves living near wildlife ever more frequently, and wildlife turns out to be often potential host of pathogens responsible for transmitting infection [10]. So, it is hardly surprising that zoonosis has been indicated as a word of the future, expected to become quite common in this century [13]. Environmental devastation provides a suitable growth medium for interspecies viral transmission, a perfect trampoline for "host jump". Three core elements have to be considered. The first is the difference between past and present human activity: nowadays Earth hosts 7 billion people, equipped with the most up to date technologies. This set far exceeds the absorption capacity of Nature. The second core element regards the notion of "virosphere", that is the remarkable viral diversity existing on our planet - a group of living organisms of exceptional size [14]. The third core element consists of the overlapping of the first two: Where wildlife and natural habitats are destroyed, there is an impressive amount of unknown pathogens prompt to assure their own survival by affecting new kind of hosts. Consequently, when we consider zoonoses, we can safely affirm that we face both an ecological and a health crisis.

Within this framework, SARS-CoV-2 is no exception. Current pandemic is the third of zoonotic origin in the twenty-first century, after severe acute respiratory syndrome coronavirus (SARS-CoV) and Middle East respiratory syndrome coronavirus (MERS-Cov) [15]. Even if the animal species at the origin of COVID-19 outbreak has yet to be determined, knowledge gained on SARS-CoV and MERS-CoV has enables scientists to identify bats as likely reservoirs of SARS-CoV-2 [2, 11, 16]. Evidences suggest that pangolins might have served as amplifiers, in a sequence of spillover from bats to pangolins and finally to humans [11, 17].

## 3. Contemporary legal shape of the precautionary principle

Emerged in German law during the 1970s, precautionary principle, in its legal declination, has since been uphold in a number of international environmental treaties and by the European Union (EU) in the Maastricht Treaty. Then, this principle has been included in the Treaty on the Functioning of the European Union (TFEU), under article 191 § 2, which provides for preservation, protection and improvement of the quality of the environment, as well as protection of human health, prudent and rational utilization of natural resources, and the promotion of measures addressing regional or worldwide environmental problems, and in particular countering climate change. Indeed, the Court of Justice of the European Union (CJEU) has classified precautionary principle as *general principle* of the EU (case Artegodan v Commission, T-74/00). In general, at EU level, precautionary principle is defined as principle enabling "decision-makers to adopt precautionary measures when scientific evidence about an environmental or human health hazard is uncertain and stakes are high" [1].

Notwithstanding, there is no universal, or European, consensus on the kind and the extension of measures that can be adopted according to precautionary principle. In fact, domestic institutions enjoy a wide discretion when defying precautionary policies, although these measures have always to be declined according to the degree of scientific uncertainty, severity of potential hazards, and costs linked to action or inaction. In this regard, a minimalist interpretation of precautionary principle does not support action to be taken as long as scientific evidence of the existence of specific hazard is provided. Instead, a maximalist interpretation advocates adoption of measures until a scientific evidence of the absence of any hazard is provided [1].

Considering pandemic spread in western contemporary societies brings to mind the notion of "risk society" immediately, that is societies facing unprecedented hazards for persons, communities, and surrounding environment [18]. Therefore, it is absolutely plain that every democratic government has a specific managing and regulatory duty towards its citizens when it comes to risk. This duty relates both to the degree of scientific uncertainty of a given phenomenon, and to the risk appetite that a given society tends to prove [19]. In this setting, precautionary principle plays a key role, whose legal nature is subject to jurisprudential and academic debate focused on the combination of risk and emergency. The first COVID-19 outbreaks in Europe, especially in Italy, have been a shining example of this combination: formerly infection containment measures have been adopted at a local level, then national governments took emergency measures.

To support the hypothesis that health emergency due to COVID-19 represents a textbook case of application of precaution, we should take into account the meaning to be attributed to scientific uncertainty. Far from suggesting that scientific uncertainty means mere ignorance, it regards "different forms of lack of information in science: the complexity of knowledge, the lack of data, the unpredictability of results, and the stochastic character of predictions" [20]. In other words, the field of action of precaution consists of complex scenarios (the case with the COVID-19 entails economic, social, health and environmental interconnection), shady risk factors (infection transmission through aerosol), and unforeseeable circumstances (acquired immunity against SARS-CoV-2).

Given complexity of scenarios and scientific uncertainty, precautionary principle may take different forms. As ethical principle, precaution is rooted in Hans Jonas' philosophical statements [21]. Precautionary principle is not a moral principle, suitable for distinguishing between good and evil, but an ethical one, that is a guiding criterion for human activity according to awareness of the uncertainty of risks and responsibility in managing hazards. At the foundation of awareness and responsibility, Hans Jonas placed the psychological element, rather than the cognitive one. That means that when facing hazards without a structure of scientific knowledge, a prudential mechanism (genus of the precautionary one) proves to be a suitable response to psychological dimension of fear, which tends to prevail over the cognitive dimension of ignorance. In legal terms, precautionary principle acknowledges a positive role to ignorance, that is it emphasizes the epistemological status of ignorance in contemporary science, by disengaging law from the submission to science and by opting for actions aimed at general safety [20]. Relationship between science and law, and between science and institutions, yields a form of science neither pure nor applied. This relationship gives rise to a policy-related science [22] required to frame problems in the light of feasible solutions identifiable through public policies. It follows that, in the case of COVID-19, precautionary principle may be declined according to different intensities under a cost–benefit analysis pertaining the adoption of more-or-less sharp containment measures. In this regard, the European Commission (EC) requires Member states to verify that measures based on precaution are proportional to chosen level of protection, consistent with eventual actions already taken, and revisable in the event that brand-new scientific evidences are acquired [1].

## 4. A precautionary approach based on the principle of responsibility

Recovery of a precautionary approach, in its ethical declination proposed by Hans Jonas, could be suggested as a theoretical and operational proposal aimed not only at managing current pandemic emergency, but also future health or environmental crises. During the 1970s, precautionary principle was enshrined in German law on environmental pollution and, particularly, degradation of air quality caused by deforestation. That law was enlivened by responsibility principle, as a cornerstone of human activity when it affected the environment. We suggest that the profile of ethical responsibility of human activity towards environment should be recovered, as proposed by Hans Jonas [21]. Consequently, it should be highlighted how human activity, and its arising environmental alterations, exceeds the related absorption capacity of Nature [23]. This is particularly true if we consider how human knowledge is, by its very definition, limited to a given time in history and, in the present, characterized by a high degree of complexity and global interconnection. Nowadays we live in risk societies wherein we have to be aware that our action on environment yields unknown and unprecedented hazards. In this context, it is often a principle of reaction, rather than precaution, which leads public health and environmental policies. That means Governments and their regulatory agencies, before they can act, find themselves in a position to have to wait until evidence of harm is established beyond all reasonable doubt [24]. Therefore, we believe that precautionary principle has to be declined both as responsibility principle and foresight, aiming at emphasizing a proactive and anticipating approach, suitable to result in actions of planning [25]. Because, if on one side human knowledge is, by its very definition, limited, on the other increasingly sophisticated technologies for assessing risks and data-processing do exist. Suffice it to refer to research project "Exscalate4CoV", dedicated to virtual screening, through supercomputing services and urgent computing, of a wide variety of molecules in order to verify their capacity to contrast SARS-CoV-2 and better the course of the disease.

Recovery of principle of precaution, with distinctive focus on human responsibility towards the environment, seems particularly profitable in the case of COVID-19. Formerly, for the zoonotic nature of the pandemic [26, 27]. Spillover phenomenon, that is a host jump from an animal species to human beings, has its deep roots in the human disruption of natural habitats, through deforestation, overfishing, natural resources extraction, intensive farming, wildlife poaching and trade. Therefore, principle of responsibility, whose archetype - according to Hans Jonas - is responsibility of human beings for human beings, and ultimately for every living, should serve as guiding criterion when it comes to foresee natural hazards and to regulate related risks. This is particularly true in so far as COVID-19 pandemic management could have taught us that, both at a domestic and international level, a governance of risks may be more effective than a governance of damages.

## 5. Bioethics in addressing zoonotic diseases

From an ethical perspective, precautionary principle and responsibility principle, which encompass not only human beings but also science, technology, and nature, may have as counterpart bioethics as a discipline. Originally, *bioethics* was a term coined and conceptualized by Van Rensselaer Potter in the 1970s, referring to the proposal to set up a new discipline able to combine ethical values with biological facts. In this sense, Potter portrayed *wisdom* as "the knowledge of how to use knowledge for the social good" and, more specifically, as a guide for action for the last decades of the twentieth century [28], when some scientists and scholars already perceived human activity's impact on nature as deadly disruptive. Indeed, until the 1970s Nature's limitlessness was taken for granted, along with its capacity to regenerate from human exploitation. Therefore, no specific questioning had been led about human responsibility for consequences of the destruction of ecosystems, natural habitats and natural resources. Beginning to sense that exploitation of nature could have resulted in human extinction, Potter suggested that an *instinct* for survival was not enough. It was more about setting a system of priorities in order to re-think how humankind related to nature, and drawing up a new "science of survival" [29]. This science had to be nourished with multidisciplinary planning: biology and ethics should have conversed progressively to create a new discipline called *bioethics*. Potter warned scholars on risks stemming from dangerous knowledge, that is knowledge acquired faster than the wisdom to manage it. Given that knowledge in itself cannot be intrinsically good or bad, dangerousness should be traced in the use made of knowledge. Particularly if knowledge is understood as technology. Potter did not suggest a radical criticism of technology, instead he highlighted the potential misuse of it, regarded as meager questioning about the consequences of its application. In this respect, a more rigorous intervention of politics was demanded, since human activity was perceived as potentially devastating to nature and hence to humankind. Indeed, amongst the priority problems of his time, Potter already identified pollution and material progress by all means.

Fifty years later, ecological instability has sharply increased and ecosystems' crisis has been drastic exacerbated. As indisputable proof of it, in the twenty-first century we faced two zoonotic epidemic due to a coronavirus, and we are currently facing the third. In this matter, the agreement on a common ethical value system and the notion of obligation to future generations assume great importance. A common ethical value system which designs responsibility principle as key factor in the relationship of human beings with nature, and precautionary principle as element capable of safeguarding when it comes to environmental hazards due to human activity. As Potter marked fifty years ago, "If the nations of the world are to find a "bridge to the future", they will have to realize that they must unite to preserve the fragile web of nonhuman life that sustains human society. From this moment on we are fighting a desperate war for survival, and we cannot indulge in fratricidal forays to uphold value systems that may no longer be relevant" [30].

## 6. COVID-19 as paradigmatic disease of the Anthropocene

To support this thesis, in recent years it has been suggested that Earth is in an epoch called Anthropocene [31, 32]. The main character of Anthropocene is a major geological and environmental force, more relevant that natural forces, which is also the most powerful species: The *Homo sapiens* [31, 33]. Human beings exhibit indeed three peculiar broad-scale ecological (macroecological) patterns: "humans spreading geographically disperse pathogens and parasites [and] visiting or settling in new areas encounter new organisms, including new pathogens, and new alternative hosts for existing pathogens and parasites; [then] increased human population density and frequency of contact substantially influence the ecology of disease" [34]. Moreover, given this deep interconnection between humans and surrounding habitats, COVID-19 outbreak will potentially have several consequences on the functioning of human population and extensive effects for human-affected ecosystems (e.g., incremented poaching, bans to wildlife trade, increased medical waste, and bad medical refuse disposal) [33, 35].

On the point of Anthropocene, and in particular of anthropogenic climate change (ACG), bioethics scholars have advocated a return to the origins of bioethics, in order to reflect about human interaction with the environment through the lens of hard sciences and humanities as well [36]. Truly, in recent years bioethics has been focusing strictly on human beings, by caring mostly about human health and clinical medical practice. Consequently, some bioethicists suggest employing public health ethics as a bridge between environmental ethics and bioethics (in its contemporary meaning) [37–43]. According to some, recovering original bioethics would mean disrupting discipline itself insofar as it would endanger its humanist character. In other words, many environmental scholars already embody Potter's perspective, mostly unconsciously, but in so doing they threaten the humanist element of the discipline [36]. This suggestion comes from a traditional understanding of humanism, as a philosophical stance placing humans at the very center of the universe, by emphasizing their experience of living and hence interpreting every phenomenon in this perspective. "Humanism involves the privileging of the human" [36]. But nowadays this angle is not consistent with precautionary principle, responsibility principle, and, even more fundamental, with a clear understanding of the environmental realm wherein we live. Given human action as a major geological force [31, 33, 44–45], whose effects will be potentially persistent for millennia, a perspective prioritizing human amongst non-human lives may be considered outdated or even dangerous. In this setting, Timothy J. LeCain notes, by addressing Dipesh Chakrabarty's work on the history of climate [45], that considering human beings as a geological force, a natural force, entails a metaphysical thesis. Thesis which consists of dissolving the traditional distinction between humans and nature, and hence suggesting an ontological flattening. LeCain's analysis is thus characterized as the "Great Ontological Collapse" [46]. In philosophical terms, it would be an authentic revolution.

Nonetheless, we may consider that addressing climate change, deforestation, natural resources exploitation, and other disruptive human activities, does not require this immediate and radical revolution. We may suggest that adopting a bioethical approach, in Potter's perspective, is feasible without thoroughly eradicating humanism as philosophical statement. Indeed, humanism may be declined differently, that is taking into account, as imperative human exigence and experience, the urgency of compressing human activity towards environment. Increasing of public environmental awareness, and consequent implementation of new international laws, would benefit both nature and human health. In other words, a new humanism might encompass the protection of the whole biotic community, since this means protecting human beings ultimately [11]. What is certain is that COVID-19 pandemic claims a new questioning about how humankind conceive its role towards the environment and, even earlier, a deep awareness of the powerful connection between humans and their surrounding habitats. We cannot pursue our action on the Earth without acquiring a "planetary health lens" [10, 47]. There can be little doubt that COVID-19 is a paradigmatic example of an Anthropocene disease, and therefore we should adopt the angle of Planetary Health, that is to say, reacting to the current pandemic being aware that we need a valid response to the crisis both for humans and the environment [9]. SARS-CoV-2 epidemic, global environmental degradation, and climate change have their roots in the very same ground, wherein we should seed a bioethical approach to face future challenges.

## 7. Conclusions

On the whole, COVID-19 pandemic provides a wake-up call for humankind. As a zoonotic disease, it represents a textbook case for scholars engaged in environmental, public health policies, ethical, medical, and legal studies. We therefore suggest that a multidisciplinary appraisal is needed. Zoonosis in itself is not a rare event, nevertheless it cannot be regarded as a random one. Indeed, zoonoses are due to many factors, such as climate change, deforestation, overfishing, natural resources extraction, intensive farming, wildlife poaching and trade. In this century, increased rates of zoonotic emerging diseases shed light on the relationship between human action and surrounding environment, and they highlight how dangerous is to conceive, even unconsciously, environment as a non-viable stage design wherein human act, concerned only by their mutual relations. Environment consists instead of a huge variety of non-human lives, increasingly affected by our exploitation of resources and transformation of habitats. Human beings and surrounding environment are inherently bound.

Nowadays, Earth is in an epoch called Anthropocene, whose main feature is a major geological force: humans. In such a context, many living beings are challenged in their habitats and fight a war, more or less consciously, for reproduction and survival. In the case of pathogens, and in particular viruses as SARS-CoV-2, we refer to unconscious living beings, which, once their habitats are disrupted, seek new organisms wherein survive, reproduce, and eventually flourish. Unfortunately, humans cannot make an analogous "host jump", as zoonosis, for their survival. For this very reason, it is unlikely that facing COVID-19 pandemic with a strictly human health perspective shall prove to be a successful strategy. Instead, it might reveal palliative care: undoubtedly relieving in short-term period, but pointless in the long one. Maybe a consistent question is not *if*, but *when* another zoonosis will occur, in the case of human action pursuing its journey of exploitation and disruption.

In this context, we would suggest that precautionary and bioethical approach would be as feasible, as effective. This means recovering and implementing precautionary principle, responsibility principle, and bioethical focus in their original meaning, as proposed by Hans Jonas and Van Rensselaer Potter. In general, that means understanding how deep is human interconnection with nature, and how relevant is human responsibility towards both other human beings and surrounding environment, conceived as a whole of living beings. In particular, at EU level precautionary principle is defined as principle enabling "decision-makers to adopt precautionary measures when scientific evidence about an environmental or human health hazard is uncertain and stakes are high" [1]. Elements depicted in this definition play a key role in contemporary society, which may be indicated as *risk societies*. Indeed, degree of technological progress and need for natural resources exceed more and more often the absorption capacity of Nature. This excess entails unavoidably increased natural hazards, particularly in the shape of ecological instability and human health crises.

If we agree that we are a major geological force, the need to implement responsibility principle ensues. Responsibility towards the whole biosphere as awareness of Nature's limitedness capacity to regenerate. Precaution as guide for action when the consequences of human activity occur. Then, prevention as perspective, instead of reaction. COVID-19 pandemic taught us how disruptive the sense of emergency can be. At the same time, we might have learnt from pandemic management, both domestic and international, that a governance of risks may be more effective than a governance of damages.

In this context, a bioethical approach appears potentially useful. We refer to the traditional understanding of bioethics, as a discipline that encompasses both biological facts (hard sciences in general) and ethical values (humanities). Contemporary bioethics scholars, in fact, focuses almost entirely on human health and clinical medical practice. Meanwhile many Anthropocene ethicists apply Van Rensselaer Potter's view, being unaware of doing so, or at least without saying it. In any case, there are many scholars who advocate a bioethical approach when it comes to natural hazards as environmental responses to human activity. Biomedical ethics, in this setting, is unquestionably needed to face effects of natural hazards such as zoonoses. But it should not be regarded as sufficient, specifically in a precaution and prevention perspective. Finally, the most urgent goal may be considered the increasing of public environmental awareness, in order to adopt and implement new international binding laws within the shortest possible time. Laws led by precautionary principle as response to natural hazards, such as zoonoses, but enlivened by a deep-rooted principle of responsibility, and nourished by scientific knowledge and ethical values. If the pandemic vanishes, we should strictly question our relationship with the environment, otherwise the precarious stability perhaps regained would result in a future - quite certain - natural catastrophe. In the end, protecting wildlife, natural habitats, and their patterns and mechanisms will also mean protecting us as living beings deeply bound with them.

## Conflict of interest

The authors declare no conflict of interest.

## Author details

Tullia Penna
Department of Law, University of Turin, Turin, Italy

*Address all correspondence to: tullia.penna@unito.it

## References

[1] Bourguignon D, EPRS - European Parliamentary Research Service European Parliamentary Research Service. The precautionary principle. 2015. Available from: https://www.europarl.europa.eu/thinktank/en/document.html?reference=EPRS_IDA(2015)573876.

[2] Reina J. The SARS-CoV-2, a new pandemic zoonosis that threatens the world. Vacunas. 2020;21:17-22. DOI: https://doi.org/10.1016/j.vacun.2020.03.001.

[3] Guarner J. Three emerging coronaviruses in two decades. AmJ Clin Pathol. 2020;153:420-421. DOI: http://dx.doi.org/10.1093/ajcp/aqaa029 .

[4] Liu SL, Saif L. Emerging viruses without borders: the Wuhan coronavirus. Viruses. 2020;12:130. DOI: http://dx.doi.org/10.3390/v12020130.

[5] Wolfe ND, Dunavan C, Diamond J. Origins of major human infectious diseases. Nature. 2007;447:279-283. DOI: https://doi.org/10.3201/eid1112.040789.

[6] Jing-An C, Fangyuan C, Shengjie F. Effect of Intermediate Hosts on Emerging Zoonoses. Vector Borne Zoonotic Dis. 2017;17(8):599-609. DOI: 10.1089/vbz.2016.2059.

[7] Quammen D. Spillover. 2nd ed. Milan: Adelphi; 2014. 39p.

[8] Morse S, editor. Emerging Viruses. New York: Oxford University Press; 1993. IX p.

[9] O'Callaghan-Gordo C, Antó JM. COVID-19: The disease of the anthropocene. Environmental Research. 2020; 187:1-2. DOI: https://doi.org/10.1016/j.envres.2020.109683

[10] Jowell A, Barry M. COVID-19: A Matter of Planetary, not Only National Health. 2020;103(1): 31-32. DOI: 10.4269/ajtmh.20-0419.

[11] Turcios-Casco MA, Cazzolla Gatti R. Do not blame bats and pangolins! Global consequences for wildlife conservation after the SARS-CoV-2 pandemic. Biodiversity and Conservation. 2020; 29:3829-3833. DOI: https://doi.org/10.1007/s10531-020-02053-y.

[12] Myers SS, Gaffikin L, Golden C D, Ostfeld R S, Redford H, Ricketts T K H, Turner W R, Osofsky SA, Human health impacts of ecosystem alteration. Proc. Natl. Acad. Sci. Unit. States Am. 2013;110: 18753-18760. DOI: https://doi.org/10.1073/pnas.1218656110.

[13] Quammen D. Spillover. 2nd ed. Milan: Adelphi; 2014. 21p.

[14] Goodman JR. Welcome to the virosphere. New Scientist. 2020; 245(3264):40-43. https://doi.org/10.1016/S0262-4079(20)30077-4.

[15] Perlman S. Another decade, another coronavirus. N Engl JMed. 2020; 382:760-762. DOI: http://dx.doi.org/10.1056/NEJMe2001126.

[16] Guo YR, Cao QD, Hong ZH, Tan YY, Chen SD, Jin HJ, Tan KS, Wang DY, Yan Y. The origin, transmission and clinical therapies on coronavirus disease 2019 (COVID-19) outbreak: an update ont he status. Mil Med Res. 2020; 7:1-10. DOI: https://doi.org/10.1186/s40779-020-00240-0.

[17] Cazzolla Gatti R. The pangolin's revenge: SARS-CoV-2 did not emerge from a lab but from wildlife exploitation. GAIA. 2020; 29:79-82. DOI: 10.14512/gaia.29.2.3.

[18] Beck U. Pioneer in Cosmopolitan Sociology and Risk Society. New York: Springer; 2014.

[19] Graziadei M. La regolazione del rischio e il principio di precauzione: Stati Uniti ed Europa a confronto. Sistemi Intelligenti. 2017; 2: 499-512.

[20] Tallacchini M. Before and beyond the precautionary principle: Epistemology of uncertainty in science and law. Toxicology and Applied Pharmacology. 2005; 207(2): 645-651.

[21] Jonas H. Il principio di responsabilità. Un'etica per la civiltà tecnologica. Torino: Einaudi; 1990.

[22] Funtowicz S, Shepherd I, Wilkinson D, Ravetz J. Science and Governance in the European Union. A Contribution to the Debate. Science and Public Policy. 2000; 27(5): 327-336.

[23] Bartolommei S. Il principio di precauzione nel diritto internazionale. Lecce: Argo; 2006, 11p.

[24] Kriebel D, Tickner J. Reenergizing public health through precaution. American Journal of Public Health. 2001; 91(9): 1351-1355.

[25] Comba P, Pasetto R. Il principio di precauzione: evidenze scientifiche e processi decisionali. Epidemiol. Prev. 2004; 28/1: 41-45.

[26] Cui J, Li F, Shi ZL. Origin and evolution of pathogenic coronaviruses. Nat. Rev. Microbiol. 2019; 17(3): 181-192. DOI: https://doi.org/10.1038/s41579-018-0118-9.

[27] Sokolow SH, Nova N, Pepin KM, Peel AJ, Pulliam JRC, Manloves K, Cross PC, Becker DJ, Plowright RK, McCallum H, De Leo GA. Ecological interventions to prevent and manage zoonotic pathogen spillover. Phil. Trans. R. Soc. 2019; 374: 1-10. DOI: https://dx.doi.org/10.6084/m9.

[28] Potter VR. Bioethics. Bridge to the Future. Englewood Cliffs: Prentice-Hall; 1971. 183p.

[29] Potter VR. Bioethics. Bridge to the Future. Englewood Cliffs: Prentice-Hall; 1971. 5p.

[30] Potter VR. Bioethics. Bridge to the Future. Englewood Cliffs: Prentice-Hall; 1971. 193p.

[31] Corlett RT. The Anthropocene concept in ecology and conservation. Trends Ecol Evol. 2015; 30:36-41. DOI: https://doi.org/10.1016/j.tree.2014.10.007.

[32] Malhi Y. The concept of the Anthropocene. Ann Rev Envir Res. 2017; 42:77-104. DOI: https://doi.org/10.1146/annurev-environ-102016-060854.

[33] Skórka P, Grzywacz B, Morón D, Lenda M. The macroecology of the COVID-19 pandemic in the Anthropocene. PLoS ONE. 2020; 15(7):1-17. DOI: https://doi.org/10.1371/journal.pone.0236856.

[34] Skórka P, Grzywacz B, Morón D, Lenda M. The macroecology of the COVID-19 pandemic in the Anthropocene. PLoS ONE. 2020; 15(7):2p. DOI: https://doi.org/10.1371/journal.pone.0236856.

[35] Buckley R. Conservation implications of COVID-19: Effects via tourism and extractive industries. Biol Conserv. 2020; 247:108640 DOI: https://doi.org/10.1016/j.biocon.2020.108640 PMID: 32501298.

[36] Cummins PJ. The Anthropocene: A challenge to humanism in bioethics?. Éthics, Medicine and Public Health. 2018; &: 105-114. DOI: 10.1016/j.jemep.2018.07.001.

[37] Lee L. A bridge back to the future: public healthethics, bioethics, and environmental ethics. Am J Bioethics. 2017;17:5—12. DOI: 10.1080/15265161.2017.1353164.

[38] Ehrlich PR. Bioethics: are our priorities right? BioScience. 2003; 53:1207—1216. https://doi.org/10.1641/0006-3568(2003)053[1207, BAOPR]2.0.CO;2

[39] Dwyer D. How to connect bioethics and environmental ethics: health, sustainability, and justice. Bioethics. 2009; 23:497—502. DOI: 10.1111/j.1467-8519.2009.01759.x

[40] Gruen L, Ruddock W. Biomedical and environmental ethics alliance: common causes and grounds. J BioethInq. 2009; 6:457—466.

[41] Macpherson CC. Climate change is a bioethics problem. Bioethics. 2013; 27:305—308. DOI: https://doi.org/10.1111/bioe.12029

[42] Richie C. What would an environmentally sustainable reproductive technology industry look like? J Med Ethics. 2015; 41:383—387.

[43] Richie C. Medical technologies, health care, and environmental conservation. Medicina e Morale. 2016; 65:759—72. DOI: 10.4081/mem.2016.465

[44] Crutzen PJ, Stoermer EF. The "Anthropocene". Global Change NewsLetter. 2000; 41:17—18.

[45] Chakrabarty D. The climate of history: four theses. Crit Inq. 2009; 35:197—222. DOI: https://doi.org/10.1086/596640

[46] LeCain TJ. Heralding a new humanism: the radical implica-tions of Chakrabarty's "Four Theses". In: Emmet R, Lekan T, editors. Whose anthropocene? Revisiting Dipesh Chakrabarty's "Four Theses". Munich: Rachel Carson Center for Environment and Society. 2016. 15—20p.

[47] Whitmee S, Haines A, Beyrer C, Boltz F, Capon AG, de Souza Dias BF, Ezeh A, Frumkin H, Gong P, Head P, Horton R, Mace GM, Marten R, Myers SS, Nishtar S, Osofsky SA, Pattanavak SK, Pongsiri MJ, Romagnelli C, Soucat A, Vega J, Yach D. Safeguarding human health in the Anthropocene epoch: report of The Rockefeller Foundation–Lancet Commission on planetary health. Lancet. 2015; 386: 1973